NUTRITION AND CANCER PREVENTION

PREVENTION

New Insights into the Role of Phytochemicals

ADVANCES IN EXPERIMENTAL MEDICINE AND BIOLOGY

Recent Volumes in this Series

Volume 483
TAURINE 4: Taurine and Excitable Tissues
Edited by Laura Della Corte, Ryan J. Huxtable, Giampietro Sgaragli, and Keith F. Tipton

Volume 484
PHYLOGENETIC PERSPECTIVES ON THE VERTEBRATE IMMUNE SYSTEM
Edited by Gregory Beck, Manickam Sugumaran, and Edwin L. Cooper

Volume 485
GENES AND PROTEINS UNDERLYING MICROBIAL URINARY TRACT
VIRULENCE: Basic Aspects and Applications
Edited by Levente Emődy, Tibor Pál, Jörg Hacker, and Gabriele Blum-Oehler

Volume 486
PURINE AND PYRIMIDINE METABOLISM IN MAN X
Edited by Esther Zoref-Shani and Oded Sperling

Volume 487
NEUROPATHOLOGY AND GENETICS OF DEMENTIA
Edited by Markus Tolnay and Alphonse Probst

Volume 488
HEADSPACE ANALYSIS OF FOODS AND FLAVORS: Theory and Practice
Edited by Russel L. Rous

Volume 489
HEMOPHILIA CARE IN THE NEW MILLENNIUM
Edited by Dougald M. Monroe, Ulla Hedner, Maureane R. Hoffman, Claude Negrier, Geoffrey F. Savidge, and Gilbert C. White II

Volume 490
MECHANISMS OF LYMPHOCYTE ACTIVATION AND IMMUNE REGULATION VIII
Edited by Sudhir Gupta

Volume 491
THE MOLECULAR IMMUNOLOGY OF COMPLEX CARBOHYDRATES—2
Edited by Albert M. Wu

Volume 492
NEUROIMMUNE CIRCUITS, DRUGS OF ABUSE, AND INFECTIOUS DISEASES
Edited by Herman Friedman, Thomas W. Klein, and John J. Madden

Volume 493
NUTRITION AND CANCER PREVENTION: New Insights into the Role of
Phytochemicals
Edited under the auspices of the American Institute for Cancer Research

NUTRITION AND CANCER PREVENTION

New Insights into the Role of Phytochemicals

Edited under the auspices of the

American Institute for Cancer Research
Washington, D.C.

KLUWER ACADEMIC / PLENUM PUBLISHERS
NEW YORK, BOSTON, DORDRECHT, LONDON, MOSCOW

Library of Congress Cataloging-in-Publication Data

Nutrition and cancer prevention: new insights into the role of phytochemicals/edited
under the auspices of the American Institute for Cancer Research.
    p. ; cm.
  Includes bibliographical references and index.
  ISBN 0-306-46545-0
    1. Cancer—Chemoprevention—Congresses. 2. Cancer—Diet therapy—Congresses. 3.
Phytochemicals—Therapeutic use—Congresses. 4. Functional foods—Congresses. I.
American Institute for Cancer Research. II. American Institute for Cancer Research.
Conference (9th: 1999: Washington, D.C.)
    [DNLM: 1. Neoplasms—prevention & control—Congresses. 2. Dietary
Supplements—Congresses. Nutrition—Congresses. 4. Plant Extracts—Congresses. 5.
Vegetarianism—Congresses. QZ 200 N97651 2001]
  RC268.15 .N88 2001
  616.99′405—dc21

                                                  2001016509

Proceedings of the Ninth Annual Research Conference of the American Institute for Cancer Research, entitled
Nutrition and Cancer Prevention: New Insights into the Roles of Phytochemicals, held September 2–3, 1999, in
Washington, D.C.

ISBN 0-306-46545-0

©2001 Kluwer Academic/Plenum Publishers, New York
233 Spring Street, New York, N.Y. 10013

http://www.wkap.nl/

10 9 8 7 6 5 4 3 2 1

A C.I.P. record for this book is available from the Library of Congress

Printed in the United States of America

FOREWORD

Recent advances have contributed to our understanding of how a plant-based diet confers many health advantages and how substances from plants may be effective in the prevention of specific cancers. The Ninth Annual Research Conference of the American Institute for Cancer Research has focused on the latest developments in several categories of nutrients of wide contemporary interest. The conference sessions included such topics as the effects of soy, green tea, selenium, wine, grapes, and spices in cancer prevention. This conference was held in Washington, D. C. on September 2nd and 3rd, 1999, and was entitled *Nutrition and Cancer Prevention: New Insights Into the Roles of Phytochemicals*.

The discussion program included a session that was devoted to the current status of herbal products in relation to cancer prevention, in recognition of the increasing attention that complementary and alternative medicine has been receiving from the scientific community as well as the general public. A separate presentation addressed the issue of nutritional supplements and cancer prevention. Furthermore, participants discussed various perspectives on the future direction of research in the field of phytochemicals and cancer prevention. Members also offered guidance toward practical application of new information both to patients who are at high risk for cancer and to the population in general.

This volume of proceedings includes nineteen formal presentations and 66 poster abstracts by key experts in the field. Each article provides current, state-of-the-art information on the subject at hand and serves as a basis for future research opportunities in dietary nutrition and cancer.

The Ninth Annual Research Conference was successfully organized by the Program Committee, which was comprised of: Richard S. Rivlin, M.D., Chair, Memorial Sloan-Kettering Cancer Center; Vay Liang W. Go, M.D., Co-Chair, UCLA Center for Human Nutrition; Judith K. Christman, Ph.D., University of Nebraska Medical Center; Richard M. Niles, Ph.D., Marshall University School of Medicine; Ritva R. Butrum, Ph.D., Vice President for Research, AICR and the Research Department of AICR.

The following conference proceedings were prepared and edited by Dr. Elizabeth Weisburger, the Research Staff of the American Institute for Cancer Research, namely Ms. Rachel Abroms, and by Dr. Vay Liang W. Go, Debra A. Wong, and David Dickinson, the Editorial Staff at the UCLA Center for Human Nutrition.

PREFACE

The conference began with an overview of the complexity surrounding soybeans, desirable for both human and animal diets, besides other applications. Trypsin inhibitors in raw soybeans make them inedible, but heat processing leads to a very useful food source; depending on the treatment, soy-based foods may contain from 5-90% protein. Important constituents of soybeans are the saponins and the isoflavones, besides other substances. An association between consumption of soy foods and lower cancer risk has led to many investigations that have emphasized the trypsin inhibitors, saponins, phytic acid, and the isoflavones. Most studies have been done in animals, but a few have advanced to the human intervention stage. As an example, soy consumption for one year reduced the labeling index and zone of proliferation in the colonic crypts of individuals at high risk for colon cancer. The data are suggestive that eating soy is protective for cancer, but other surveys led to inconsistent results. Further, use of soy products may be an indicator of a healthier lifestyle, and reductions in risk should not be attributed only to soy.

Cancer and food containing antioxidants were explored in further presentations. Lycopene from tomato products has the highest antioxidant capacity of any dietary carotenoid; consumption was correlated with a reduced risk of prostate cancer. Eating heat-processed tomato products and the presence of some fat caused a several-fold increase in serum lycopene levels, but raw tomatoes had no effect. Beneficial changes in prostate cell histology were noted in patients using a tomato-based juice product.

On the other hand, several large trials with beta-carotene supplementation showed neither harm nor benefit for cardiovascular disease or cancer. Also, beta-carotene supplementation for smokers led to higher lung cancer death rates than in the control smokers. However, subjects who had higher beta-carotene serum levels due to dietary sources developed fewer lung tumors. The complexities of these intervention trials are still being analyzed.

Although tea is not usually considered as a chemopreventive agent, it contains many polyphenols, which have been highly effective against cancer in animal models. These compounds, the catechins and derivatives, can sequester metal ions, scavenge reactive oxygen and nitrogen species, and reduce damage to cellular constituents. Despite the effectiveness in animal models, in humans the results are suggestive and also conflicting. Mechanistically, tea polyphenols can influence the signal transduction pathways that are involved in tumor promotion.

Other tumor inhibitory compounds are those in garlic, especially the allyl sulfides. Garlic has been considered as desirable to reduce hypertension and to lower the risk of heart disease and stroke. In animal models, garlic has shown protection against various cancers; studies in humans are equivocal. However, garlic compounds can inhibit nitroso compound formation both in animals and humans, and block the bioactivation of N-nitroso compounds. This is not through changes in P450 enzymes, but through inhibition of cyclooxygenases. Mechanistic studies indicate that garlic compounds can suppress the growth of transformed cells, inhibit signal transduction and protein kinases and modify steroid hormone responsiveness.

The periodic table analog of sulfur, selenium and its compounds can alter carcinogen metabolism/activation, enhance immune surveillance and apoptosis, and thus influence carcinogenesis. The active forms of selenium are probably selenated amino acids, but methyl selenol had perhaps the best chemopreventive activity. Methyl selenol leads to apoptosis in cancer cells without evidence of genotoxicity, and also acts to regulate angiogenesis. Deficiency in dietary selenium may contribute to cancer; one human intervention study with a selenium supplement did reduce the risks of some cancers, but not of others.

The attention then turned to resveratrol, a trihydroxystilbene phytoalexin occurring in grapes, peanuts, spruce trees, and some plants used in folk medicine. Resveratrol synthesis is induced by UV-irradiation, trauma and fungal infection; the gene responsible can be transferred to other plants. Resveratrol modulates a number of the metabolic and enzymatic pathways leading to inflammatory responses and atheroscelerosis; it inhibits COX enzymes, prostaglandin synthase and blocks protein kinase activation.

Resveratrol acts as an antiproliferative agent in vitro and in vivo; one mechanism may be through induction of apoptosis. It also inhibits the P450 enzymes, GYPIAI and GYPIA2, which are responsible for activation of various polycyclic aromatic hydrocarbons and dioxin. It had antioxidant properties, and in some cases attached to estrogen receptors. However, it did not appear in blood to any great extent after an oral dose; it apparently is cleared rapidly from circulating blood. Thus, attempts to increase the level by supplementation may not be useful.

The matter of the increasing use of herbal materials, either as dietary supplements or alternative medicine, was discussed. Many phytochemicals present in herbal materials can be grouped according to four mechanisms of chemopreventive action: antioxidant or anti-inflammatory, modifier of carcinogen metabolism, modifier of tumor biology, or inducer of differentiation. In human studies, anti-inflammatory compounds have shown some promise in reducing colon cancer risk. Some botanicals are good sources of anti-inflammatory compounds and may become natural agents for cancer prevention.

The background on approval of botanicals as dietary supplements was presented, along with the requirements that must be met in order that a product may be marketed. Use of these products has grown dramatically, and it is estimated that 100 million people use dietary supplements; diet and health professionals are among these groups. Government agencies are conducting clinical trials for some botanicals with some promising leads. Further study is needed on toxicity and adverse effects, interactions of active constituents, and use by patients without informing their physicians. In Europe, botanicals are more likely to be standardized and be regarded as medicinals.

An additional presentation emphasized that although research has been founded on results with single chemical entities, the whole diet needs to be considered for cancer intervention, due to interactions between various dietary components. Thus, food groups, rather than single components and possible synergistic actions, should be examined. As an example, the differing effects of various flaxseed fractions as inhibitors of mammary cancer in rats given DMBA were mentioned.

The problems of doing human intervention studies, the many diet choices, the need for consideration of whether supplements are high or low energy, and many other issues involved were discussed. More rapid communication of results may aid in defining effective agents.

A final paper also emphasized that populations consume food that is a combination of nutrients, and deficiencies or excesses of one can influence results. More effective biomarkers for human cancer are needed to assess the efficacy of interventions, but animal models can be utilized to establish mechanisms of action. Leads from alternative or complementary medicine may be useful. Diets high in phytochemicals from fruits and vegetables, besides being useful in prevention of cancer, are also effective against heart disease, which is still the leading cause of death.

In addition to the full papers, there were 66 poster abstracts, representing research efforts from 14 countries.

CONTENTS

1. Soybeans and Cancer Prevention: A Complex Food and a
   Complex Disease 1
   Diane F. Birt

2. Dietary Soy Reduces Colon Carcinogenesis in Humans
   and Rats 11
   Maurice R. Bennink

3. Soy and Risk of Hormone-Related and Other Cancers 19
   Anna H. Wu

4. Role of Tomatoes, Tomato Products and Lycopene in Cancer
   Prevention 29
   David Heber, Qing-Yi Lu, and Vay Liang W. Go

5. Tea and Tea Polyphenols in Cancer Prevention 39
   Chung S. Yang, Guang-yu Yang, Jee Y. Chung,
   Mao-Jung Lee, and Chuan Li

6. Effects of Tea Polyphenols on the Signal Transduction
   Pathways 55
   Zigang Dong, Masaaki Nomura, Chuanshu Huang, and
   Wei-ya Ma

7. Mechanisms by Which Garlic and Allyl Sulfur Compounds
   Suppress Carcinogen Bioactivation 69
   John A. Milner

8. Antiproliferative Effects of Garlic-Derived and Other Allium
   Related Compounds 83
   John T. Pinto, Sameer Lapsia, Amy Shah, Harsha Santiago,
   and Grace Kim

9. Considering the Mechanisms of Cancer Prevention by
   Selenium 107
   Gerald F. Combs, Jr.

10. Selenium Metabolism and Mechanisms of Cancer Prevention 119
    Howard E. Ganther

11. Apoptosis and Angiogenesis in Cancer Prevention by
      Selenium 131
   Junxuan Lu

12. Resveratrol Inhibits the Expression of Cyclooxygenase-2
      in Mammary Epithelial Cells 147
   Kotha Subbaramaiah and Andrew J. Dannenberg

13. The World of Resveratrol 159
   George J. Soleas, Eleftherios P. Diamandis and
   David M. Goldberg

14. The Effects of Resveratrol on *CYP1A1* Expression and
      Aryl Hydrocarbon Receptor Function *In Vitro* 183
   Henry P. Ciolino and Grace Chao Yeh

15. Herbals and Cancer 195
   Michael J. Wargovich

16. The Role of Dietary Supplements in Health 203
   Bernadette M. Marriott

17. The Beta-Carotene Story 219
   Peter Greenwald and Sharon S. McDonald

18. Dietary Intervention Strategies: Validity, Execution and
      Interpretation of Outcomes 233
   Phyllis E. Bowen

19. Nutrition and Cancer Prevention: New Insights Into the
      Role of Phytochemicals. Future Directions 255
   Richard S. Rivlin

20. Chemoprevention: Progress and Opportunity 263
   Elizabeth C. Miller, Zhiming Liao, Yanping Guo,
   Swati M. Shah, and Steven K. Clinton

Abstracts 275

Index 345

SOYBEANS AND CANCER PREVENTION:
A COMPLEX FOOD AND A COMPLEX DISEASE

Diane F. Birt, Ph.D.

Department of Food Science and Human Nutrition and
Center for Designing Foods to Improve Nutrition
2312 Food Sciences Building
Iowa State University
Ames, IA 50011-1061

INTRODUCTION

There is a human tendency to simplify complex and chaotic relationships so that we can better communicate information. This is certainly true with public health information. In considering soybeans and cancer prevention, this has resulted in attempts to translate the associations between dietary intake and disease as being due to single compounds, and the influences of complex biological processes as being through single or simple mechanisms. We anticipate that the series of three papers on the impact of soybeans on cancer will demonstrate the complexity of the soybean and the complexity of the impact of soybeans and constituents from soybeans on carcinogenesis. The first of these three papers will provide a foundation for considering the complexity of soybeans and the complexity of the cancer process in attempting to understand and to optimize strategies for the use of dietary soybeans or soybean constituents in the prevention of human cancer.

Nutrition and Cancer Prevention, edited under the auspices of AICR
Kluwer Academic / Plenum Publishers, New York, 2000.

THE COMPLEXITY OF SOYBEAN COMPOSITION

Numerous varieties of soybeans have been developed through standard plant breeding and more recently through genetic engineering. These varieties differ appreciably in environmental, insect and herbicide tolerance. However, overall gross compositional characteristics demonstrate high protein (35%) and relatively high oil (19%), with soluble carbohydrate (24%), fiber (5%), ash (5%) and moisture (12%). This composition has provided a basis for multiple uses in human and animal foods and more recently in extensive non-food value-added applications.

Soybean protein is important not only in its abundance but also in its adaptability to the human diet. The amino acid ratios in soybean protein have been shown to be particularly appropriate for growth and development of human and other mammalian species, including domestic animals. Protein contents of selected human foods and food ingredients are shown in Table 1. It is notable that soybean protein content differs considerably between widely consumed soybean foods. Soybean proteins include the major proteins glycinin and β-conglycinin (comprising 65-80% of the protein), and minor fractions including

Table 1. Protein Content of Soy Foods

Soybean	35%
Concentrates	70%
Isolates	90%
Tofu (packaged)	5%
Tempeh	18%
Miso	13%
Soy Curd	17%

From: Wilson, L.A. et al.[1]

Kunitz soybean trypsin inhibitor and Bowman-Birk trypsin inhibitor (BBI).[2] There is currently considerable interest in the role of soybean proteins or other soybean constituents on the reduction of circulating cholesterol and on the prevention of cancer, as will be discussed below.

The trypsin inhibitors in soybeans make the raw soybean, with its high trypsin inhibitor activity, inedible.[3] However, it is well known that heat processing destroys a significant amount of the trypsin inhibitor activity and makes for a most edible bean. For example, raw soy flour had 99 units of trypsin inhibitor activity/mg while soyprotein isolate had from 8.5-20.9 units/mg.[3] It is important to note that heat treatment does not destroy all of the trypsin inhibitor activity, and it is believed by many, as discussed below, that this residual activity is important in the prevention of cancer by soybeans.

Isoflavones are an ethanol extractable soybean constituent that have been studied extensively for their role in health and disease, and for their content in foods and food ingredients. The biological effects of these compounds have been discussed by Dr. Steven Barnes, and thus I will not address the extensive investigations on the potential mechanism of action in cancer prevention by these compounds. Instead I will provide some background for this discussion. The laboratory of Dr. Patricia Murphy has conducted extensive studies on the forms and levels of isoflavones in soybean foods and food ingredients.[4-6] Her studies demonstrated the importance of soybean variety and processing on the isoflavone content of the food or food ingredient. Different soybean varieties can vary in isoflavone content by a factor of 5. Further, heat treatment decreases the content of malonylglucosides, and water exposure, as in making tempeh or tofu, increased the concentration of aglycones. Furthermore, extraction with ethanol reduced the content of all isoflavones. Fermented soybean foods contained higher concentrations of aglycone while non-fermented foods were richer in glycosides. Murphy and her collaborators have quantitated the content of 12 isoflavones in soyfoods and 4 of these are shown in Table 2. An extensive data base was developed by Murphy and colleagues, and since this class of compounds is complex and varied, the data base will continue to grow.

Table 2. Isoflavone Contents of Representative Soyfoods

Product	Aglycone		Glucoside	
	Daidzen	Genistein	Daidzin	Genistin
Roasted soybeans	44	77	474	568
Tofu	116	140	453	562
Roasted soyflour	18	16	470	584
Tempeh	318	518	117	346
Miso	61	39	157	122
Soy Isolate (high isoflavone)	12	36	133	382

From: Murphy, P.A. et al.[4-6]

Unfortunately, less is known regarding agents such as saponins and their complexity is expected to hinder the accrual of information on their content in human foods.

THE ROLE OF SOYBEAN FOODS AND SOYBEAN CONSTITUENTS IN CANCER PREVENTION

Early observations on the role of soybeans in the prevention of human cancer developed from correlative investigations that were seeking hypotheses for the global differences in cancer between the western and Asian cultures. In the data redrawn from Hirayama[7] in Figure 1, it is apparent that the rate of

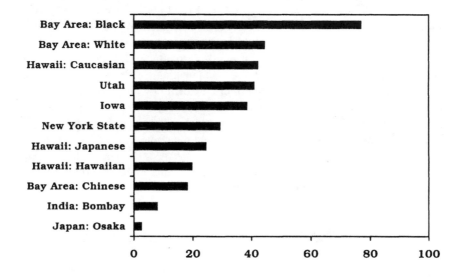

Figure 1. Age-standardized incidence rates of prostate cancer. Adapted from: Hirayama, T.[7]

prostate cancer was far lower in Japan than in the US and further, that Japanese who were living in the US had rates that approached those in US whites. However, it was impossible to separate the impact of soyfoods on this relationship from the impact of other dietary factors. For example, in another study people who had lower rates of breast cancer and ate more soyfoods, also consumed more green tea and seaweed, and less meat and butter, than populations with higher cancer rates.[8] Furthermore, in reviewing the literature on associations between soybean consumption and cancer, Messina[9] noted that associations suggesting soy food protection against human cancer were more often seen with non-fermented soybean products than with fermented products, e.g. bean paste and miso soup. In general, the population based epidemiological investigations into soybeans and cancer risk are compromised by difficulties separating classes of soy foods and problems categorizing the soybean genetics. This is complicated by our limited knowledge on the active constituents and the influence of cooking and processing on these constituents. Plus, the influence of human genetics or gender on the impact of soybean constituents and cancer is not adequately explored. Further, a limited number of prospective studies have been conducted and no intervention trials have been conducted with a long enough duration for a cancer endpoint. Dr. Anna Wu will present recent and ongoing epidemiological investigations into the role of soybeans on cancer in a later chapter.

A large number of animal investigations have provided strong evidence for a role of soyfoods and soy ingredients in the prevention of cancer. This data was reviewed by Messina in 1994, and he reported that 65% (17 of 26 studies) of the studies provided evidence of protection.[9] A later evaluation by Fournier et al. in 1998 found that 94% of the studies that were reported between 1990 and 1998 supported protection by soyfoods or soyfood components.[10] It is interesting that many of the studies reviewed in this later evaluation used isoflavones as the intervention strategy and the majority of the studies were with models of mammary, colon and prostate cancer.[10]

CONSTITUENTS IN SOYBEANS THAT MAY CONTRIBUTE TO CANCER PREVENTION

Trypsin inhibitor

A soybean bioactivity that has been extensively studied for cancer prevention potential is protease inhibitor activity. The research on soybean protease inhibitors and cancer prevention was recently reviewed by Kennedy and clearly suggests that these constituents contribute to cancer prevention by soybeans.[11] The primary soybean trypsin inhibitors are Bowman-Birk protease inhibitor (BBI) and soybean trypsin inhibitor (Kunitz inhibitor). BBI is a polypeptide with seven disulfide bonds and a M_r of 8,000. It has been studied as the purified protein PBBI and as a concentrate from soybeans enriched for BBI, BBI concentrate (BBIC). BBI acts against both trypsin and chymotrypsin. In contrast, Kunitz inhibitor suppresses primarily trypsin with only weak activity against chymotrypsin.

Human intervention studies are currently underway because of the strength of the data in animal and cell culture systems. In particular, soybean Bowman-Birk protease inhibitor was found to prevent chemically induced mouse lung, liver, and colon carcinogenesis; rat liver, and esophagus, and hamster oral cancer.[11] Further, genetically induced colon adenomas in mice carrying a truncated adenomotosis polyposis coli (APC) were also inhibited by Bowman-Birk protease inhibitor.[12] In addition, protease activity in an isolated soybean protein was associated with reduced spontaneous mouse liver cancer. Inhibition of carcinogenesis was also observed for numerous other protease inhibitors.[11]

Several hypotheses have been put forward to explain the inhibition of carcinogenesis by protease inhibitors. It is particularly noteworthy that the observed inhibition correlates strongly with protease inhibitor activity.[11] Further, protease inhibitor activity was shown to suppress carcinogen induced malignant transformation in cultured cells using radiation, 3-methylcholanthrene, N-methyl-N'-nitro-N-nitroso-guanidine, benzo(a)pyrene, and β-propiolactone.[11]

It appears that protease inhibitor prevention of carcinogenesis may be through several mechanisms. For example, Bowman-Birk protease inhibitor has strong anti-inflammatory activity. Further, carcinogen induced protease activity was inhibited by Bowman-Birk protease inhibitor. Recent studies from the Kennedy laboratory have focused on the ability of BBI to block expression of the proto-oncogene c-myc, and it is believed that this blockage is important in the suppression of cellular proliferation. In research by St. Clair et al.[13] the induction of c-myc in the irradiated colon was completely blocked in animals gavaged daily with BBI. These results suggest that soybean trypsin inhibitors may play an important role in the prevention of cancer in humans.

Another series of experiments on soybean trypsin inhibitors has focused on their bioavailability. In a recent review Ann Kennedy summarized the results by stating that "approximately 50% of the BBI from dietary sources is taken up into the blood stream and distributed throughout the body. . . ."[11] However, this view is not held by all scientists in this area, since Fournier et al. in their review noted that ". . . intake of large dietary quantities of BBI may result in high levels in the colon lumen without a simultaneous increase in internal organ levels."[10]

A serious problem in monitoring the role of protease inhibitor exposure as a potential contributor to cancer prevention is the absence of exposure markers for protease inhibitor intake and the difficulties in quantitating protease inhibitor concentration in soyfoods. Because of these limitations nutritional epidemiologists usually use isoflavone levels in blood and or urine as exposure markers for soybean intake (A. Wu, 2000, this volume). This results in the erroneous conclusion that soybean cancer prevention is causally associated with isoflavone intake.

Saponins

Legumes are a primary dietary source of saponins. Saponins are amphiphilic glucoside compounds that consist of a steroid or a triterpene moiety bound with sugar residues providing the hydrophilic characteristics. Intake of saponins has been associated with diets that support lowered rates of cancer, and heart disease, and saponins have been found to be immunostimulatory, hypocholesterolemic, and anticarcinogenic.[10, 14] In a recent investigation, the impact of soybean dietary saponins (3%) on the incidence of aberrant crypt foci

(ACF) was determined in mice treated with the colon carcinogen azoxymethane (AOM).[14] The group receiving the saponin supplement developed one-third the number of ACF/colon in comparison with the AOM treated mice that did not receive saponins. It is noteworthy that the dietary concentration of saponins in this study (3% by weight of the diet) was higher than would be possible with a legume rich diet, since it has been estimated that soy foods contain 0.3-0.4% saponins.

Phytic Acid (Inositol hexaphosphate)

Early studies on inositol phosphate focused on the interference of this agent with divalent mineral absorption.[15] Inositol phosphate occurs naturally as a salt with monovalent and divalent cations. More recent investigations have demonstrated potential for cancer prevention by inositol phosphate. In particular, studies have demonstrated the inhibition of growth and differentiation of the human colon carcinoma cell line HT-29[16] and the prevention of colon carcinogenesis in rats by inositol hexaphosphate supplemented in the drinking water.[17] Several mechanisms have been assessed for cancer prevention by inositol phosphate, including reductions in cellular proliferation, increasing differentiation and incorporation into and modification of the inositol phosphate-signaling pathway.[16,18]

Isoflavones

Publications by Dr. Stephen Barnes are focused on the cancer prevention potential of isoflavones and on the potential mechanisms of action of these compounds.

CONSIDERATION OF THE COMPLEXITIES RELATED TO THE IMPACT OF SOYBEAN CONSTITUENTS ON CANCER PREVENTION

All soybean constituents that are implicated in the prevention of cancer have also been associated with some potential toxicity. The toxicity of raw soybeans has long been known to be associated with soybean trypsin inhibitor activity. The most severe toxicity was observed in some rat strains that developed pancreatic hyperplasia and cancer.[3] It has been suggested that this severe toxicity is species specific and does not predict human toxicity.[3] Since the soybean trypsin inhibitors are heat labile, dietary intake can be controlled by thermal processing strategies.

Soybean isoflavones have been extensively studied because of their structural relationship with estrogens and their ability to act as estrogen agonists and antagonists.[19] While several investigators have found compelling evidence that the dietary phytoestrogens of soybeans have activity in the prevention of carcinogenesis in animal models, it is important to note that these chemicals, like estrogen, can promote hormone sensitive cancer models such as mammary cancer. For example, Hsieh et al.[20] used an estrogen-sensitive estrogen receptor positive human breast cancer (MCF-7) model to demonstrate a strong enhancement of growth of the tumor cells by genistein. MCF-7 cells were implanted into ovariectomized athymic mice that were treated with genistein. They also demonstrated that genistein enhanced growth of cultured MCF-7 cells and induced the induction of the estrogen responsive gene pS2.[20] It is possible that this is an organ specific phenomena since parallel observations have not been made with other models. Furthermore, some scientists have been concerned that the MCF-7 implant model does not adequately represent human breast cancer. However, it is notable that this model has been used extensively to assess antiestrogens that are used for human breast cancer prevention and therapy.

Saponins have been shown to increase permeability of the small intestine in limited studies with high doses, but the relevance to humans is not clear. Phytic acid is a well-known antagonist to the absorption of di-and tri-valent metals and there is evidence that this toxicity is relevant to human mineral bioavailability.[10]

FUTURE RESEARCH NEEDS TO OPTIMIZE CANCER PREVENTION BY SOYBEANS

Cancer studies will be strengthened by better information on the constituents in soybeans and the biology of these constituents; doses, metabolism, and mechanisms of action. Research should address combinations of soybean constituents in disease prevention. Research on soybeans should use new models of cancer, such as prostate intervention models in humans (following prostate specific antigen) and transgenic or knock out models in animals. We need more relevant animal models of human breast cancer. Gender and genetic differences between people may be important in the efficacy of soybeans (or constituents) against cancer. More emphasis is needed on intervention studies to assess the role of soybeans and disease in humans. Research on the relationship of isoflavones to cancer will benefit from a better understanding of the role of estrogens and estrogen metabolites in cancer. Strategies are needed to decrease genotoxic estrogens (or estrogen metabolites) and enhance non-genotoxic estrogens. We need a better understanding of the role of estrogens (and phytoestrogens) at different times during life. The data on soybeans and cancer presently offer considerable promise, however, research on several fronts will be required to develop sound strategies for the prevention of human cancer through soybean based foods or soybean constituents.

In considering the potential for future cancer prevention by soybeans, it is important that we identify the optimal intake of all constituents that interact in cancer prevention. This will require considerable investigation on the independent and interactive ability of soybean constituents in cancer prevention and the optimization of the combination. Furthermore, it is highly likely that the efficacy of cancer prevention by soybeans will be dependent on the genetics of cancer susceptibility in the population consuming the soybean-based food. Thus, we need to consider the optimization of the constituents of soybeans for disease prevention. It is probable that the optimization of the soybeans will differ depending on the cancer susceptibility of the population consuming the soybeans. The optimization process will involve both the genetics that control constituent levels, the processing of the soybeans, the time of harvest and other factors that have been found to be important in the control of the constituents that impact on cancer risk.

ACKNOWLEDGMENTS

This research was supported by the Iowa Soybean Promotion Board, the Iowa State University Agricultural and Home Economics Experiment Station and the USDA Award to the Center for Designing Foods to Improve Nutrition at Iowa State University.

REFERENCES

1. Wilson, L.A., Murphy, P.A., and Gallagher, P. Japanese Soyfoods: Markets and Processes 1, 1-63. 1991. Iowa State University, Ames, IA, CCUR. Ref Type: Report
2. Hammond, E.G., Johnson, L.A., and Murphy, P.A. (1993) Properties and Analysis. In Caballero, B., Trugo, L.C., and Finglas, P. (eds.) *Enclyclopedia of Food Science, Food Technology and Nutrition*. Academic Press, New York City, pp 4223-5.3
3. Liener, I.E. (1995) Possible adverse effects of soybean anticarcinogens. *American Institute of Nutrition*, 744S-750S.
4. Wang, H.J. and Murphy, P.A. (1996) Mass balance of isoflavones study in soybean processing. *J. Agric. Food Chem.*, 44, 2377-2383.
5. Song, T., Barua, K., Buseman, G., and Murphy, P.A. (1998) Soy isoflavone analysis: quality control and new internal standard. *Am. J. Clin. Nutr*, 68 (Suppl), 1474S-1479S.
6. Wang, H.J. and Murphy, P.A. (1994) Isoflavones of commercial soybean foods. *J. Agric. Food Chem.*, 42, 1666-1673.
7. Hirayama, T. (1979) Epidemiology of prostate cancer with special reference to the role of diet. *Natl. Cancer Inst. Monogr.*, 53, 149-155.
8. Nomura, A., Henderson, B.E., and Lee, J. (1978) Breast cancer and diet among the Japanese in Hawaii. *Am. J. Clin. Nutr.*, 31, 2020-2025.
9. Messina, M.J., Persky, V., Setchell, K.D.R., and Barnes, S. (1994) Soy intake and cancer

risk: A review of the *in vitro* and *in vivo* data. *Nutr. Cancer*, 21, 113-131.

10. Fournier, D.B., Erdman, J.W., Jr., and Gordon, G.B. (1998) Soy, its components, and cancer prevention: A review of the *in vitro*, animal, and human data. *Cancer Epidemiol. Biomarkers Prev.*, 7, 1055-1065.

11. Kennedy, A.R. (1998) Chemopreventive agents: Protease Inhibitors. *Pharmacology and Therapeutics*, 78, 167-209.

12. Sorensen, I.K., Kristiansen, E., Mortensen, A., Nicolaisen, G.M., Wijnandes, J.A.H., Van Kranen, H.J., and Van Kreijl, C.F. (1998) The effect of soy isoflavones on the development of intestinal neoplasia in Apc^{Min} mouse. *Cancer Letters*, 130, 217-225.

13. St.Clair, W.H., Billings, P.C., and Kennedy, A.R. (1990) The effects of the Bowman-Birk protease inhibitor on c-myc expression and cell proliferation in the unirradiated and irradiated mouse colon. *Cancer Letters*, 52, 145-152.

14. Koratkar, R. and Rao, A.R. (1997) Effect of Soya Bean Saponins on Azoxymethane-Induced Preneoplastic Lesions in the Colon of Mice. *Nutr. Cancer*, 27, 206-209.

15. Thompson, L.U. (1993) Potentional health benefits and problems associated with antinutrients in foods. *Food Res. Intl.*, 26, 131-149.

16. Yang, G.Y. and Shamsuddin, A.M. (1995) IP$_6$-induced growth inhibition and differentiation of HT- 29 human colon cancer cells: Involvement of intracellular inositol phosphates. *Anticancer Res.*, 15, 2479-2487.

17. Ullah, A. and Shamsuddin, A.M. (1990) Dose-dependent inhibition of large intestinal cancer by inositol hexaphosphate in F344 rats. *Carcinogenesis*, 11, 2219-2222.

18. Shamsuddin, A.M. (1995) Inositol phosphates have novel anticancer function. *J. Nutr.*, 125, 725S-732S.

19. Clarke, R., Hilakivi-Clarke, L., Cho,E., James, M.R., and Leonessa, F. (1996) Estrogens, phytoestrogens, and breast cancer. *Adv. Exp. Med. Biol.*, 401, 63-85.

20. Hsieh, C.Y., Santell, R.C., Haslam, S.Z., and Helferich, W.G. (1998) Estrogenic effects of genistein on the growth of estrogen receptor-positive human breast cancer (MCF-7) cells *in vitro* and *in vivo*. *Cancer Res.*, 58, 3833-3838.

2

DIETARY SOY REDUCES COLON CARCINOGENESIS IN HUMAN AND RATS
Soy and Colon Cancer

Maurice R. Bennink

Michigan State University
106 G. M. Trout Building
East Lansing, MI 48824

INTRODUCTION

The anti-cancer activity of individual soy phytochemicals (non-nutritive plant components with biological activity) have been extensively studied *in vitro* and *in vivo*. There is much less data relating soy consumption and colon cancer. This chapter will summarize epidemiologic studies and discuss the animal experiments and one intervention study that have evaluated the potential of dietary soy to inhibit colon carcinogenesis.

EPIDEMIOLOGIC STUDIES

Messina and Bennink (1) reviewed two ecological and eight case control studies that examined the relationship between soy food intake and colorectal cancer. Soy intake was not associated with a statistically significant reduction in colon cancer risk in any of the studies. Three studies did report lower risks. However, some studies also reported higher risks for some soy products and colon cancer. Overall, these studies do not support the hypothesis that soy intake reduces the risk of colorectal cancer. However, these studies were not designed specifically to determine if a relationship existed between soy consumption and risk of colon cancer, so it is still possible that such a relationship exists.

ANIMAL STUDIES

Although the epidemiologic data did not suggest that soy ingestion would reduce colon cancer risk, soy phytochemicals had been shown to inhibit growth of colon cancer cells and to inhibit chemically induced colon cancer. This prompted us to determine if soy could deliver sufficient quantities of anti-cancer phytochemicals to inhibit chemically induced colon cancer. Colon cancer was initiated in male F344 rats by injecting azoxymethane (15 mg/kg) at 22 and 29 days of age (2). The control diet was fed to all rats from 21 - 35 days of age and feeding of experimental diets began on day 36. We felt that the entire soybean would contain all of the anti-cancer phytochemicals and as soy was processed, some anti-cancer phytochemicals could be lost. In the first experiment we tested the anti-cancer potential of (a) full-fat soy flour (the entire soybean), (b) defatted soy flour (full-fat soy flour minus the oil and oil soluble phytochemicals), and (c) soy concentrate (defatted soy flour minus ethanol soluble phytochemicals). Feeding full fat soy flour and defatted soy flour reduced aberrant crypt formation compared to casein (2). However, feeding soy concentrate did not reduce aberrant crypt formation.

Since feeding full fat soy flour and defatted soy flour decreased the formation of precancerous lesions, we felt encouraged to determine if soy would inhibit tumor formation. Removing oil and oil soluble phytochemicals from full fat soy flour did not diminish the anti-cancer potential of soy (2), so we chose to test only defatted soy flour and soy concentrate in the second study. Diet composition and cancer induction were similar to the first experiment. After feeding the experimental diets for 7 months, we found that feeding defatted soy flour decreased tumor incidence by 44% and average tumor weight by 75% compared to casein (Table 1). Feeding soy concentrate did not reduce tumor incidence, number, or weight. These results suggested that ethanol soluble phytochemicals were the anti-cancer phytochemicals in defatted soy flour (3).

Since isoflavones are ethanol soluble, a third study was designed to determine if genistin or a mixture of genistin, daidzin, and glycitin, (the three major isoflavone glucosides in soy) would inhibit colon tumor formation. Tumor formation was measured in rats fed (a) defatted soy flour, (b) soy concentrate, (c) soy concentrate plus genistin, and (d) soy concentrate plus genistin, daidzin, and glycitin (4).

The isoflavones were added to soy concentrate to equal the amounts found in defatted soy flour. Feeding defatted soy flour decreased tumor incidence by 34% (Table 2). Feeding the mixture of isoflavones did not affect tumor incidence, but adding genistin increased tumor incidence (P=0.06). This result confirms the study by Rao et al. (5) where they fed 250 ppm genistein and

Table 1. Colon tumor incidence, number and weight in rats fed casein, soy concentrate or defatted soy flour

Diet	N	Tumor Incidence	Number of tumors/rat	Tumor weight (mg/rat)
Casein	19	61[a] %	1.05[a]	64[a]
Soy concentrate	40	64[a] %	1.06[a]	108[a]
Defatted soy flour	39	35[b] %	0.45[b]	16[b]

Means within a column with different superscripts are different (P≤0.05).

increased azoxymethane induced colon cancer. The genistin content of the diet in study three (Table 2) was equivalent to 500 ppm genistein. It should be noted that adding genistin or an isoflavone mixture to soy concentrate or feeding defatted soy flour decreased average tumor weight by about 50% (Table 2). These results suggest that genistin by itself is sufficient to inhibit tumor growth but not tumor incidence.

Table 2. Colon tumor incidence, number and weight in rats fed soy concentrate, defatted soy flour, genistin, or a mixture of isoflavones

Diet	N	Tumor Incidence	Number of tumors/rat	Tumor weight (mg/rat)
Soy concentrate	30	73[b] %	1.20[a]	209[a]
Defatted soy flour	29	48[a] %	0.83[b]	105b
Soy concentrate plus genistin	26	89[c] %	1.54[b]	103[b]
Soy concentrate plus isoflavone mixture	24	63[b] %	1.29[a]	81[b]

Means within a column with different superscripts are different (P≤0.05) except tumor incidence for the soy concentrate plus genistin group was different at P=0.06.

The overall conclusions from our animal studies were: (a) defatted soy flour inhibits colon carcinogenesis; (b) soy protein per se does not inhibit colon carcinogenesis; (c) ethanol soluble phytochemicals are the anti-cancer components in defatted soy flour; (d) genistin and other isoflavones are not the ethanol soluble phytochemicals that inhibit colon tumor incidence; and (e) genistin inhibits tumor growth.

There are two studies that report results contradictory to ours. McIntosh et al. (6) compared 1,2-dimethylhydrazine induced colon carcinogenesis in Spraque-Dawley rats fed defatted soybean meal, meat, casein and whey. There were no statistically significant difference in tumor incidence or tumor mass. When the dairy protein groups were combined (casein + whey) and compared to the meat plus soybean meal fed groups, there was a lower tumor burden in the groups fed dairy protein. The main difference between soybean meal and soybean flour is particle size (meal vs flour) and particle size is not likely to cause the discrepancy in our results. Other differences between their protocol and ours is strain of rat (Sprague-Dawley vs Fisher 344), carcinogen (1,2-dimethylhydrazine vs azoxymethane) and they fed the experimental diets prior to and during carcinogen administration whereas we start feeding the experimental diets one week after carcinogen administration. Barrett et al. (7) compared 1,2-dimethylhydrazine induced colon carcinogenesis in CF_1 male mice fed soybean meal, crambe meal or rapeseed meal. Mice fed soybean meal had a higher tumor incidence and more tumors than mice fed crambe or rapeseed meals. They did not include a casein control as a reference protein and they used a very high dosage of carcinogen. Differences in protocols most likely explain the discrepancy in results between defatted soy flour vs meal.

Soy protein isolate processed to retain isoflavones (Supro™) is used in many carcinogenesis studies. We have not used this soy protein source in our animal studies, but we used it in an human intervention study. However, Badger et al. (8) have conducted azoxymethane induced colon cancer studies in rats and report that feeding soy protein isolate (Supro™) inhibited colon carcinogenesis.

HUMAN INTERVENTION STUDY

We wanted to know if soy consumption would reduce colon cancer in a group of subjects identified as being "at risk". Our goal was to have subjects consume as much soy as possible for one year with minimum inconvenience and kcal to encourage compliance. We decided to use a soy protein isolate with relatively high levels of isoflavones (Supro™). Protein Technologies International kindly provided Supro™ and casein in unlabeled packets so that a double blind, prospective study could be conducted. The supplements provided 39 g of isolated soy protein or casein and 204 kcal per day (9). There was no other dietary intervention imposed on the free living subjects. The subjects self-reported supplement consumption and compliance was monitored by measuring isoflavone excretion in bimonthly urine samples.

Although it would be ideal to use tumor incidence as the endpoint, such a study would be very costly and would require a long time interval (probably more than 10 - 15 yr). Therefore, it was necessary to use a biomarker that would reflect colon cancer risk to evaluate effectiveness of dietary treatment. Epidemiologic and genetic studies have demonstrated that certain diseases or conditions significantly increase the risk for developing colon cancer. People with sporadic adenomatous polyps are known to have a significantly increased risk for developing colon cancer compared to the general U.S. population (10,11). People with a high risk for colon cancer, people with colon cancer and animals treated with colon carcinogens all have a relatively high number of mitotic cells in the top one third of the colon crypt (12-15). Humans with low risk for colon cancer and control animals have few or no mitotic cells in the upper one-third of the colon crypt (12,13,15). A downward shift in the proliferative zone of colon crypts appears to be the best indicator that a treatment has reduced the risk for colon cancer.

Subjects with a history of colon polyps or colon cancer (an "at risk"population) were randomly assigned to treament. Colon mucosa biopsies were obtained before and after consuming the supplement for a year. More than 92% of the urine samples from subjects consuming the soy supplement contained isoflavones which indicates a high degree of compliance. Immunohistochemical detection of proliferative cell nuclear antigen (PCNA) was used to detect crypt cell proliferation patterns in the biopsies. There was a statistically significant reduction in labeling index (P=0.02) and proliferation zone (P=0.06) in subjects that consumed the soy supplement (Table 3). The labeling index and proliferation zone were unchanged (P>0.95) for subjects that consumed casein. Since the presence of nuclear PCNA indicates that a cell is capable of division, lack of nuclear PCNA implies that the cell has terminally differentiated. These results suggest that eating soy protein isolate enhances cell differentiation in colon mucosa and reduces risk of colon cancer in a 'at risk' population. We have also measured the labeling index and proliferation zone in subjects with no known intestinal diseases (16). Both the labeling index and the proliferation zone increased linearly with age from 20 to 70 yr. The beginning proliferation patterns for the subjects consuming soy (Table 3) were typical of a 75 yr old whereas the ending values were typical of a 55-60 yr old. The percentage of people developing malignant colon cancer

Table 3. Cell proliferation in colon mucosa biopsies before and after consuming casein or soy supplements for one year

	Casein (N=13)		Soy Protein Isolate (N=29)	
	before	after	before	after
Labeling index	0.285	0.282	0.308	0..257[*]
Proliferation zone	0.486	0.473	0.528	0.4.52[*]

Labeling index and proliferation zone decreased for the group consuming the soy supplement (P≤0.05), but not for the group consuming casein.

at 55-60 yr is much less than for 75 yr old. Thus, we interpret the downward shift in proliferative zone and the decrease in labeling index as meaningful decrease in colon cancer risk.

CONCLUSIONS

Soy flour reduces azoxymethane induced colon cancer in rats. The reduction of colon carcinogenesis with soy feeding is not due to soy protein per se, but appears to be due to ethanol soluble components other than the isoflavones found in soy flour. The isoflavone genistin reduced tumor growth but increased tumor incidence. Subjects with a history of adenomatous polyps or colon cancer consumed 39g of isolated soy protein for one year and had a significant reduction in labeling index and proliferation zone in their colonic crypts. Overall, our results strongly suggest that eating soy flour or isolated soy protein will reduce colon cancer risk.

ACKNOWLEDGMENTS

The following have made substantial contributions to the research reported above: L.D. Bourquin, J.E. Mayle, A.S. Om, and D.G. Thiagarajan.

REFERENCES

1. Messina, M., Bennink, M. Soyfoods, isoflavones and risk of colon cancer: A review of the in vitro and in vivo data. *Bailliere's Clin. Endocrin. Metab.* 1998; 12:707-28.

2. Thiagarajan, D.G., Bennink, M.R., Bourquin, L.D., Kavas, F.A. Prevention of precancerous colonic lesions in rats by soy flakes, soy flour, genistein, and calcium. *Am. J. Clin. Nutr.* 1998; 68:1394S-9S.

3. Bennink, M.R., Om, A.S. Inhibition of colon cancer (CC) by soy phytochemicals but not by soy protein. FASEB J 1998; 12:A655.

4. Bennink, M.R, Om, AS, Miyagi Y. Inhibition of colon cancer (CC) by soy flour but not by genistin or a mixture of isoflavones. FASEB J 1999; 13:A50.

5. Rao, C.V., Wang, C.-X., Simi, B., Lubet, R., Kelloff, G., Steele, V., Reddy, B.S. Enhancement of experimental colon cancer by genistein. *Cancer Res* 1997; 57:3717-22.

6. McIntosh, G.H., Regester, G.O., Leu Le, R.K, Royle, P.J., Smithers, G.W. Dairy proteins protect against dimethylhydrazine-induced intestinal cancers in rats. *J. Nutr.* 1995; 125:809-16.

7. Barrett, J.E., Klopfenstein, C.F., Leipold, H.W. Protective effects of cruciferous seed meals and hulls against colon cancer in mice. *Cancer Lett* 1998; 127:83-8.

8. Badger, T., Hakkak, R., Korourjian, S., Ronis, M., Rowlands, C., Shelnutt, S. Differential and tissue specific protective effects of diets formulated with whey or soy proteins on chemically-induced mammary and colon cancer in rats. FASEB J 1999; 13:A583.

9. Thiagarajan, D., Bennick, M.R., Bourquin, L.D., Mayle, J.E., Seymour, E.M., Mridvika. Effect of soy protein consumption on colonic cell proliferation in humans. FASEB J 1999; 13: A370.

10. Lofti, A.M. and Spencer, R.J., Ilstrup, D.M., Melton, J. Colorectal polyps and the risk of subsequent carcinoma. *Mayo Clin. Proc.* 1986; 61: 337-43.

11. Cole, J.W., McKalen, A. Studies on the morphogenesis of adenomatous polyps in the human colon. Cancer (Phila) 1963; 16: 998.

12. Lipkin, M. Biomarkers of increased susceptibility to gastrointestinal cancer: New applications to studies of cancer prevention in human subjects. *Cancer Res* 1988; 48: 235-45.

13. Lipkin, M. and Higgins, P. Biological markers of cell proliferation and differentiation in human gastrointestinal diseases. *Adv Cancer Res* 1998; 50: 1-22.

14. Deschner, E.E. "The relationship of altered cell proliferation to colonic neoplasia". In *Colonic Carcinogenesis: Falk Symposium 31*, R.A. Malt and R.C. Williamson, ed. Lancaster, UK: MTP Press Ltd. 1982, pp. 25-30.

15. Lipkin, M., Blattner, W.E., Fraumeni, J.F., Lynch, H., Deschner, E. and Winawer, S. Tritiated thymidine (O_p, O_h) labeling distribution as a marker for hereditary predisposition to colon cancer. *Cancer Res* 1983; 43:1899-1904.

16. Thiagarajan, D., Bennink, M.R., Srinivasan, R., Mayle, J.E., Bourquin, L.D. Epithelial cell proliferation in colonic crypts of humans at varying risks for colon cancer (CC). FASEB J 1998; 12: A567.

3

SOY AND RISK OF HORMONE-RELATED AND OTHER CANCERS

Anna H. Wu, Ph.D.

University of Southern California,
Department of Preventive Medicine
1441 Eastlake Avenue, MS#44
Los Angeles, CA 90089

INTRODUCTION

For the last presentation in this session on soy and cancer, I will cover the epidemiologic evidence on soy and several hormone-related and other cancers. My comments will focus on breast, endometrium and prostate cancers, three hormone-related cancer sites. The role of soy has been also investigated in several non-hormone related cancers including colorectal, stomach and lung cancer. As Dr. Maurice Bennink has just given an excellent presentation on colorectal cancer, my remarks will be limited to stomach and lung cancers.

Soy foods are the main source of isoflavones, one of two main classes of phytoestrogens important in the human diet. The analytic epidemiologic studies I have included are those that have data on dietary soy intake or urinary excretion of isoflavones on an individual level (isoflavone excretion is used as a marker of soy intake). Cross-sectional studies,

Nutrition and Cancer Prevention, edited under the auspices of AICR
Kluwer Academic / Plenum Publishers, New York, 2000.

19

dissertations, abstracts and articles in languages other than English are excluded in this discussion.

ASSESSMENT OF SOY INTAKE IN EPIDEMIOLOGIC STUDIES

Before describing the epidemiologic evidence, it is important to review the types of soy foods that were included in the published epidemiologic studies. These studies were primarily concerned with the intake of the traditional Asian soy foods. The whole soybeans may be consumed although this is not a very common form of soy food in the Asian diet (Adlercreutz et al., 1990; Wakai et al., 1999a; Chen et al., 1999). More commonly consumed are various fermented (e.g., miso, natto) and nonfermented soy foods (e.g., tofu, soymilk, fried or dried bean curd). In addition, select processed foods or meat-based mixed dishes may contain varying amounts and various types of soy ingredients (e.g., soy protein, soy flour) that have been added as an extender (Lampe et al., 1999; Horn-Ross et al., 2000). It is difficult to accurately assess exposure to these 'hidden' sources of soy isoflavones as the manufacturers' practice of adding soy ingredients may be brand- and product-specific and variable over time. However, these 'hidden' sources of soy intake are unlikely to be important in epidemiologic studies conducted in populations that consume traditional Asian soy foods because Asian soy foods would account for most of the isoflavones consumed. In the last few years, a growing number of second-generation soy foods have been introduced (e.g., soy burger, soy hot dog, soy yogurt, soy cheese). The isoflavone contents in these second- generation soy foods are highly variable and tend to be lower than those in Asian soy foods (Coward et al., 1993; Wang and Murphy, 1994; Kirk et al., 1999; Murphy et al., 1999). These second-generation soy foods are not relevant in the epidemiologic studies published to date but they may become more important in future studies if the intake of these foods increases and they become an integral part of the American diet.

BREAST CANCER

A role of diet, particularly, dietary fat has been long suspected in the etiology of breast cancer but its role remains controversial (Greenwald 1999; Hunter 1998). In recent years, high intake of soy has been suggested to explain in part, the traditionally much lower risk of breast cancer in Asia (Adlercreutz 1990). Many hormonal and non-hormonal properties (Barnes 1999) have been associated with genistein, one of the three isoflavones, providing compelling biologic plausibility that soy foods may indeed have a role in the etiology of breast and other cancers.

Since 1990, three case-control (Lee et al., 1991; Hirose et al., 1995; Yuan et al., 1995) and two cohort studies (Hirayama 1990; Key et al., 1999) conducted in Asia have evaluated the association between soy intake and risk of breast cancer. Results from two hospital-based case-control studies (Lee et al., 1991; Hirose et al., 1995) suggest a decreased risk associated with high soy intake, but this was limited to premenopausal women only (details of these studies are provided in Wu et al., 1998 and Key et al., 1999). Soy intake was not associated with risk of breast cancer in three other studies including a large and well-conducted population-based case-control study conducted in China that considered many potential dietary and non-dietary confounders (Yuan et al., 1995). In two prospective studies conducted in Japan, intake of miso (Hirayama, 1990; Key et al., 1999) and bean curd (Key et al., 1999) was not significantly associated with risk of breast cancer (results on soy were not presented separately by menopausal status).

The role of soy foods and breast cancer risk was evaluated in two case-control studies conducted in the US. In a small study of bilateral breast cancer in premenopausal women, Witte et al (1997) reported that weekly intake of tofu was associated with a reduced risk (odds ratio (OR)=0.5) that was not statistically significant. In a large multi-center study of breast cancer conducted among Asian-Americans residing in California and Hawaii, high intake of tofu ($\geq$120 times per year) was associated with a statistically significant 30% reduced risk compared to low intake (<13 times per year). This finding was observed after adjustment of migration status and select dietary and non-dietary risk factors and was present in both pre- and postmenopausal women. However, the inverse association was stronger and statistically significant only among women born in Asia and not among US born Asian women (Wu et al., 1996).

Two other studies, comparing urinary excretion of phytoestrogens (as a marker of dietary intake) in breast cancer patients and healthy control women, further suggested that soy may have a protective role (Ingram et al., 1998; Zheng et al., 1999). In an Australian study, risk of breast cancer was reduced by more than 50% among women whose urinary excretion of equol (an isoflavone metabolite) was in the upper three quartiles (p=0.009) (Ingram et al., 1998). In a study conducted in China (Zheng et al., 1999), women who had total urinary isoflavone levels in the upper two tertiles showed a statistically nonsignificant 50% reduction in risk of breast cancer compared to those in the lowest tertile. Risk was lowest (RR=0.14, p<0.05) for those who displayed high excretion levels of both isoflavones and phenol (a surrogate marker of fruit and vegetable intake) (Zheng et al., 1999). Despite these intriguing results, both biomarker studies are limited in that the urine specimens from breast cancer patients were obtained after their diagnosis. Thus the results are meaningful only if the intake of phytoestrogen-rich foods did not change after cancer diagnosis. In addition, soy intake was not available in the Australian study and was described only for controls in the Chinese study (Chen et al., 1999). In the Australian study, level of isoflavone excretion was also low, even among those in the highest excretion category whereas level of lignan excretion was relatively high, even among those in the low excretion category. It is unclear whether the effects of lignans and isoflavone were independent of each other.

ENDOMETRIAL CANCER

We are aware of only one study with specific data on soy intake and risk of endometrial cancer (Goodman et al., 1997). In this population-based case-control study conducted among Asians (65% were Japanese) and Whites in Hawaii (332 cases and 511 controls), increasing intakes of tofu, tofu and other soy products, and all legumes combined (which included tofu) were associated with statistically significant decreased risks of endometrial cancer after adjustment of total calories and select non-dietary risk factors. For example, the odds ratios for endometrial cancer associated with the three upper quartiles compared with the lowest quartile of tofu intake were 0.65, 0.70, and 0.53, respectively. The inverse associations with soy (and legumes) were observed in both Asians and non-Asians in this study. In contrast, intake of legumes was not associated with risk of endometrial cancer in a case-control study conducted in Shanghai, China (Shu et al., 1993). The intake level of legumes was not provided in this Chinese population and it is unclear whether soy foods were specifically included under 'legumes' in this study.

PROSTATE CANCER

The effect of soy intake on prostate cancer risk was investigated in three cohort (Severson et al., 1989; Hirayama 1990; Jacobsen et al., 1998) and four case-control (Oishi et al., 1988; Lee et al., 1998; Strom et al., 1999; Kolonel et al, 2000) studies. Data from the three studies conducted in Asia are not supportive of a reduction in risk in association with soy intake (Hirayama 1990; Oishi et al., 1988; Lee et al., 1998). In both studies from Japan, the risk of prostate cancer increased in association with high intake of miso (Hirayama 1990; Oishi et al., 1988); the result was statistically significant in one (relative risk = 1.45, 95% CI = 1.09-1.94) (Hirayama 1990). Intake of non-fermented soy foods was not assessed in these two Japanese studies. In a 13 city case-control study conducted in China, mean daily intake of soy (based on 7 soy foods) was lower among prostate cancer cases compared to population controls (71 versus 83 gm per day, respectively) (no other details regarding soy intake were provided) (Lee et al., 1998).

In contrast, results from two cohort and two case-control studies conducted in the US are supportive of an inverse association with non-fermented soy foods. Among Seventh Day Adventists in California, high daily intake of soymilk compared to no intake was associated with a statistically significant 70% reduction in risk (Jacobson et al., 1998). High (5+ times per week) intake of tofu compared to less than weekly intake was also associated with a statistically significant 65% reduction in risk of prostate cancer in a cohort of Japanese in Hawaii (Severson et al., 1989). However, high intake of miso (5+ times per week vs less than weekly intake) was associated with a small increased risk among Japanese in Hawaii (OR=1.29), similar to the increased risk reported among native Japanese men (Oishi et al., 1988; Hirayama 1990). In this study of Japanese in Hawaii, the results on tofu and miso were not simultaneously adjusted for each other. In a small, hospital-based case-control study conducted among white men in Texas, intake of genistein and daidzen was reported to be lower among prostate cancer cases compared to controls. However, the intake of isoflavones was extremely low in this population, less than 0.1 mg per day (daily intake of isoflavones in Japan and China ranges between 20 to 40 mg (Wakai et al., 1999a; Chen et al., 1999)). Thus, the significance of this study's findings is questionable. In a large and well-conducted case-control study of African-Americans, whites, and Asians residing California, Hawaii and British Columbia, Canada, highest quintile intake of tofu (>39.4 gm per day versus no intake) was associated with a 38% lower risk of prostate cancer (p trend=0.06). However, the inverse association in this study may be due to intake of all legumes and not specifically to intake of soy foods (Kolonel et al., 2000).

STOMACH CANCER

Data on soy intake and risk of stomach cancer are available from some twenty studies which were conducted to investigate reasons for the high risk of this cancer among Chinese, Japanese, and Koreans (Wu et al., 2000). Fermented soy foods are known to be high in salt; high salt intake is a well-established risk factor for stomach cancer (Nomura 1996). On the other hand, high intake of non-fermented soy foods may be associated with intake of plant-based foods which is associated with a reduced risk of stomach cancer (Nomura 1996). Thus, we conducted a meta-analysis to examine the separate effects of fermented and non-fermented soy foods on risk of stomach cancer (Wu et al., 2000).

In our pooled analysis which included over 8000 stomach cancers with data on intake of miso or other fermented soy foods, high intake was associated with a statistically significant 11% reduction in stomach cancer risk. However, this inverse association was due solely to the reduced risk observed in a single study (Hirayama 1990) which accounted for some 65% of the stomach cancers in the pooled analysis. Exclusion of this single study yielded a statistically significant 24% increased risk in association with high intake of miso and stomach cancer risk. When we conducted a pooled analysis that included 11 studies with data on intake of non-fermented soy foods, risk of stomach decreased statistically significantly by 28% in association with high intake of non-fermented soy foods. However, because of the potential confounding effects of other dietary factors such as intake of salt and plant foods, the role of fermented and non-fermented soy foods cannot be determined based on the published data (Wu et al., 2000).

LUNG CANCER

Intake of soy foods and risk of lung cancer has been investigated in a Japanese cohort (Hirayama 1990) and in case-control studies conducted in Japan (Wakai et al., 1999b) and among Chinese residing in Hong Kong (Koo et al., 1998) and in select lung cancer high-risk areas in China (Wu-Williams et al., 1990; Swanson et al., 1992; Hu et al., 1997). In two studies, risk of lung cancer was not associated with intake of miso (Hirayama 1990) or soybean products (Wu-Williams et al., 1990). In three other studies conducted among Chinese subjects, a 40 to 60% reduction in lung cancer risk was found in association with the highest level of tofu / soybean intake (Koo et al., 1998; Swanson et al., 1992; Hu et al., 1997); the result was statistically significant in one study (Swanson et al., 1992). In a Japanese case-control study, the association between risk of lung cancer and soy intake differed for fermented and nonfermented soyfoods (Wakai et al., 1999b). In this study, lung cancer risk increased statistically significantly in association with daily intake of miso, but the risk decreased statistically significantly in association with daily or almost daily intake of tofu / soybeans. As discussed above (see Stomach Cancer), intake of fermented and nonfermented soyfoods may be correlated with other dietary factors that are causally important in lung cancer development. For example, high intake of vegetables was associated with a statistically significantly lowered risk of lung cancer in the studies by Swanson et al (1992) and Koo et al (1988); the findings on soy were not adjusted for the effects of vegetable intake in these studies.

SUMMARY

The collective evidence on the role of soy food and the cancer sites discussed above is inconclusive. For breast cancer, five studies conducted in Asia with dietary soy data produced inconsistent results. In contrast, an inverse association was found in two US studies with data on tofu intake and in two other studies with urinary isoflavone levels on breast cancer cases and controls. In several studies, a lowered risk associated with soy intake was observed primarily in premenopausal women.

High intake of miso was associated with an increased risk of prostate cancer in all three studies conducted among native Japanese or those residing in Hawaii. On the other hand, there is some support from studies conducted in China and the US that the risk of prostate cancer may be lowered in association with high intake of non-fermented soy foods (i.e., not miso). A role of non-fermented soy food may be related to a general inverse association with high intake of legumes.

Results based on a single study conducted in Hawaii suggest that high intake of soy may lower the risk of endometrial cancer. As in prostate cancer, the lowered risk associated with soy intake may be related to the protection conferred by high intake of legumes.

Our meta-analysis suggests that high intake of fermented soy foods may be associated with an increased risk of stomach cancer whereas high intake of non-fermented soy foods may be associated with a reduced risk. Because intake of soy foods is correlated with other dietary factors that are known to influence risk of stomach cancer, the role of fermented and non-fermented soy foods cannot be determined until the roles of these potential confounders are considered.

There is some suggestion that intake of nonfermented soy foods may be lower in lung cancer cases compared to controls. However, as in the studies of stomach cancer, intake of plant based foods should be, but has not been considered in these analyses. Adequate adjustment for smoking is also critical in studies of lung cancer and soy intake.

Sources of inconsistencies in the studies published to date

It is important to emphasize that almost all the published studies on soy and cancer were not designed specifically to investigate the role of this food group. Thus, the assessment of soy intake varied and was often incomplete. These studies, however, have the advantage in that respondent recall bias is unlikely since there was little or no interest in the soy hypothesis when these studies were conducted. In fact, in many of the studies, results on soy were not even described or discussed by the investigators but were presented as one of the many dietary factors assessed. In most of the studies conducted in China, almost all asked about the intake of more than one soy food and the risk of cancer was determined in relation to total soy intake. In contrast, studies conducted in Japan often only asked about intake of miso when this single food represents approximately 25% of the soy intake; tofu represents approximately 45% of the total soy intake in Japan (Adlercreutz et al., 1990; Nagata et al., 1998; Wakai et al., 1999a). Thus, in studies conducted in Japan, misclassification of soy intake is likely when assessment was based solely on miso consumption. Most of the studies conducted in the US used tofu as a marker of total soy intake. Misclassification of exposure may also exist since tofu eaten by itself or in mixed dishes represents the primary source, but only about 60%, of the total soy intake among Asians residing in Los Angeles County (Wu, unpublished). Since not all soyfoods are the same, it is important that future studies distinguish between fermented and nonfermented soyfoods in the assessment and analysis. Because of the generally high consumption of soy in Asia, the comparison in these studies is between very high versus less high, but still substantial, soy intake. On the other hand, studies conducted in the US cover much lower soy consumption; the baseline group is usually represented by no intake. Data on dose-response relationships are sparse and they are clearly needed as different parts of the dose-response curve are examined in the studies conducted in Asia and those outside of Asia. Finally, published studies are also varied in terms of adjustment of potential confounders. Because soy was not a primary dietary factor under investigation, many studies presented only the sex- and/or age-adjusted risk estimates associated with soy intake. Only some studies considered both potential dietary and non-dietary confounders in the analyses. Our pooled analysis on soy intake and stomach cancer illustrates clearly that adequate adjustment of dietary confounders is essential in studies of soy and cancer (Wu et al., 2000). The extent to which 'soy' is a marker of acculturation cannot be discounted in studies conducted in Asian-Americans. Soy intake may also be a marker of a 'healthier' lifestyle; this needs to be considered.

REFERENCES

1. Adlercreutz, H. Western diet and western disease: some hormonal and biochemical mechanisms and associations. *Scand. J. Clin. Lab Invest. Suppl.* 1990; 50:3-23.
2. Barnes, S. Phytoestrogens and breast cancer. *Bailliere's Clinical Endo. Metab.* 1998; 12: 559-79.
3. Chen, Z., Zheng, W., Custer, L.J., Dai, Q., Shu, X.O., Jin, F., Franke, A.A. Usual dietary consumption of soy foods and its correlation with the excretion rate of isoflavonoids in overnight urine samples among Chinese women in Shanghai. *Nutr. Cancer* 1999; 33: 82-7.

4. Coward, L., Barnes, N.C., Setchell, K.D.R., Barnes, S. Genistein, daidzein, and their b-glycoside conjugates: Antitumor isoflavones in soybean foods from American and Asian diets. *J. Agric. Food Chem.* 1993; 4: 1961-7.

5. Goodman, M.T., Wilkens, L.R., Hankin, J.R., Lyu, L.C., Wu, A.H., Kolonel, L.N. Association of soy and fiber consumption with the risk of endometrial cancer. *Am. J. Epidemiol.* 1997; 146: 294-306.

6. Greenwald, P. Role of dietary fat in the causation of breast cancer: Point. *Cancer Epidemiology, Biomarkers and Prev* 1999; 8: 3-7.

7. Horn-Ross, P.L., Barnes, S., Lee, M., Coward, L., Mandel, E., Koo, J., John, E.M., Smith, M. Assessing phytoestrogen exposure in epidemiologic studies: development of a database (United States). Cancer Causes and Control 2000; 11: 289-298.

8. Hirayama, T. Life-style and mortality. A large-scale census-based cohort study in Japan. In: *Contributions to Epidemiology and Biostatistics.* Vol 6. Wahrendorf, J. (eds). Karger, Basel. 1990.

9. Hirose, K., Tajimak, K., Hamajimak, N., Inouek, M., Takezaki, T., Kuroishi, T., Yoshida, M., Tokudome, S. A large-scale, hospital-based case-control study of risk factors of breast cancer according to menopausal status. *Jpn. J. Cancer Res.* 1995; 86: 146-154.

10. Hu, J., Johnson, K.C., Mao, Y., Xu, T., Lin, Q., Wang, C., Zhao, F., Wnag, G., Chen, Y., Yang, Y. A case-control study of diet and lung cancer in Northeast China. *Int. J. Cancer* 1997; 71: 924-31.

11. Hunter, D.J. Role of dietary fat in the causation of breast cancer: Counterpoint. *Cancer Epidemiology, Biomarkers and Prev* 1999; 8: 9-14.

12. Ingram, D., Sanders, K., Kolybaba, M. Case-control study of phyto-estrogens and breast cancer. *Lancet* 1997; 350: 990-4, 1997.

13. Jacobsen, B.K., Knutsen, S.F., Fraser, G.E. Does high soy milk intake reduce prostate cancer incidence? The Adventist Health Study (United States). *Cancer Causes and Control* 1998; 9: 553-557.

14. Key, T.J., Sharp, G.B., Appleby, P.N., Beral, V., Goodman, M.T., Soda, M., Mabuchi, K. Soya foods and breast cancer risk: A prospective study in Hiroshima and Nagasaki, Japan. *Br. J. Cancer* 1999; 81: 1248-1256.

15. Kirk, P., Patterson, R.E., Lampe, L. Development of a soy food frequency questionnaire to estimate isoflavone consumption in US adults. *J. Am Diet Assoc.* 1999; 99: 558-563.

16. Kolonel, L.N., Hankin, J.H., Whittemoore, A.S., Wu, A.H., Gallagher, R.P., Wilkens, L.R., John, E.M., Howe, G.R., Dreon, D.M., West, D.W., Paffenbarger, R.S., Jr. Vegetables, fruits, legumes and prostate cancer: A multiethnic case-control study. *Cancer Epidemiol., Biomarkers and Prev* 2000; 9:795-804.

17. Koo, L.C. Dietary habits and lung cancer risk among Chinese females in Hong Kong who never smoked. *Nutr. Cancer* 1988; 11: 155-72.

18. Lampe, J.W., Gustafson, D.R., Hutchins, A.M., Martini, M.C., Li, S., Wahala, K., Grandits, G.A., Potter, D.J., Slavin, J.L. Urinary isoflavonoid and lignan excretion on a Western diet: relation to soy, vegetable and fruit intake. *Cancer Epidemiol, Biomarkers and Prev* 1999; 8:699-707.

19. Lee, H.P., Gourley, L., Duffy, S.W., Esteve, J., Lee, J., Day, N.E. Dietary effects on breast-cancer risk in Singapore. *Lancet* 1991;331:1197-200.

20. Lee, M.M., Wang, R.T., Hsing, A.W., et al. Case-control study of diet and prostate cancer in China. *Cancer Causes and Control* 1998; 9: 545-552.

21. Murphy, P.A., Song, T.T., Buseman, G., Barua, K., Beecher, G.R., Trainer D, Holden J. Isoflavones in retail and institutional soy foods. *J. Agric. Food Chem.* 1999; 47:2697-2704.

22. Nagata, C., Takatsuka, N., Inaba, S., Norito, K. and Shimizu, H. Effect of soymilk consumption on serum estrogen concentrations in premenopausal Japanese women. *J. Natl. Cancer Inst.* 1998; 90:1980-1985.

23. Nomura, A. "Stomach Cancer." *In Cancer Epidemiology and Prevention*, D.Schottenfeld, J.F. Fraumeni, Jr, eds. New York, Oxford Press, 1996.

24. Oishi, K., Okada, K., Yoshida, O., Tamaba, H., Ohno, Y., Hayes, R.B., Schroeder, F.H. A case-control study of prostatic cancer with reference to dietary habits. *The Prostate* 1988; 12: 179-190.

25. Severson, R.K., Nomura, A.M.Y., Grove, J.S., Stemmermann, G.N. A prospective study of demographics, diet, and prostate cancer among men of Japanese ancestry in Hawaii. *Cancer Res.* 1989; 49: 1857-1860.

26. Shu, X.O., Zheng, W., Potischman, N., Brinton, LA., Hatch, M.C., Gao, Y.T., Fraumeni, J.F., Jr. A population-based case-control study of dietary factors and endometrial cancer in Shanghai, People's Republic of China. *Am. J. Epidemiol.* 1993; 137: 155-165.

27. Strom, S.S., Yamamura, Y., Duphorne, C.M., Spitz, M.R., Babaian, R.J., Pillow, P.J., Hursting, S.D. Phytoestrogen intake and prostate cancer: A case-control study using a new database. *Nutr. Cancer* 1999; 33: 20-5.

28. Swanson, C.A., Mao, B.L., Li, J.Y., Lubin, J.H., Yao, S.X., Wang, J.Z., Cai, S.K., Hou, Y., Luo, Q.S., Blot, W.J. Dietary determinants of lung cancer risk: Results from a case-control study in Yunnan Province, China. *Int. J. Cancer* 1992; 50: 876-80.

29. Wakai K., Egami, I., Kato, K., Kawamura, T., Tamakoshi, A., Lin, Y., Nakayama, T., Wada, M. and Ohno, Y. Dietary intake and sources of isoflavones among Japanese. *Nutr. Cancer* 1999a; 33: 139-145.

30. Wakai, K., Ohno, Y., Genka, K., Ohmine, K., Kawamura, T., Tamakoshi, A., Lin, Y., Nakayama, T., Aoki, K., Fukuma, S. Risk modifications in lung cancer by a dietary intake of preserved foods and soyfoods: findings from a case-controlled study in Okinawa, Japan. *Lung Cancer* 1999b; 25:147-159.

31. Wang, H.J. and Murphy, P.A. Isoflavone content in commercial soybean foods. *J. Agric. Food Chem.* 1994; 42: 1666-1673.

32. Witte, J.S., Ursin, G., Siemiatycki, J., Thompson, W.D., Paganini-Hill, A., Haile, R.W. Diet and premenopausal bilateral breast cancer: a case-control study. *Breast Cancer Res. Treat.* 1997; 42: 243-551.

33. Wu, A.H., Ziegler, R.C., Horn-Ross, P.L., Nomura, A.M.Y., Weot, D.W., Kolonel, L.N., Rosenthal, J.F., Hoover, R.N., Pike, M.C. Tofu and risk of breast cancer in Asian-Americans. *Cancer Epidemiol. Biomarkers Prev.* 1996; 5: 901-6.

34. Wu, A.H., Yang, D., Pike, M.C. A meta-analysis of soy foods and risk of stomach cancer: The problem of potential confounders. Cancer Epidemiol., Biomarkers and Prev 2000; 9: 1051-1058.

35. Wu-Williams, A.H., Dai, X.D., Blot, W., Xu, Z.Y., Sun, X.W., Xiao, H.P., Stone, B.J., Yu, S.F., Feng, Y.P., Ershow, A.G., Sun, J., Fraumeni, J.R., Jr., Henderson, B.E. Lung cancer among women in north-east China. *Br. J. Cancer* 1990; 62: 982-7.

36. Yuan, J.M., Wang, Q.S., Ross, R.K., Henderson, B.E., Yu, M.C. Diet and breast cancer in Shanghai and Tianjin, China. *Br. J. Cancer* 1995; 71: 1353-8.

37. Zheng, W., Dai, Q., Custer, L.J., Shu, X.O., Wen, W.Q., Jin, F., Franke, A.A. Urinary excretion of isoflavonoids and the risk of breast cancer. *Cancer Epidemiol. Biomark Prev.* 1999; 8: 35-40.

4

ROLE OF TOMATOES, TOMATO PRODUCTS AND LYCOPENE IN CANCER PREVENTION

David Heber, Qing-Yi Lu, and Vay Liang W. Go

UCLA Center for Human Nutrition
Los Angeles, CA 90095

A great deal of evidence from international epidemiological studies indicates that diets high in fruit and vegetable intake are associated with a lower risk of many common forms of cancer[1-3]. Dietary recommendations emphasize increasing total fruit and vegetable intake from diverse sources such as citrus fruits, cruciferous vegetables, and green and yellow vegetables.[3] It is assumed that each of these classes of plant-derived foods has unique phytochemicals which interact with the host to confer a preventive benefit by upregulation of enzymes important in metabolizing xenobiotics and carcinogens, by direct effects on nuclear receptors and cellular signaling of proliferation and apoptosis, and indirectly through antioxidant actions which reduce proliferation and protect DNA from damage.[4]

Lycopene, the predominant carotenoid in tomatoes and tomato products has the highest antioxidant activity of any dietary carotenoid.[5] Giovanucci et al.[6] found that increased dietary intake of lycopene was associated with a reduced risk of prostate cancer. Other carotenoids such as lutein, β-cryptoxanthin, and α- and β-carotene were not correlated with decreased risk in this epidemiological study. Earlier epidemiologic studies on the relationship of the intake of tomatoes or tomato products to cancer incidence results were equivocal, while studies where serum levels of lycopene were measured demonstrated a clear association between cancer

Nutrition and Cancer Prevention, edited under the auspices of AICR
Kluwer Academic / Plenum Publishers, New York, 2000.

incidence and serum levels of lycopene (see Figure 1).[6] One possible explanation for these disparate findings is that the bioavailability of lycopene is greater from heat-processed tomato products such as soups, mixed vegetable juices, and pasta sauces than from raw tomato.[7]

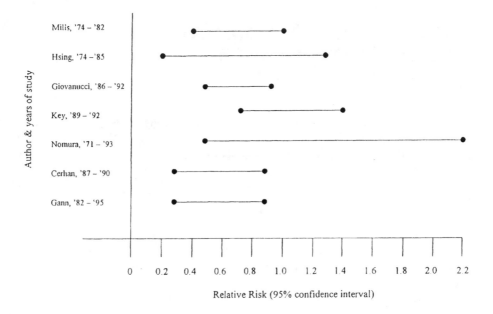

Figure 1. Epidemiological studies of tomato or lycopene intake and relative risk of prostate cancer. (Modified from Table 4, Ref. 8)

In studies of the bioavailability of lycopene, the uptake of lycopene into chylomicrons was found to be greater from heat-processed tomato juice than from unprocessed tomato juice. Ingestion of tomato juice cooked in an oil medium resulted in a two- to three-fold increase in lycopene serum concentrations one day after ingestion, but an equivalent consumption of unprocessed tomato juice caused no rise in plasma concentrations.[9] Cooking or chopping are thought to increase bioavailability by breaking down sturdy cell walls, thus making carotenoids more bioavailable.

A typical high-pressure liquid chromatography profile of carotenoids in human plasma is shown in Figure 2A and can be compared to the carotenoid pattern in fresh tomatoes or tomato paste (Figures 2B and 2C).

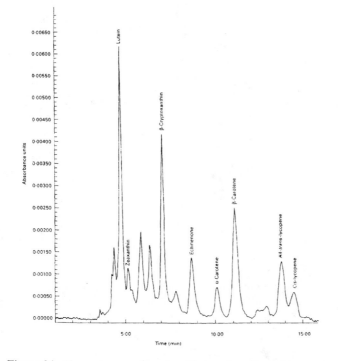

Figure 2A. Chromatogram of carotenoids in a plasma sample. (With permission, Ref. 10)

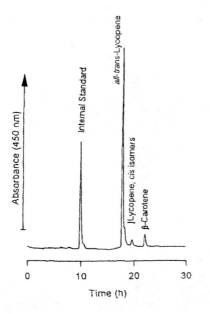

Figure 2B. Carotenoid pattern in fresh tomatoes. (With permission, Ref. 7)

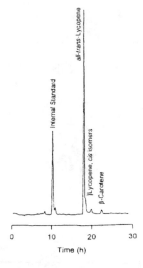

Figure 2C. Carotenoid pattern in tomato paste. (With permission, Ref. 7)

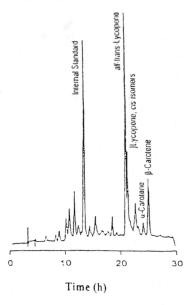

Figure 2D. Carotenoid pattern in the chylomicron fraction of one volunteer four hours after consumption of tomato paste. (With permission, Ref. 7)

     The key difference that can be noted on close examination of the chromatograms above is that lycopene undergoes cis-isomerization during the process of absorption into plasma. Tomatoes and tomato products have predominantly all-trans lycopene, but once lycopene appears in chylomicrons a significant fraction has been isomerized and that pattern remains when plasma samples are analyzed for lycopene.

Lycopene is the predominant carotenoid in the prostate gland and the profile of lycopene metabolites found in prostatic tissue differs from the profile found in plasma samples.[11] There are suggestions that the local metabolism of lycopene in the prostate may be important in determining its preventive effects on prostate cancer growth and development. Previous work had shown that the levels of lycopene in plasma could be increased by tomato or tomato puree over a seven day period (Figure 3). Elevations in total lycopene, all-trans lycopene and cis-lycopene were greater with the tomato puree than with raw tomato.

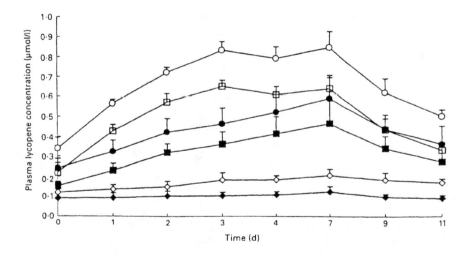

Figure 3. Plasma lycopene concentrations over time in subjects consuming daily portions of raw tomato or tomato puree over seven days of study. (With permission, Ref. 10)

   In order to determine whether a mixed vegetable juice (V-8, Campbell's Soup Company) would be a feasible means of elevating serum lycopene levels in prostate cancer patients, we studied 38 prostate cancer patients ages 52 to 79 who were not under active treatment.[12] Patients had prostate cancer in stages T1C to T2C. Over a three-month period, patients were instructed to eat a very low fat diet (15% of energy from fat), which was also high in fiber (18 gm/1000 kcal) and high in fruits, vegetables, and soy protein. Subjects were also given a six-ounce serving per day of mixed vegetable juice (V-8, Campbell's Soup Company). Food frequency questionnaires were administered at baseline and after three months of intervention.

   The mixed vegetable juice was extracted in hexane and subjected to high-pressure liquid chromatography (Figure 4).

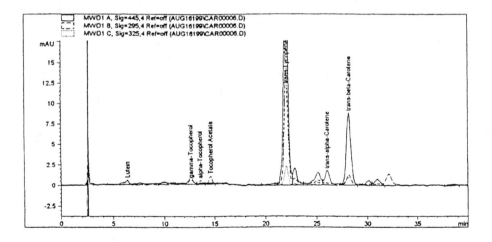

Figure 4. HPLC chromatogram of mixed vegetable juice extracted with hexane.

   The juice contained not only all-trans-lycopene, but also significant amounts of trans-alpha-carotene and trans-beta-carotene. After three months of supplementation, there was a significant increase in lycopene and alpha-carotene as shown in Table 1 below. In fact, lycopene concentrations were increased by 46% (p=0.002), alpha-carotene was increased by 46% (p=0.0109), beta-carotene by 30% (p=0.0268) and beta-cryptoxanthin increased by 36% (p=0.0391) compared to baseline.

Table 1. Plasma lycopene and carotene changes after V-8 supplementation

Plasma Lycopene and Carotene Changes
after V-8 Supplementation

	Baseline		3 months	
	Mean	SD	Mean	SD
Lycopene	0.24	0.12	0.35	0.18
α-Carotene	0.18	0.12	0.27	0.17
β-Carotene	0.86	0.85	1.12	0.83
β-Cryptoxanthin	0.15	0.13	0.20	0.15

This study demonstrated that supplementation with a mixed vegetable juice could significantly increase serum carotenoids when administered over a 12 week period. Based on food frequency analysis at baseline and at three months, the intake of beta-carotene was not changed significantly (Table 2), suggesting strongly that the increases observed in carotenoids were the result of supplementation with the mixed vegetable juice.

Table 2. Dietary beta-carotene intake at baseline and 3 months

Dietary Beta Carotene Intake at
Baseline and 3 Months

	Baseline		3 months	
	Mean	SD	Mean	SD
Beta Carotene	3392.8	1727.9	3085.8	1379.0

The significant increase seen is consistent with the enhanced bioavailability of lycopene from processed tomato products. However, the magnitude of the increase is remarkable and reflects some special properties of lycopene. While it undergoes isomerization during the process of uptake in the gastrointestinal tract, the plasma levels of lycopene do not appear to be tightly regulated. The cis-lycopene is reminiscent in structure to 9-cis retinoic acid and there are suggestions that lycopene may be able to act as a cell signal as well as an antioxidant. The metabolism of lycopene locally in the prostate and its concentration in the prostate are additional areas which require more investigation to enable us to understand the local gene-nutrient interactions in the prostate gland that may mediate some of the effects of lycopene on prostatic cells in vitro and in vivo. While the clinical observations in humans of the effects of lycopene supplementation are only preliminary,[13] these findings indicate changes in prostate cell histology in a direction consistent with decreased proliferation and increased apoptosis.

Our observation that lycopene in mixed vegetable juice can lead to such a significant increase makes it feasible to study the effects of dietary supplementation with mixed carotenoids in a number of nutrition intervention studies relevant to cancer prevention. In fact, mixed carotenoids may have different effects from a high dose of a single purified carotenoid such as beta-carotene or lycopene. Until these scientific issues are addressed, diet recommendations must be made to the public. Based on our current knowledge of the potential benefits of lycopene from tomato products, processed tomato sauces, soups, seasoning, and juices should be considered as an important part of a plant-based diet in which fruit and vegetable intake is encouraged for cancer prevention.

Supported by CaPCure (The Association for the Cure of Prostate Cancer) and the National Cancer Institute Grant No. CA 42710.

REFERENCES

1. Steinmetz KA, Potter JD. Vegetables, fruits, and cancer. I. *Epidemiol. Cancer Causes Control*; 2:325-337, 1991.
2. Block G, Patterson B, Subar A. Fruit, vegetables, and cancer prevention. A review of the epidemiological evidence. *Nutr Cancer*; 18:1-29, 1992.
3. World Cancer Research Fund, American Institute for Cancer Research. Food, nutrition, and the prevention of cancer: A global perspective. Washington, DC: American Institute for Cancer Research, 1997.
4. Heber D, and Go VLW. "Gene-Nutrient Interaction and the Xenobiotic Hypothesis of Cancer." In: *Nutritional Oncology*, Heber D, Blackburn GL, Go VLW, eds. San Diego, CA: Academic Press, 1999.
5. Di Mascio P, Kaiser S, Sies H. Lycopene as the most efficient biological carotenoid singlet oxygen quencher. *Arch Biochem Biophys*; 274:532-538, 1989.
6. Giovanocci E, Ascherio A, Rimm EB, Stampfer MJ, Colditz GA, Willett WC. Intake of carotenoids and retinol in relation to risk of prostate cancer. *J Natl Cancer Inst*; 87:1767-1776, 1995.
7. Gartner C, Stahl W, Sies H. Lycopene is more bioavailable from tomato paste than from fresh tomatoes. *Am J Clin Nutr*; 66:116-122, 1997.
8. Giovannucci E. Tomatoes, tomato-based products, lycopene, and cancer: Review of the epidemiologic literature. *J Natl Cancer Inst*; 91:317-331, 1999.

9. Stahl W, Sies H. Uptake of lycopene and its geometrical isomers is greater from heat-processed than from unprocessed tomato juice. *J Nutr*; 122:2161-2168, 1992.

10. Porrini M, Riso P, Testolin G. Absorption of lycopene from single or daily portions of raw and processed tomato. *Brit J Nutr*; 80:353-361, 1998.

11. Clinton SK, Emenhiser C, Schwartz SJ, Bostwick DG, Williams AW, Moore BJ, et al. Cis-trans lycopene isomers, carotenoids, and retinol in the human prostate. *Cancer Epidemiol Biomarkers Prev*; 5:823-833, 1996.

12. Heber D, Yip I, Go VLW, Liu W, Elashoff RM, Lu Q-Y. Plasma Lycopene and Carotenoid Profiles in Prostate Cancer Patients Supplemented with Mixed Vegetable Juice. American Institute for Cancer Research 9th Annual Research Conference, September, 1999 (abstract).

13. Kucuk O, Sakr W, Sarkar F, Djuric Z, Li YW, Khachik F, Velazquez F, Heilbrun L, Bertram JS, Crissman JD, Pontes E and Wood DP. Lycopene supplementation in men with prostate cancer (Pca) reduced grade and volume of preneoplasia (PIN) and tumor, decreases serum prostate specific antigen (PSA) and modulates biomarkers of growth and differentiation. International Carotenoid Meeting; Cairns, Australia, August, 1999 (abstract).

5

TEA AND TEA POLYPHENOLS IN CANCER PREVENTION

Chung S. Yang, Guang-yu Yang, Jee Y. Chung, Mao-Jung Lee, and Chuan Li

Laboratory for Cancer Research, College of Pharmacy
Rutgers, The State University of New Jersey
Piscataway, New Jersey 08854

Abbreviations used: EGCG, (–)-epigallocatechin-3-gallate; EGC, (–)-epigallocatechin; ECG, (–)-epicatechin-3-gallate; EC, (–)-epicatechin; NNK, 4-(methylnitrosamino)-1-(3-pyridyl)-1-butanone; EGF, epidermal growth factor; regulated protein kinase; NFκB, nuclear factor κB; DGT, decaffeinated green tea; C_{max}, maximal plasma concentrations; PGE_2, prostaglandin E_2.

INTRODUCTION

The inhibitory action of tea (*Camellia sinensis*) and tea components against cancer formation has been demonstrated in different animal models in many laboratories. The public press heralds tea as a cancer-prevention beverage. The preventive activity of tea against cancer in humans, however, has been suggested by some epidemiological studies, but not by others. A critical question is whether the information obtained from animal studies is

Nutrition and Cancer Prevention, edited under the auspices of AICR
Kluwer Academic / Plenum Publishers, New York, 2000.

39

applicable to humans. The quantities of tea used in animal studies and those consumed by humans are different. The mechanisms of carcinogenesis in animal models may differ from those in humans in many aspects. This presentation will review these issues in the light of the results from studies with animals, cell lines, and humans as well as discuss the possible cancer inhibitory mechanisms that may apply to human cancer prevention.

CHEMISTRY AND BIOCHEMICAL PROPERTIES OF TEA CONSTITUENTS

Tea is usually prepared by infusing dried green or black tea leaves in hot water. A typical tea beverage, prepared in a proportion of 1 g of tea leaves to 100 ml water in a 3-minute brew, usually contains 250 to 350 mg tea solids. A cup of tea is usually made from 2 to 3 g of dried tea leaves in 200 to 300 ml of water. Green tea is manufactured by drying fresh tea leaves. Its composition resembles that of fresh tea leaves in that it contains characteristic polyphenolic compounds, (–)-epigallocatechin-3-gallate (EGCG), (–)-epigallocatechin (EGC), (–)-epicatechin-3-gallate (ECG), and (–)-epicatechin (EC). These compounds, commonly known as catechins, usually account for 30-42% of the dry weight of the solids in brewed tea.[1] The structures of the major catechins and some black tea polyphenols are shown in Figure 1. EGCG is the most abundant catechin and has received a great deal of attention among researchers. Flavonols such as quercetin and their glycosides exist at lower levels. Caffeine usually accounts for 3-6% of the dry weight of brewed tea. In the manufacture of black tea, the tea leaves are crushed to release the polyphenol oxidase which catalyzes the oxidation of catechins, leading to the polymerization of these compounds, in a process known as "fermentation". Some of the catechins still remain and may account for 3-10% of the dry weight in brewed black tea. Theaflavins, which include theaflavin, theaflavin-3-gallate, theaflavin-3'-gallate, and theaflavin-3,3'-digallate, are key to the characteristic color and taste of black tea, and account for 2-6% of the dry weight in brewed black tea. The major fractions of black tea polyphenols, generally known as thearubigens, have higher molecular weights and are poorly characterized chemically; they account for more than 20% of the solid weight of brewed black tea.[1]

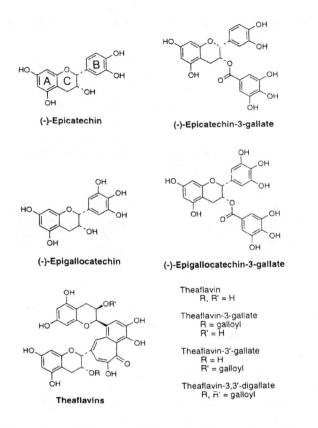

(-)-Epicatechin

(-)-Epicatechin-3-gallate

(-)-Epigallocatechin

(-)-Epigallocatechin-3-gallate

Theaflavins

Theaflavin
R, R' = H

Theaflavin-3-gallate
R = galloyl
R' = H

Theaflavin-3'-gallate
R = H
R' = galloyl

Theaflavin-3,3'-digallate
R, R' = galloyl

Figure 1. The structures of the major catechins and black tea polyphenols.

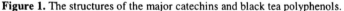

The most widely recognized properties of tea polyphenols are the antioxidant properties due to their ability to sequester metal ions and to scavenge reactive oxygen species.[2]   Green and black tea polyphenols have been shown to scavenge reactive oxygen and nitrogen species and reduce their damage to lipid membranes, proteins, and nucleic acids in cell-free systems. Tea polyphenols are known to bind to proteins, as exemplified by their binding to the proline rich salivary proteins[3] as well as to the plasma proteins fibronetin, fibrinogen, and histidine-rich glycoprotein.[4]   At low concentrations of tea polyphenols, this binding property may specifically affect certain enzymes, receptors, and membrane activities, resulting in the different biological activities observed by different investigators.

INHIBITION OF CANCER FORMATION BY TEA IN ANIMAL MODELS

The inhibition of cancer formation by tea preparations has been demonstrated by different investigators in many animal models, including those for the skin, lung, esophagus, stomach, liver, duodenum and small intestine, pancreas, colon, bladder, prostate, and mammary gland.[5-9] Inhibition of lung tumorigenesis by tea preparations has been demonstrated in A/J mice that have been treated with the tobacco carcinogen, 4-(methylnitrosamino)-1-(3-pyridyl)-1-butanone (NNK). Administration of decaffeinated green or black tea to mice during or after the NNK treatment period markedly reduced the number of tumors formed in the mice.[10] The inhibitory activity of black tea theaflavins was also demonstrated in this model.[11] When the mice were given black tea 16 weeks after the NNK injection, at which time almost all of the mice had developed adenomas, the progression of these tumors to adenocarcinomas was significantly inhibited.[11] Brewed black tea and green tea infusions, when given to A/J mice as the sole source of drinking fluid, also inhibited spontaneous lung tumorigenesis.[12] In this experiment, the body weights of the mice in the tea-treated groups were significantly (10-16%) lower than in the control group, and the differences in the fat-pad weights were even more dramatic. We believe this effect was mainly due to the caffeine in tea. The inhibitory action of caffeine against lung tumorigenesis has been demonstrated previously in mice[13] and in rats.[14] In the latter study, caffeine, at a concentration corresponding to that in a 2% black tea extract, displayed inhibitory activity comparable to, or stronger than, that of 2% black tea. The above experiments indicate that tea has broad inhibitory activity against both spontaneous and chemically-induced lung tumorigenesis, and it is effective when administered during the initiation, promotion, or progression stages of carcinogenesis.

This conclusion may also apply to other animal models such as chemically and UV light-induced skin carcinogenesis.[8, 15-17] Based on studies with this model with green tea, decaffeinated green tea, and caffeine, Conney *et al.* postulated that the "lowering of body fat levels", mainly by caffeine, is an important factor in the reduction of tumor multiplicity.[9, 15, 18]

Conflicting results have been reported concerning the effects of tea on colon and mammary carcinogenesis. Colon cancer formation induced by azoxymethane in rats and by 1,2-dimethylhydrazine in mice was inhibited by low concentrations of green tea polyphenols (0.01 or 0.1% solution as drinking fluid) and EGCG (reviewed in [19]). On the other hand, treatment of rats with black tea (0.6 to 2.5% solution) in drinking fluid did not inhibit azoxymethane-induced colon carcinogenesis.[20] One possible interpretation of these different results is that green tea polyphenols inhibit colon carcinogenesis whereas some black tea constituents are much less effective. The inhibitory effect of tea on mammary carcinogenesis was not demonstrated in several studies. In a recent study, black tea (1.25 or 2.5% solution) did not inhibit 7,12-dimethylbenz[a]anthracene-induced mammary gland tumorigenesis in rats fed an AIN-76A diet (containing 5% corn oil), but reduced mammary tumorigenesis in rats on a high fat diet.[21] Again the effect of tea consumption on fat metabolism may be a factor in the anti-carcinogenicity in this model.

STUDIES WITH CELL LINES

Green and black tea polyphenols have inhibited the growth of many cell lines derived from cancers of the lung (PC-9, A-427, H441, H661), skin (A431, HaCat, VACC-375), colon (CaCo-2, HT-29), stomach (KA70III), breast (MCF7), prostate (DU145), blood (Molt-43), and oral cavity (1483 HNSCC) (reviewed in [22]). The efficacy of inhibition varied depending on the polyphenols and cell lines used. EGCG was usually the best inhibitor in most of the cell lines tested, with IC_{50} values ranging between 18-130 μM. EGC and ECG were less effective and EC had even lower activity. Our laboratory has shown that EGCG and EGC inhibit the growth of H661 and H1299 cells with IC_{50} values of 22 μM. The growth inhibition of Ha-ras transformed 21 BES cells by the black tea polyphenol, theaflavin-3,3'-digallate, was similar to the growth inhibition caused by green tea polyphenols, EGCG and EGC.[23] These studies demonstrated the biological activities of tea polyphenols in the inhibition of cancer cell growth, but the effective concentrations observed were generally 1-2 orders of magnitude higher than the peak human plasma concentrations in humans and animals after tea consumption (see subsequent sections). The lowest effective concentration of EGCG (1-2 μM) observed was in the inhibition of the transformation of pre-neoplastic human mammary epithelial cells by benzo[a]pyrene.[24]

Tea polyphenols may inhibit cell growth through a variety of mechanisms. One such mechanism is through the induction of apoptosis. Human cancer cell lines which have shown changes indicative of apoptosis after EGCG or EGC treatment are PC-9, H661, KATO III, DU 145, A431, HaCat, and Molt-43.[23, 25-28] Higher concentrations of tea polyphenols are usually needed for induction of apoptosis than growth inhibition. In some studies, EGCG may also act as a pro-oxidant through H_2O_2 production to induce apoptosis, because addition of catalase to the culture media inhibited EGCG-induced apoptosis.[23] In combination with other chemopreventive drugs such as sulindac and tamoxifen, EGCG induced a synergistic apoptotic effect.[29]

Concerning the prevention of cancer, the inhibition of tumor promotion related activities by tea polyphenols is probably more relevant than inhibition of cancer cell growth. For example, EGCG and theaflavins (in the range of 1-20 µM) significantly inhibited epidermal growth factor (EGF)- or 12-*O*-tetradecanoylphorbol-13-acetate-induced transformation of JB6 cells. This inhibition was correlated to the inhibition of AP-1 (activator protein 1)-dependent transcriptional activity, but caffeine (up to 40 µM) was inactive.[30] The inhibition of AP-1 activation occurs through the inhibition of a c-jun NH2-terminal kinase (JNK)-dependent pathway. EGCG has also been shown to interfere with the binding of epidermal growth factor and 12-*O*-tetradecanoylphorbol-13-acetate to their respective receptors.[31,32] In H-ras transformed JB6 (the 30.7b Ras 12 cells), in which activation of membrane receptor is not involved, the AP-1 activation was inhibited by many tea polyphenols, of which EC had the lowest activity. EGCG and theaflavin-3,3'-digallate inhibited the phosphorylation of both c-jun and extracellular signal-regulated protein kinase (Erk), but did not change the level of phospho-JNK.[33] A key issue under investigation is on the mechanisms and specificity of the inhibition. Preliminary results indicated that there is specificity in the inhibition. In the inhibition of phosphorylation of Elk by isolated Erk, EGCG appeared to compete with Elk rather than with ATP.

All the anti-proliferative, anti-promotion, and apoptosis-induction activities may be due to the inhibition of signal transduction pathways involving AP-1 and NFκB (nuclear factor κB).[25,26,30,34] Other mechanisms for the growth inhibition of cancer cells may be through the induction of cell cycle arrest by EGCG. EGCG and other tea polyphenols have been shown to inhibit the phosphorylation of Rb by Cdk2/4,[35] which may affect cell cycle regulation.

POSSIBLE ACTIVE COMPONENTS FOR THE INHIBITION OF CARCINOGENESIS

Many authors have considered EGCG as the active component of green tea because EGCG is the most abundant catechin, and the cancer inhibitory activity of EGCG has been demonstrated. The *in vitro* studies discussed in the previous section suggest that other tea polyphenols could also be active. The inhibitory activity of EGCG against skin, stomach, colon, and lung carcinogenesis[8, 13, 14, 36] as well as the growth of human prostate and breast tumors in athymic mice has been reported.[37] Theaflavins (a mixture of theaflavin and theaflavingallates) have been shown to inhibit lung and esophageal carcinogenesis.[38, 39] EGCG and theaflavins, when given 24 hr after a dose of NNK, inhibited the bronchiolar epithelial cell hyperproliferation in mice measured 4 days after the NNK dose ([39] and unpublished). Short term studies showed that EGC has similar anti-proliferative activity as EGCG (unpublished results). ECG is expected to have similar activity. In many studies, black tea has comparable or slightly lower inhibitory activities. It is possible that the remaining catechins in black tea, theaflavins, and other components in black tea all contribute to the cancer inhibitory activity. The bioavailability and bioactivity of thearubigens in animals are just being studied. Preliminary results from our lab indicate that a crude preparation of thearubigens, when administered orally, inhibited NNK-induced brochiolar hyperproliferation (unpublished results).

Current results suggest that both tea polyphenols and caffeine are the components responsible for the anti-carcinogenic activity in tea. The relative importance of these compounds may depend on the different carcinogenesis models used. The possible activities of the metabolites of tea polyphenols and caffeine, and the possible interactions between these two groups of compounds, need further investigation.

BIOAVAILABILITY AND BIOTRANSFORMATION OF TEA POLYPHENOLS AND CAFFEINE

The absorption and tissue distribution of tea catechins have been studied only recently. Following *i.v.* injection of decaffeinated green tea (DGT) to rats, most of the plasma catechins were in the glucuronide and sulfate conjugated forms; the total amount (free plus conjugated forms) of each catechin was used for pharmacokinetic analysis.[40] The plasma concentration-time curves of EGCG, EGC, and EC could be fitted into a two-compartment model. The β elimination half-lives ($t_{1/2}(\beta)$) were 212, 45, and 41 min for EGCG, EGC, and EC, respectively. After *i.g.* administration of DGT, about 14% of EGC and 31% of EC appeared in the plasma, but less than 1% of EGCG was bioavailable in rats. After *i.v.* administration of DGT, the highest level of EGCG was in the intestines, and the highest levels of EGC and EC were observed in the kidney. When 0.6% green tea polyphenols were administered through the drinking fluid, the rat plasma blood levels of EGC and EC were much higher than that of EGCG, even though the amounts of EGCG to EGC were at a 5:1 ratio in the drinking fluid.[41] Substantial amounts of EGC and EC were found in the rat esophagus (185-195 ng/g tissue), large intestine (300-930), kidney (400-500), bladder (800-810), lung (190-230), and prostate (240-250), but the concentrations of EGC and EC were low in the liver, spleen, heart, and thyroid. The levels of EGCG were higher in the esophagus and large intestine than in other organs because of poor systemic absorption of EGCG by the rat. A sizable amount of EGCG was found in the feces. In mice, after consuming a 0.6% solution of green tea polyphenols, the plasma level of EGCG was much higher than that in rats. This species difference was probably due to the poor absorption of EGCG by the rats; i.p. injection of green tea produced much higher plasma levels of EGCG, and the plasma EGCG to EGC ratio approximated their concentrations in the green tea preparation. The highest levels of these catechins were in the low micromolar range.[41]

In a pharmacokinetic study in human volunteers, administration of 1.5, 3.0, and 4.5 g of DGT (in 500 ml of water) resulted in maximal plasma concentrations (C_{max}) of 0.71, 1.80, and 0.65 μM EGCG, EGC, and EC (free plus conjugated forms), respectively.[23] These C_{max} values were observed at 1.4 to 2.4 hr after the ingestion of the tea preparation. The $t_{1/2}$ of EGCG (5.0-5.5 hr) appeared to be higher than those of EGC and EC (2.5-3.4 hr). EGC and EC, but not EGCG, were excreted in the urine with over 90% of the total urinary EGC and EC (mostly in the conjugated forms) excreted within 8 hr. Substantial amounts of the catechins were detected in colon mucosa and prostate tissues in surgical samples from patients who consumed green tea 12 hrs before surgery. After drinking green tea, peak saliva levels of EGC (11.7-43.9 μg/ml), EGCG (4.8-22 μg/ml), and EC (1.8-7.5 μg/ml) were observed after a few minutes in human volunteers {Yang, 1999 #312}. These levels were two orders of magnitude higher than those in the plasma. The $t_{1/2}$s of the salivary catechins were 10-20 min, much shorter than in the plasma.

The catechins are readily conjugated as glucuronides and sulfates; the conjugated forms may account for 60 to 80% of the catechins found in the plasma or urine. *O*-Methyl EGC (mostly in the glucuronide or sulfated forms) has recently been found by our laboratory to be a major metabolite, present at levels 4-5 times higher than EGC in human plasma and urine (unpublished results). *O*-Methylated EGCG derivatives, with methylation occurring at the one or two of the 3', 4', 3" and 4" positions, have been detected in the bile of the rat.[42] The conversion of EGCG to EGC (and presumably ECG to EC) by esterase is known to take place in the oral cavity and the intestine.[43] This catechin esterase activity is probably of microbial origin; administration of EGCG to rats by *i.v.* injection and gastric intubation did not produce EGC in the plasma or urine.[40] Substantial amounts of catechins are degraded by microorganisms in the intestine of humans and animals leading to the formation of M4 [5-(3',4'-dihydroxyphenyl)-γ-valerolactone] and M6 [5-(3',4,',5'-trihydroxyphenyl)-γ-valerolactone].[44] These metabolites are the ring fusion products of EGC and EC, respectively. It is also expected that the intestinal microbial esterase can convert EGCG to EGC and ECG to EC, leading to the formation of M4 and M6, respectively. Both M4 and M6 (mainly in the glucuronide and sulfate forms) have been detected in the urine and plasma; in some individuals the amounts of urinary M4 and M6 were several fold higher than their respective precursors. These metabolites, apparently present in higher quantities than their parent compounds, are expected to exist in various tissues. The biological activities of these catechin metabolites are, therefore, an important topic for future studies.

The presence of theaflavins and thearubigens in the plasma and urine has not been reported, but these compounds have certain biological activities. It is possible that these black tea polyphenols are degraded by the microflora in the intestine and the metabolites are absorbed by animals and humans. This hypothesis remains to be tested and the possible bioactive metabolites need to be identified.

The absorption, distribution, metabolism, and excretion of caffeine have been well characterized,[45, 46] but the pharmacokinetic properties of the caffeine in tea in our animal model systems are not known. It remains to be determined whether these parameters are affected by the presence of polyphenols in tea and whether caffeine affects the pharmacokinetic behavior of tea polyphenols.

POSSIBLE MECHANISMS FOR THE INHIBITION OF CARCINOGENESIS IN HUMANS

Although the inhibition of tumor formation has been demonstrated in animal models and many different mechanisms have been proposed, the reduction of human cancer risk by tea consumption has only been demonstrated in some but not in other studies.[6, 8, 47, 48] For example, in a case-control study in Shanghai, frequent consumption of green tea has been associated with a lower incidence of esophageal cancer, especially among non-smokers and non-alcohol-drinkers.[49] The protective effect against gastric cancer by tea has also been suggested from studies in Kyushu (Japan), northern Turkey, and central Sweden, but not from many other studies in different geographic areas (reviewed in [19]). In studies in Saitama, Japan, women consuming more than 10 cups of green tea daily had a lower risk for cancer (all sites combined) and increased tea consumption was associated with lower risk for breast cancer metastasis and recurrence.[50, 51] On the other hand, in the Netherlands Cohort Study on Diet and Cancer, consumption of black tea did not affect the risk for stomach, colorectal, lung, and breast cancers.[52] A recent study on middle aged Finnish men has indicated a positive association between increased tea consumption and colon cancer risk.[53]

Although there are many confounding factors associated with the life-styles of the subjects, the different etiological factors and different mechanisms of pathogenesis of various cancers may determine whether tea consumption can have an effect. For example, if N-nitroso compounds are risk factors for stomach cancer in Japan, but not in the Netherlands, then tea consumption may only inhibit stomach cancer in Japan, because of the inhibition of endogenous nitrosation by tea polyphenols. The type and quantity of tea consumed are likely important factors. Studies in Saitama, Japan imply that a daily consumption of >10 cups of green tea is needed to produce a protective effect;[50] whereas studies in Shanghai suggested 2 to 3 cups of green tea may be effective.[49] These quantities are estimated to be lower than those used in most studies in which tea preparations were given to animals as the sole source of drinking fluid.

Many mechanisms have been proposed concerning the inhibitory action of tea against tumorigenesis. As was pointed out previously,[19, 54] in the search for relevant mechanisms, it is necessary to consider the tissue concentrations of the effective components. Inhibitory activities elicited by low micromolar or lower concentrations are likely to be more relevant than activities demonstrated with higher concentrations of tea constituents. The anti-carcinogenic activities of tea polyphenols are generally believed to be related but not entirely due to, their antioxidative properties. Finding that green tea polyphenol fractions inhibited 12-*O*-tetradecanoylphorbol-13-acetate-induced hydrogen peroxide formation in mouse epidermis[55] and 8-hydroxydeoxyguanosine formation in different systems[13,56] is consistent with this concept. The concentrations of tea polyphenols in the blood and tissue (estimated to be at the low μM levels), however, appear to be much lower that those of vitamin E, vitamin C, and other natural antioxidants; the actual physiological antioxidative function of tea constituents is a subject of debate.

It is likely that other mechanisms are also involved, which may be more important in the possible anti-carcinogenic actions of tea. The anti-proliferative effects, inhibition of cell transformation, and induction of apoptosis are promising mechanisms to be investigated in humans and appropriate animal models. The concept that caffeine, by itself or acting synergistically with tea polyphenols, inhibits tumor formation by lowering the body fat levels of mice[9,15,18] is very interesting and deserves more investigation in humans. The recent report that consumption of green tea extract can increase the 24-hr energy expenditure in humans[57] will encourage further studies on this topic pertaining to the reduction of cancer risk.

The inhibition of lipoxygenase and cyclooxygenase by tea polyphenols has been demonstrated,[58, 59] and is also under investigation in our own laboratory (results unpublished). Recently, we have demonstrated that green tea administration to normal human subjects resulted in a rapid decrease in prostaglandin E_2 (PGE_2) levels in rectal biopsy tissues,[60] a possible mechanism for the inhibition of human colorectal cancer. A recent study by Cao *et al.* demonstrated that EGCG can inhibit angiogensis by suppressing the growth of endothelial cells and that administration of 1.25% green tea as the drinking fluid to mice reduced significantly VEGF (vascular endothelial growth factor)-induced corneal neovascularization.[61] If the angiogenesis activity could be demonstrated in humans, it would be an important mechanism for the inhibition of cancer growth.

CONCLUDING REMARKS

Judging from the diverse inhibitory activities observed in different animal carcinogenesis systems and different cancer cell lines, it is likely that there are multiple mechanisms by which tea constituents elicit their inhibitory effects against carcinogenesis. The challenge is to determine which mechanisms are applicable to human cancer prevention. In this context, only the biochemical and physiological effects that are achievable in humans through tea consumption are important. Therefore, information on the bioavailability and tissue levels of tea constituents and their biological effect should be a vital part of future research. The recently gained knowledge on the tissue levels and biological activities of tea polyphenols will be useful in the planning of future epidemiological studies and human cancer prevention trials. Further studies are needed to determine the best dosage and route to deliver particular tea constituents to a certain organ.

ACKNOWLEDGMENT

This research is supported by US NIH grant CA56673.

REFERENCES

1. Balentine, D. A., Wiseman, S. A., Bouwens, L. C. M., The chemistry of tea flavonoids, *Crit. Rev. Food Sci. Nutr.* 37:693-704 (1997).
2. Wiseman, S. A., Balentine, D. A., Frei, B., Antioxidants in tea, *Crit. Rev. Food Sci. Nutr.* 37:705-718 (1997).
3. Haslam, E., Natural polyphenols and vegetable tannins as drugs: possible modes of action, *J. Nat. Prod.* 59:205-215 (1996).
4. Sazuka, M., Itoi, T., Suzuki, Y., Odani, S., Koide, T., Isemura, M., Evidence for the interaction between (-)-epigallocatechin gallate and human plasma proteins fibronectin, fibrinogen, and histidine-rich glycoprotein, *Biosci. Biotechnol. Biochem.* 60:1317-1319 (1996).
5. Yang, C. S., Kim, S., Yang, G.-Y., Lee, M.-J., Liao, J., Chung, J. Y., Ho, C.-T., Inhibition of carcinogenesis by tea: bioavailability of tea polyphenols and mechanisms of actions, *Proc. Soc. Exptl. Biol. Med.* 220:213-217 (1999).
6. Yang, C. S., Wang, Z.-Y., Tea and cancer: A review, *J. Natl. Cancer Inst.* 58:1038-1049 (1993).
7. Dreosti, I. E., Wargovich, M. J., Yang, C. S., Inhibition of carcinogenesis by tea: The evidence from experimental studies, *Crit. Rev. Food Sci. Nutr.* 37:761-770 (1997).
8. Katiyar, S. K., Mukhtar, H., Tea in chemoprevention of cancer: epidemiologic and experimental stuides (review), *Intl. J. Oncology* 8:221-238 (1996).
9. Conney, A. H., Lu, Y.-P., Lou, Y.-R., Xie, J.-G., Huang, M.-T., Inhibitory effect of green and black tea on tumor growth, *Proc. Soc. Exptl. Biol. Med.* 220:229-233 (1999).

10. Wang, Z. Y., Hong, J.-Y., Huang, M.-T., Reuhl, K. R., Conney, A. H., Yang, C. S., Inhibition of N-nitrosodiethylamine- and 4-(methylnitrosamino)-1-(3-pyridyl)-1-butanone-induced tumorigenesis in A/J mice by green tea and black tea, *Cancer Res.* 52:1943-1947 (1992).

11. Yang, C. S., Inhibition of carcinogenesis by tea, *Nature* 389:134-135 (1997).

12. Landau, J. M., Wang, Z.-Y., Yang, G.-Y., Ding, W., Yang, C. S., Inhibition of spontaneous formation of lung tumors and rhabdomyosarcomas in A/J mice by black and green tea, *Carcinogenesis* 19:501-507 (1998).

13. Xu, Y., Ho, C.-T., Amin, S. G., Han, C., Chung, F.-L., Inhibition of tobacco-specific nitrosamine-induced lung tumorigenesis in A/J mice by green tea and its major polyphenol as antioxidants, *Cancer Res.* 52:3875-3879 (1992).

14. Chung, F.-L., Wang, M., Rivenson, A., Iatropoulos, M. J., Reinhardt, J. C., Pittman, B., Ho, C.-T., Amin, S. G., Inhibition of lung carcinogenesis by black tea in Fischer rats treated with a tobacco-specific carcinogen: caffeine as an important constituent, *Cancer Res.* 58:4096-4101 (1998).

15. Huang, M.-T., Xie, J.-G., Wang, Z.-Y., Ho, C.-T., Lou, Y.-R., Wang, C.-X., Hard, G. C., Conney, A. H., Effects of tea, decaffeinated tea, and caffeine on UVB light induced complete carcinogenesis in SKH-1 mice: demonstration of caffeine as a biologically important constituent of tea., *Cancer Res.* 57:2623-2629 (1997).

16. Wang, Z.-Y., Huang, M.-T., Lou, Y.-R., Xie, J.-G., Reuhl, K. R., Newmark, H. L., Ho, C.-T., Yang, C. S., Conney, A. H., Inhibitory effects of black tea, green tea, decaffeinated black tea, and decaffeinated green tea on ultraviolet B light-induced skin carcinogenesis in 7,12-dimethylbenz[a]anthracene-initiated SKH-1 mice, *Cancer Res.* 54:3428-3425 (1994).

17. Wang, Z. Y., Huang, M.-T., Ferraro, T., Wong, C. Q., Lou, Y.-R., Reuhl, K., Latropoulos, M., Yang, C. S., Conney, A. H., Inhibitory effect of green tea in the drinking water on tumorigenesis by ultraviolet light and 12-O-tetradecanoylphorbol-13-acetate in the skin of SKH-1 mice, *Cancer Res.* 52:1162-1170 (1992).

18. Lou, Y.-R., Lu, Y.-P., Xie, J.-G., Huang, M.-T., Conney, A. H., Effects of oral administration of tea, decaffeinated tea, and caffeine on the formation and growth of tumors in high-risk SKH-1 mice previously treated with ultraviolet B light, *Nutr. Cancer* 33:146-153 (1999).

19. Yang, C. S., Chen, L., Lee, M.-J., Landau, J. M., Effects of tea on carcinogenesis in animal models and humans (edited under the auspices of the American Institute for Cancer Research), In: *Dietary Phytochemicals in Cancer Prevention and Treatment*, pp. 51-61, Plenum Press, New York, (1996).

20. Weisburger, J. H., Rivenson, A., Reinhardt, J., Aliaga, C., Braley, J., Pittman, B., Zang, E., Effect of black tea on azoxymethane-induced colon cancer, *Carcinogenesis* 19:229-232 (1998).

21. Rogers, A. E., Hafer, L. J., Iskander, Y. S., Yang, S., Black tea and mammary gland carcinogenesis by 7,12-dimethylbenz[a]anthracene in rats fed control or high fat diets, *Carcinogenesis* 19:1269-1273 (1998).

22. Yang, C. S., Chung, J. Y., Growth inhibition of human cancer cell lines by tea polyphenols, *Curr. Pract. Med.* 2:163-166 (1999).

23. Yang, G.-Y., Liao, J., Kim, K., Yurkow, E. J., Yang, C. S., Inhibition of growth and induction of apoptosis in human cancer cell lines by tea polyphenols, *Carcinogenesis* 19:611-616 (1998).

24. Katdare, M., Osborne, M. P., Telang, N. T., Inhibition of aberrant proliferation and induction of apoptosis in pre-neoplastic human mammary epithelial cells by natural phytochemicals, *Oncol. Rep.* 5:311-315 (1998).

25. Okabe, S., Suganuma, M., Hayashi, M., Sueoka, E., Komori, A., Fujiki, H., Mechanisms of growth inhibition of human lung cancer cell line, PC-9, by tea polyphenols, *Jpn. J. Cancer Res.* 88:639-643 (1997).

26. Ahmad, N., Feyes, D. K., Nieminen, A.-L., Agarwal, R., Mukhtar, H., Green tea constituent epigallocatechin-3-gallate and induction of apoptosis and cell cycle arrest in human carcinoma cells, *J. Natl. Cancer Inst.* 89:1881-1886 (1997).

27. Hibasami, H., Achiwa, Y., Fujikawa, T., Komiya, T., Induction of programmed cell death (apoptosis) in human lymphoid leukemia cells by catechin compounds, *Anticancer Res.* 16:1943-1946 (1996).

28. Hibasami, H., Komiya, T., Achiwa, Y., Ohnishi, K., Kojima, T., Nakanishi, K., Akashi, K., Hara, Y., Induction of apoptosis in human stomach cancer cells by green tea catechins, *Oncol. Rep.* 5:527-529 (1998).

29. Suganuma, M., Okabe, S., Kai, Y., Sueoka, N., Sueoka, E., Fujiki, H., Synergistic effects of (-)-epigallocatechin gallate with (-)-epicatechin, sulindac, or tamoxifen on cancer-preventive activity in the human lung cancer cell line PC-9, *Cancer Res.* 59:44-47 (1999).

30. Dong, Z., Ma, W.-Y., Huang, C., Yang, C. S., Inhibition of tumor promoter-induced AP-1 activation and cell transformation by tea polyphenols, (-)-epigallocatechin gallate and theaflavins, *Cancer Res.* 57:4414-4419 (1997).

31. Liang, Y.-C., Lin-Shiau, S.-Y., Chen, D.-F., Lin, J.-K., Suppression of extracellular signals and cell proliferation through EGF receptor binding by (-)-epigallocatechin gallate in human A431 epidermoid carcinoma cells, *J. Cell. Biochem.* 67:55-65 (1997).

32. Kitano, K., Nam, K. Y., Kimura, S., Fujiki, H., Imanishi, Y., Sealing effects of (-)-epigallocatechin gallate on protein kinase C and protein phosphatase 2A, *Biophys. Chem.* 65:157-164 (1997).

33. Chung, J. Y., Huang, C., Meng, X., Dong, Z., Yang, C. S., Inhibition of activator protein 1 activity and cell growth by purified green tea and black tea polyphenols in H-*ras*-transformed cells: structure-activity relationship and mechanisms involved, *Cancer Res.* 20:1810-1807 (1999).

34. Lin, Y.-L., Lin, J.-K., (-)-Epigallocatechin-3-gallate blocks the induction of nitric oxide synthase by down-regulating lipopolysaccharide-induced activity of transcription factor nuclear factor-kB, *Am. Society Pharmacol. Exp. Ther.* 52:465-472 (1997).

35. Liang, Y. C., Lin-Shiau, S. Y., Chen, C. F., Lin, J. K., Inhibition of cyclin-dependent kinases 2 and 4 activities as well as induction of Cdk inhibitors p21 and p27 during growth arrest of human breast carcinoma cells by (-)-epigallocatechin-3-gallate, *J. Cell. Biochem.* 75:1-12 (1999).

36. Yamane, T., Takahashi, T., Kuwata, K., Oya, K., Inagake, M., Kitao, Y., Suganuma, M., Fujiki, H., Inhibition of *N*-methyl-*N'*-nitro-*N*-nitrosoguanidine-induced carcinogenesis by (-)-epigallocatechin gallate in the rat glandular stomach, *Cancer Res.* 55:2081-2084 (1995).

37. Liao, S., Umekita, Y., Guo, J., Kokontis, J. M., Hiipakka, R. A., Growth inhibition and regression of human prostate and breast tumors in athymic mice by tea epigallocatechin gallate, *Cancer Lett* 96:239-243 (1995).

38. Morse, M. A., Kresty, L. A., Steele, V. E., Kelloff, G. J., Boone, C. W., Balentine, D. A., Harbowy, M. E., Stoner, G. D., Effects of theaflavins on *N*-nitrosomethylbenzylamine-induced esophageal tumorigenesis, *Nutr Cancer* 29:7-12 (1997).

39. Yang, G.-Y., Wang, Z.-Y., Kim, S., Liao, J., Seril, D., Chen, X., Smith, T. J., Yang, C. S., Characterization of early pulmonary hyperproliferation, tumor progression and their inhibition by black tea in a 4-(methylnitrosamino)-1-(3-pyridyl)-1-butanone (NNK)-induced lung tumorigenesis model with A/J mice, *Cancer Res.* 57:1889-1894 (1997).

40. Chen, L., Lee, M.-J., Li, H., Yang, C. S., Absorption, distribution, and elimination of tea polyphenols in rats, *Drug Metab. Dispos.* 9:1045-1050 (1997).

41. Kim, S., Lee, M.-J., Hong, J., Li, C., Smith, T. J., Yang, G.-Y., Seril, D. N., Yang, C. S., Plasma and tissue levels of tea catechins in rats and mice during chronic consumption of green tea polyphenols, (submitted)

42. Nanjo, F., Kida, K., Suzuki, M., Matsumoto, N., Hara, Y., Identification of metabolites of (-)-epigallo-catechin gallate in the rat bile, In: *Chemistry and Health Promotion. 2nd International Conference on Food Factors*, Abstract no. P013, Kyoto, Japan, (1999).

43. Yang, C. S., Lee, M.-J., Chen, L., Human salivary tea catechin levels and catechin esterase activities: implication in human cancer prevention studies, *Cancer Epidemiol. Biomark. Prev.* 8:83-89 (1999).

44. Li, C., Lee, M.-J., Sheng, S., Prabhu, S., Winnik, B., Huang, B., Meng, X., Chung, J. Y., Yan, S., Ho, C.-J., Yang, C. S., Structural identification and characterization of two metabolites of catechins in human urine and blood after tea ingestion, *Chem. Res. Toxicol.* (accepted)

45. Dan-Shya Tang-Liu, D., Williams, R. L., Riegelman, S., Disposition of caffeine and its metabolites in man, *J. Pharmacol. Exp. Ther.* 224:180-185 (1983).

46. Ullrich, D., Compagnone, D., Munch, B., Brandes, A., Hille, H., Bircher, J., Urinary caffeine metabolites in man: age-dependent changes and pattern in various clinical situations, *Clin. Pharmacol.* 43:167-172 (1992).

47. Blot, W. J., McLaughlin, J. K., Chow, W.-H., Cancer rates among drinkers of black tea, *Crit. Rev. Food Sci. Nutr.* 37(8):739-760 (1997).

48. Buschman, J. L., Green tea and cancer in humans: a review of the literature, *Nutr. Cancer* 31:151-159 (1998).

49. Gao, Y. T., McLaughlin, J. K., Blot, W. J., Ji, B. T., Dai, Q., Fraumeni, J. J., Reduced risk of esophageal cancer associated with green tea consumption, *J. Natl. Cancer Inst.* 86:855-858 (1994).

50. Imai, K., Suga, K., Nakachi, K., Lead Article: Cancer-preventive effects of drinking green tea among a Japanese population, *Prev. Med.* 26:769-775 (1997).

51. Nakachi, K., Suemasu, K., Suga, K., Takeo, T., Imai, K., Higashi, Y., Influence of drinking green tea on breast cancer malignancy among Japanese patients, *Jpn. J. Cancer Res.* 89:254-261 (1998).

52. Goldbohm, R. A., Hertog, M. G. L., Brants, H. A. M., van Poppel, G., van den Brandt, P. A., Consumption of black tea and cancer risk: a prospective cohort study, *J. Natl. Cancer Inst.* 88:93-100 (1996).

53. Hartman, T. J., Tangrea, J. A., Pietinen, P., Malila, N., Virtanen, M., Taylor, P. R., Albanes, D., Tea and coffee consumption and risk of colon and rectal cancer in middle-aged Finnish men, *Nutr. Cancer* 31:41-48 (1998).

54. Yang, G.-Y., Liu, Z., Seril, D. N., Liao, J., Ding, W., Kim, S., Bondoc, F., Yang, C. S., Black tea constituents, theaflavins, inhibit 4-(methylnitrosamino)-1-(3-pyridyl)-1-butanone (NNK)-induced lung tumorigenesis in A/J mice, *Carcinogenesis* 18:2361-2365 (1997).

55. Huang, M.-T., Ho, C.-T., Wang, Z. Y., Ferraro, T., Finnegan-Olive, T., Lou, Y.-R., Mitchell, J. M., Laskin, J. D., Newmark, H., Yang, C. S., Conney, A. H., Inhibitory effect of topical application of a green tea polyphenol fraction on tumor initiation and promotion in mouse skin, *Carcinogenesis* 13:947-954 (1992).

56. Bhimani, R., Troll, W., Grunberger, D., Frenkel, K., Inhibition of oxidative stress in HeLa cells by chemopreventive agents, *Cancer Res.* 53:4528-4533 (1993).

57. Dulloo, A. G., Duret, C., Rohrer, D., Girardier, L., Mensi, N., Fathi, M., Chanire, P., Vandermander, J., Efficacy of a green tea extract rich in catechin polyphenols and caffeine in increasing 24-h energy epxenditure and fat oxidation in human, *Am. J. Clin. Nutr.* 70:1040-1045 (1999).

58. Katiyar, S., Agarwal, R., Wood, G. S., Inhibition of 12-*O*-tetradecanoylphorbol-13-acetate-caused tumor promotion in 7,12-dimethylbenz(a)anthracene-initiated SENCAR mouse skin by a polyphenolic fraction isolated from green tea, *Cancer Res.* 52:6890-6897 (1992).

59. Lou, F. Q., A study of prevention of atherosclerosis with tea-pigment, *The Int. Tea-Quality-Human Health Symp. (China), Abstract* 141-143 (1987).
60. August, D. A., Landau, J. M., Caputo, D., Hong, J., Lee, M., Yang, C. S., Ingestion of green tea rapidly decreases prostaglandin E_2 levels in rectal mucosa in humans, *Cancer Epidemiol. Biomark. Prev.* (in press) (1999).
61. Cao, Y., Cao, R., Angiogenesis inhibited by drinking tea, *Nature* 398:381 (1999).

6

EFFECTS OF TEA POLYPHENOLS ON THE SIGNAL TRANSDUCTION PATHWAYS

Zigang Dong, Masaaki Nomura,
Chuanshu Huang, and Wei-ya Ma

University of Minnesota
Hormel Institute
801 16th Avenue NE
Austin, MN 55912

SIGNAL TRANSDUCTION PATHWAYS IN THE TUMOR PROMOTION PROCESS

Mitogenic stimulation is likely to be an important component of tumor promotion. However, that alone is not sufficient for transformation, and changes in gene expression are required to avoid growth regulation or differentiation. In general, alterations in the transcription of a specific set of cellular genes are mediated by specific regulatory DNA binding proteins or transcription factors that regulate gene expression directly by binding to specific DNA sequences in promoter regions (1-9). The expression of genes transcriptionally induced by 12-*O*-tetradecanoylphorbol-13-acetate (TPA) and other tumor promoters such as UV irradiation are thought to be required in tumor promotion (4-10).

UV irradiation from the sun is the most important environmental carcinogen and is responsible for a high incidence of non-melanoma skin cancers (NMSC) in humans. Mechanistically, UV induces both genotoxic effects such as DNA damage and mutations including p53 or ras mutations. Such a DNA-damaging effect is proposed as the mechanism of UV-induced initiation and UV-induced signal transduction is believed to be related to tumor promotion. UV-enhanced gene expression mediated by the initiation of a transcriptional induction response is known as the "UV response". Two transcription factors are implicated in the "UV response", AP-1 and NFκB (6).

The 7,12-dimethylbenz(a)anthracene-TPA mouse skin model is a well-characterized model for the study of tumor promotion *in vivo*. Our understanding of multi-stage carcinogenesis is based largely on data generated from this model. Recently, we showed that AP-1 is induced (11) and that inhibition of AP-1 also represses tumor promotion in this model.

The JB6 mouse epidermal cell system of clonal genetic variants that are promotion-sensitive (P⁺) or promotion-resistant (P⁻) allows the study of genetic susceptibility to transformation, promotion and progression at the molecular level (5, 10-17). The P⁻, P⁺ and transformed (Tx) variants are a series of cell lines representing "earlier-to-later" stages of preneoplastic-to-neoplastic progression. P⁻ variants gain P⁺ phenotype upon transfection with mutated p53 (18, 19). The P⁺ cells gain Tx phenotype irreversibly upon treatment with TPA, epidermal growth factor (EGF) or other tumor promoters with c-Jun overexpression (20, 21). Transformed variants grow under anchorage-independent (AI) conditions and are tumorigenic in nude or BALB/c mice in the absence of tumor promoting conditions. One of the few molecular events known to distinguish P⁻ or P⁺ cellular responses to tumor promoters is the activation of AP-1-driven transcriptional activity in P⁺ cells but not in P⁻ cells (10-17).

This model is a well-developed cell culture system for studying tumor promotion and anti-tumor promotion *in vitro*. We generated stable AP-1-luciferase or NFκB-luciferase transfectants in JB6 cells and used these cell lines for the study of signal transduction pathways for tumor promotion.

Through comparison of promotion sensitive (P⁺) and promotion-resistant (P⁻) derivatives of the mouse epidermal JB6 cell line, we found that transcriptional factor AP-1 plays a critical role in tumor promotion (Figure 1) (5, 10, 12). AP-1 is only activated in P⁺ cells, but not in P⁻ cells (13). Furthermore, blocking the tumor promoter-induced AP-1 activity inhibited neoplastic transformation (5, 10). Overexpression of a dominant negative mutant of Jun caused carcinoma cells to lose their tumorigenicity in nude mice (14, 15). Inhibition of AP-1 activity in transformed JB6 RT101 cells caused reversion of tumor phenotype (16, 17). Through the mechanism of protein-protein interaction of Jun with one retinoic acid receptor, retinoids block AP-1 activity in these cells. Because only those retinoids that inhibit AP-1 activity also inhibit tumor promoter-induced transformation, and the retinoic acid response element (RARE) activation-specific retinoid did not inhibit tumor promoter-induced transformation, we believe that inhibition of tumor promoter-induced transformation is an AP-1-dependent and not a RARE-dependent event. We used a more specific AP-1 inhibitor, dominant negative mutant of c-Jun (TAM67) in JB6 cells. All stable TAM67 transfectants blocked TPA-induced AP-1 activity and transformation (10). Because AP-1 DNA binding is not always correlated with AP-1 transcription activity, the best way to study AP-1 activity *in vivo* is to use transgenic animals expressing an AP-1 reporter gene such as luciferase. We used an AP-1 luciferase transgenic mouse model to study the role of AP-1 activity in tumor promotion *in vivo*. Our data indicated that AP-1 inhibitory retinoids, but not RARE activation-specific retinoid, repressed skin tumor promotion (11).

As discussed above, tumor promoters (e.g., TPA, TNFα or UV irradiation) also induce activation of transcription factor NFκB in many cell systems. In JB6 cells, inhibition of NFκB activation by antisense or pentoxifylline also blocks tumor promoter-induced cell transformation (22).

Three classes of MAPKs are known and they include extracellular-signal-regulated protein kinases (ERKs), c-Jun N-terminal kinases/stress-activated protein kinases (JNKs/SAPKs), and p38 kinases (Figure 1) (23-26). The activation of MAPKs may occur by translocation to the nucleus, where these kinases phosphorylate target transcription factors such as AP-1 (25-28). ERKs are believed to be strongly activated and to play a critical role in transmitting signals initiated by TPA and growth factors such as epidermal growth factor (EGF) and platelet-derived growth factor (PDGF) (29-30). On the other hand, JNKs/SAPKs and p38 kinases are potently activated by various forms of stress, including UV irradiation (26, 31). However, the activation of these pathways is not mutually exclusive. For example, heat shock and UV irradiation partially activate the ERKs cascade and EGF partially activates the JNKs/SAPKs pathway (25, 30). The UVC-induced activation of the AP-1 complex involves altered phosphorylation of the c-Jun protein. In unstimulated cells, the c-Jun protein is phosphorylated in the C-terminal half on a tryptic peptide, 227-252, located just upstream of the basic region of the DNA binding domain (32). UVC irradiation of cells causes enhanced DNA binding activity of Jun and the net phosphorylation of peptide 227-252 is decreased. The mechanism for the UVC-induced decrease in phosphorylation of this basic domain near the DNA binding region is not known. All of the stimuli including UVC that increase the transactivating potential of Jun cause hyperphosphorylation of two amino acids, serine-63 and serine-73 on the N-terminus (33-35). Hyperphosphorylation of serines 63 and 73 of c-Jun is suggested to prolong the interaction between Jun and p52/54 intermediary factors leading to more stable assembling of the pre-initiation complex and enhanced initiation of transcription (51).

Because different tumor promoters stimulate the activation of distinct MAP kinases, we proposed that the tumor promotion process induced by these different tumor promoters may depend on specific MAP kinase pathways. Indeed, we found that ERK is required for TPA- or EGF-induced cell transformation in JB6 cells (36-37). Shortage of ERK is responsible for resistance to AP-1 transactivation and transformation in JB6 P cells (36). Blocking MAP kinase activation by dominant negative mutant (DMN) ERK1 blocks TPA-induced AP-1 transactivation in JB6 P^+ cells and DNM-ERK also block arsenic-induced cell transformation (38). On the other hand, JNK activation is required for JB6 cell transformation induced by TNFα but not by TPA (39).

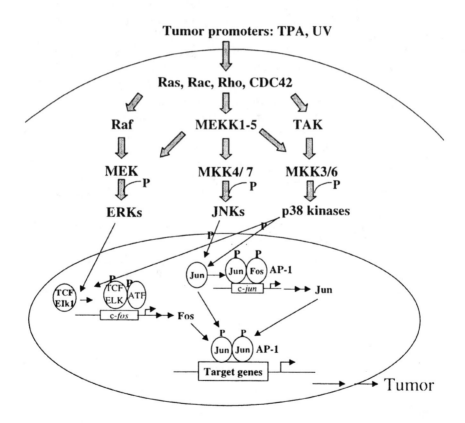

Figure 1. Tumor promoter-induced signal transduction.

ANTI-CARCINOGENESIS EFFECTS OF TEA AND TEA CONSTITUENTS

Prevention of carcinogenesis is one of the major strategies for cancer control.   Many studies have shown that green tea, black tea, and tea polyphenol preparations have inhibitory effects on carcinogenesis in rodent models (40-43). These include cancers of the skin, lung, esophagus, stomach, liver, duodenum and small intestine, pancreas, and colorectum.   Skin carcinogenesis induced by chemicals, UV light, and TPA is one of the most extensively studied systems (44-55). The anti-promoting effect of a green tea constituent, (-)-epigallocatechin 3-gallate (EGCG), has been demonstrated (44, 47, 49, 51). However, other tea components may also be effective anti-promoting agents. The underlying mechanisms responsible for these cancer-preventive activities have not been clearly elucidated.

Polyphenols are the most abundant group of compounds in tea leaves, and EGCG is the best studied tea polyphenol. A cup of green tea (2.5 g of dried green tea leaves brewed in 200 ml of water) usually contains about 90 mg of EGCG. In addition, it contains a similar or slightly smaller amount (65 mg) of (-)-epigallocatechin (EGC), about 20 mg each of (-)-epigallocatechin 3-gallate (ECG) and (-)-epigallocatechin (EC), and about 50 mg of caffeine (51). In black tea, these polyphenols are reduced to about one fourth of those in green tea, and theaflavins account for 1 to 2% of the total dry matter (1, 13, 16). About 10 to 20% of the dry weight of black tea is due to thearubigins which are not well characterized chemically (40, 52, 55). One cup of black tea (2.5 g of dried black tea leaves brewed in 200 ml of water) usually contains 12 to 15 mg theaflavins (50). These tea polyphenols are generally considered to be the effective components for the inhibition of carcinogenesis, but the mechanisms are not well characterized (40, 41).   However, a commonly discussed mechanism is the antioxidative activity of these polyphenolic compounds (40, 53).   The inhibitory activities of tea polyphenols on the growth of tumor cell lines were shown (54, 55, 56) and antioxidative and antimutagenic effects of theaflavins were reported (57, 58). The anti-promotion activity of EGCG was demonstrated and its possible effects on signal transduction pathways were suggested (47). Recently, Yu *et al.* reported that tea polyphenols may regulate antioxidant-response element (ARE)-mediated phase II enzyme expression through a mitogen-activated protein kinase C pathway (59). Jankun *et al.* reported that EGCG (2-10 mM) inhibits urokinase activity (60). As discussed in previous publications (41, 61), much work is needed to assess the importance of different proposed mechanisms in the inhibition of carcinogenesis by EGCG and theaflavins *in vivo*. The tissue concentrations of these compounds used *in vitro* may not be relevant to the anti-carcinogenesis process.

EFFECTS OF TEA POLYPHENOLS ON TUMOR PROMOTER-INDUCED SIGNAL TRANSDUCTION PATHWAYS

AP-1 and NFκB signal transduction pathways are known to be important in tumor promoter-induced transformation and tumor promotion. Both AP-1 and NFκB are activated by various tumor promoters. Therefore, the inhibitory effect of tea and tea constituents on the tumor promoter-induced signal transduction leading to the activation of AP-1 or NFκB may be important in the anti-tumor promotion activity of these compounds. We, therefore, investigated the inhibition of these signal transduction pathways as molecular mechanisms for the anti-tumor promotion activity of tea polyphenols EGCG and theaflavins.

EGCG and Theaflavins Inhibited TPA- or EGF-induced Cell Transformation

As shown in Table 1, EGF- or TPA-induced JB6 cell transformation was significantly inhibited by EGCG or theaflavins at the concentration range from 5 to 20 µM.

Table 1. Inhibition of TPA- or EGF-induced Cell Transformation, AP-1 Activity and JNK Activity by EGCG and Theaflavins

	Cell Transformation Activity	AP-1 Transactional Activity	AP-1 DNA Binding Activity	JNK Activity
Control	-	+/-	+/-	+/-
TPA	+++	+++	++	++
EGF	+++	+++	++	++
TPA + EGCG	+/-	+/-	+/-	+/-
TPA + theaflavins	+/-	+/-	+/-	+/-
EGF + EGCG	+/-	+/-	+/-	+/-
EGF + theaflavins	+/-	+/-	+/-	+/-

At this concentration range, EGCG or theaflavins did not inhibit cell proliferation as measured by $[H^3]TdR$ incorporation. Interestingly, EGCG and theaflavin inhibited TPA- or EGF-induced AP-1 activity in a similar dose range seen for inhibition of cell transformation. This suggests that inhibition of AP-1 activity by EGCG and theaflavins may be important for their inhibitory effect on cell transformation (62).

EGCG and Theaflavins Inhibited JNK Activity and Sequence Specific AP-1 DNA Binding Activity

To study the molecular basis of the inhibition of AP-1 transactivation by EGCG and theaflavins, we considered the possibilities that sequence specific AP-1 DNA binding activity and/or MAP kinases, upstream activator kinases responsible for the phosphorylation of AP-1/c-Jun proteins, might be altered by these tea polyphenols. Our results showed that EGCG or theaflavins inhibited TPA-induced AP-1 DNA binding activity (Table 1). Further, these two tea compounds also inhibited TPA- or EGF-induced JNK activation. Therefore, the inhibition of AP-1 transactivation by EGCG and theaflavins occurs through an inhibition of AP-1 DNA binding activity and a JNK-dependent pathway (62).

EGCG and Theaflavins Inhibited UVB-induced AP-1 Activity, NFκB Activity and Phosphorylation of P44/42 MAP Kinase and IκBα

The ultraviolet (UV)B portion of solar light is an important causative factor for human skin cancers. UV-induced signal transduction pathways play a critical role in tumor promotion. We, therefore, investigated the effect of EGCG and theaflavins on UVB-induced AP-1 and NFκB activity. As shown in Table 2, pretreatment of JB6 cells with EGCG or theaflavins inhibited UVB-induced AP-1 and NFκB activity. At a similar concentration range (1-20 μM), EGCG and theaflavins also inhibited UVB-induced phosphorylation of P44/42 MAP kinase, while phosphorylation of p38 kinases was not affected. Furthermore, IκBα phosphorylation, a critical step for the activation of NFκB transactivation, was significantly inhibited by EGCG and theaflavins.

EGCG Inhibited UVB-induced AP-1 Activity in an AP-1-luciferase Transgenic Mouse Model

Since DNA binding activity measured by gel-shift assay does not always correspond with AP-1 or NFκB transcription activity, the best way to study transcription activity *in vivo* is by using the transgenic mouse model containing a reporter gene. Recently, our laboratory used a B6D2 transgenic

Table 2. Inhibition of UVB-induced AP-1 Activity, NFκB Activity, Phosphorylation of MAP Kinase and IKBα

	AP-1 Activity	P44/42 MAP Kinase Phosphorylation	NFκB Activity	IKBα Phosphorylation
Control	+/-	+/-	+/-	+/-
UVB	++++	+++	+++	+++
UVB + EGCG	+/-	+/-	+/-	+/-
UVB + theaflavins	+/-	+/-	+/-	+/-

mouse expressesing the luciferase reporter gene under the control of four TREs (AP-1 binding sequences) to study the role of AP-1 activity in tumor promotion and progression (11).

Mice were treated topically three times a week with 5 mg of EGCG in acetone. The area of the skin treated was ~12 cm^2. The mice were then irradiated with 10 kJ/M^2 of UVB, followed 30 min later by a final application of 5 mg EGCG. One day later, skin epidermis was harvested for luciferase activity. In mouse skin epidermis, UVB irradiation induced a nearly 40-fold increase in luciferase activity, as compared with acetone treated controls. Treatment with topical EGCG reduced this UVB-induction of AP-1 transactivation activity by 60%. By inhibiting AP-1 activity in UVB-irradiated mouse skin, EGCG may be preventing non-melanoma skin cancer at the level of tumor promotion (63).

CONCLUSIONS

Studies by others and us demonstrated that tumor promoter-induced signal transduction pathways are critical in tumor promotion. These signaling molecules can be used as targets for development of cancer preventative agents. As shown in Figure 2, we demonstrated that:

(a)   tea polyphenols EGCG and theaflavins inhibit cell transformation;
(b)   EGCG and theaflavins inhibit AP-1, NFκB, phosphorylation of MAP kinases and IκBα;
(c)   inhibition of AP-1, NFκB, and other signal transduction pathways may explain the anti-tumor promotion action of tea polyphenols.

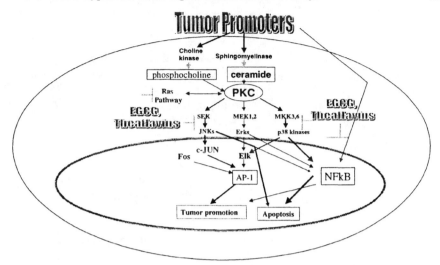

Figure 2. Possible Targets of Tea Polyphenols in Tumor Promoter-induced Signal Transduction Pathways

FUTURE DIRECTIONS

Figure 2 summarizes the possible role of EGCG and theaflavins in signal transduction pathways and tumor promotion. This work also opened up intriguing new questions that need to be addressed in the future. For example, how do these signaling molecules coordinate responses from different stimuli, and how do the cells make the decision to activate one signaling pathway or another? Which pathway is more critical in tumor promotion induced by one tumor promoter over another? Other specific directions include studies of (a) direct binding target(s) for the tea polyphenols, (b) detailed mechanisms of inhibition of tumor formation by EGCG and theaflavins, (c) mechanisms of other tea components, such as caffeine, on the inhibition of carcinogenesis, (d) effect of combinations of tea polyphenols and other chemopreventive agents, and (e) the administration of clinical trials of tea polyphenols for their chemoprevention effect in humans. These studies will provide insight into the anti-cancer effect of tea and tea polyphenols and the molecular basis for the development of new chemopreventive agents for human cancer.

ACKNOWLEDGMENTS

We thank Drs. C. S. Yang, G. Tim Bowden, Ann Bode, and H.H.O. Schmid for scientific discussion and editorial advice and Andria Percival for secretarial assistance. This work was supported by grants CA81064, CA77646, CA74916, and CA27502 from the National Cancer Institute.

REFERENCES

1. Beckman HH, Chen JL, O'Brien T, Tjian R. Coactivator and promoter-selective properties of RNA polymerase I TAFS. Science 1995; 270:1505-1509
2. O'Brien T, Lis JT. Rapid changes in Drosophila transcription after an instantaneous heat shock. Mol Cell Biol 1993; 13:3456-3463
3. Matrisian LM, McDonnel S, Miller DB, Navre M, Seftor EA, Hendrix MJC. The role of the matrix metalloproteinase stromelysin in the progression of squamous cell carcinomas. Am J Med Sci 1991; 302:157-162
4. Angel P, Baumann I, Stein B, Delius H, Rahmsdorf HJ, Herrlich P. 12-*O*-tetradecanoyl-phorbol-13-acetate induction of the human collagenase gene is mediated by an inducible enhancer element located in the 5'-flanking region. Mol Cell Biol 1987; 7:2256-2266
5. Dong Z, Colburn NH. AP-1: a molecular target for prevention of carcinogenesis. In: S Srivastava, SM Lippman, WK Hong, and JL Mulshine (eds.), Early Detection of Cancer, pp. 123-130, Futura Publishing Corp, Armonk, NY, 1994
6. Angel P. The role and regulation of Jun proteins in response to phorbol ester and UV light.   In: PA Baeurle (ed.), Induced Gene Expression, Vol. 1, pp. 62-92, Birkhauser, Boston, 1995
7. Derijard B, Hibi M, Wu IH, Barrett T, Su B, Deng T, Karin M, Davis RJ. JNK1: a protein kinase stimulated by UV light and Ha-Ras that binds and phosphorylates the c-Jun activation domain. Cell 1994; 76:1025-1037
8. Devary Y, Gottlieb RA, Lau LF, Karin M. Rapid and preferential activation of the c-Jun gene during the mammalian UV response. Mol Cell Biol 1991; 11:2804-2811
9. Devary Y, Rosette C, DiDonato JA, Karin M. NFκB activation by ultraviolet light not dependent on a nuclear signal. Science 1993; 261:1442-1445
10. Dong Z, Birrer MJ, Watts RG, Matrisian LM, Colburn NH. Blocking tumor promoter induced AP-1 activity inhibits transformation in JB6 cells. Proc Natl Acad Sci USA 1994; 91:609-613
11. Huang C, Ma WY, Dawson MI, Rincon M, Flavell RA, Dong Z. Blocking AP-1 activity, but not activating RARE, is required for anti-tumor promotion effects by retinoic acid. Proc Natl Acad Sci USA 1997; 94:5826-5830
12. Dong Z, Watts SG, Sun Y, Colburn NH. Progressive elevation of AP-1 activity during preneoplastic-to-neoplastic progression as modeled in mouse JB6 cell variants. Int J Oncol 1995; 7:359-364
13. Bernstein LR, Colburn NH. AP-1/Jun function is differentially induced in promotion-sensitive and resistant JB6 cells. Science 1989; 244:566-569
14. Domann FE, Levy JP, Birrer MJ, Bowden GT. Stable expression of c-Jun deletion mutant in two malignant mouse epidermal cell lines blocks cellular AP-1 activity and tumor formation in nude mice. Cell Growth & Diff 1994; 5:9-16

15. Bowden GT, Schneider B, Domann R, Kuleszmartin M. Oncogene activation and tumor suppressor gene inactivation during multistage mouse skin carcinogenesis. Cancer Res 1994; 54:S1882-S1885

16. Dong Z, Lavrovsky V, Colburn NH. Induction of reversion transformation in JB6 RT101 cells by AP-1 inhibitors. Carcinogenesis 1995; 16:749-759

17. Lavrovsky V, Dong Z, Ma W, Colburn NH. Drug induced reversion of progression phenotype is accompanied by reversion of AP-1 phenotype in JB6 cells. In Vitro Cell & Develop Biol 1996; 32:234-237

18. Huang C, Schmid PC, Ma WY, Schmid HHO, Dong Z. Phosphatidylinositol-3 kinase is necessary for 12-O-tetradecanoylphorbol-13-acetate-induced transformation of AP-1 activation. J Biol Chem 1997; 272:4187-4194

19. Sun Y, Nakamura K, Hegamyer G, Dong Z, Colburn N. No point mutation of Ha-ras or p53 genes expressed in preneoplastic-to-neoplastic progression as modeled in mouse JB6 cell variants. Mol Carcinogenesis 1993; 8:49-57

20. Colburn NH, Wandel E, and Srinivas L. Responses of preneoplastic epidermal cells to tumor promoters and growth factors: use of promoter-resistant variants for mechanism studies. J Cell Biochem 1982; 18:261-270

21. Colburn NH, Former BF, Nelson KA, Yuspa SH. Tumor promoter induces anchorage independence irreversibly. Nature(London) 1979; 281:589-591

22. Li JJ, Westergaard C, Ghosh P, Colburn NH. Inhibitors of both nuclear factor-kappaB and activator protein-1 activation block the neoplastic transformation response. Cancer Res 1997; 57:3569-3576

23. Boulton TG, Nye SH, Robbins DJ, Ip NY, Radziejewska E, Morgenbesser SD, DePinho RA, Panayotatos N, Cobb MH, Yancopoulos GD. ERKs: A family of protein-serine/threonine kinases that are activated and tyrosine phosphorylated in response to insulin and NGF. Cell 1991; 65:663-675

24. Kyriakis JM, Banerjee P, Niolakaki E, Dai T, Rubie EA, Ahmad MF, Avruch J, Woodgett JR. The stress-activated protein kinase subfamily of c-Jun kinases. Nature(London) 1994; 369:156-160

25. Davis RJ. MAP kinases: a new JNK expands the group. Trends Biochem Sci 1994; 19:470-473

26. Kallunki T, Su B, Tsigelny I, Sluss HK, Derijard B, Moore G, Davis RJ, Karin M. JNK2 contains a specificity-determining region responsible for efficient c-Jun binding and phosphorylation. Genes Dev 1994; 8:2996-3007

27. Angel P, Hattori K, Smeal T, Karin M. The jun proto-oncogene is positively autoregulated by its product, Jun/AP-1. Cell 1988; 55:875-885

28. Sanchez I, Hughes RT, Mayer BJ, Yee K, Woodgett JR, Avruch J, Kyriakis JM, Zon LI. Role of SAPK/ERK kinase-1 in the stress-activated pathway regulating transcription factor c-Jun. Nature 1994; 372:794-798

29. Cowley S, Paterson H, Kemp P, Marshall CJ. Activation of MAP kinase kinase is necessary and sufficient for PC12 differentiation and for transformation of NIH 3T3 cells. Cell 1994; 77:841-852

30. Minden A, Lin A, McMahon M, Lange-Carter C, Derijard B, Davis RJ, Johnson GL, Karin M. Differential activation of ERK and JNK mitogen-activated protein kinases by Raf-1 and MEKK. Science 194; 266:1719-1723

31. Angel P. The role and regulation of the Jun proteins in response to phorbol ester and UV light. In: PA Baeuerle (ed.), Inducible Gene Expression, pp. 62-92, Birkhauser, Boston, 1995

32. Boyle WJ, Smeal T, Defize LHK, Angel P, Woodgett JR, Karin M, Hunter T. Activation of protein kinase C decreases phosphorylation of c-Jun at sites that negatively regulate its DNA-binding activity. Cell 1991; 64:573-584

33. Smeal T, Binetruy B, Mercola D, Grover-Bardwick A, Heidecker G, Rapp UR, Karin M.   Oncoprotein mediated signaling cascade stimulates c-Jun activity by phosphorylation of serines 63 and 73. Mol Cell Biol 1992; 12:3507-3513

34. Devary Y, Gottleib RA, Smeal T, Karin M. The mammalian ultraviolet response is triggered by activation of Src tyrosine kinases. Cell 1992; 71:1081-1091

35. Radler-Pohl A, Sachsenmaier C, Gebel S, Auer HP, Bruder JT, Rapp U, Angel P, Rahmsdorf HJ, Herrlich P.   UV-induced activation of AP-1 involves obligatory extranuclear steps including Raf-1 kinase. EMBO J 1993; 12:1005-1012

36. Huang C, Ma WY, Young C, Colburn NH, Dong Z. The shortage of mitogen-activated protein (MAP) kinase is responsible for the tumor promotion resistant (P⁻) phenotype of JB6 cells. Proc Natl Acad Sci USA 1998; 95:156-161

37. Watts RG, Young MR, Huang C, Li JJ, Dong Z, Pennie WD, Colburn NH. Erk is required AP-1 mediated transcriptional activity and neoplastic transformation. Oncogene 1998; in press

38. Huang C, Ma WY, Li J, Goranson A, Dong Z. Requirement of Erks, but not JNKs, for arsenite-induced cell transformation. J Biol Chem 1999; 274:14595-14601

39. Huang C, Li J, Ma WY, Dong Z. JNKs activation is required for JB6 cell transformation induced by TNFα but not by TPA. J Biol Chem 1999; in press

40. Yang CS, Wang ZY. Tea and cancer: a review. J Natl Cancer Inst 1993; 58:1038-1049

41. Yang CS, Yang GY, Lee ML, Chen L. Mechanistic considerations of the inhibition of carcinogenesis by tea. In: H Ohigashi (ed.). Proceedings of the International Conference on Food Factor in Cancer Prevention, pp. 113-117, Springer-Verlag, Tokyo, 1997

42. Katiyar SK, Mukhtar H. Tea in chemoprevention of cancer: epidemiologic and experimental studies. Int J Oncology 1996; 8:221-238

43. Dreosti IE, Wargovich MJ, Yang CS. Inhibition of carcinogenesis by tea: The evidence from experimental studies. Crit Rev Food Sci & Nutr 1997; 37:761-770

44. Yoshizawa S, Horiuchi T, Fukiji H, Yoshida T, Okuda T, Sugimura T. Antitumor promoting activity of (-)-epigallocatechin gallate, the main constituent of "tannin" in green tea. Photother Res 1987; 1:44-47

45. Wang ZY, Khan WA, Bickers DR.   Protection against polycyclic aromatic hydrocarbon-induced skin tumor initiation in mice by green tea polyphenols. Carcinogenesis (Lond.) 1989; 10:411-415

46. Gensler HL, Timmermann BN, Valcic S, Wachter GA, Dorr R, Dvorakova K, Alberts DS. Prevention of photocarcinogenesis by topical administration of pure epigallocatechin gallate isolated from green tea. Nutr Cancer 1996; 26:325-335

47. Huang MT, Ho CT, Wang ZY, Ferraro T, Finnegan-Olive T, Lou YR, Mitchell JM, Laskin JD, Newmark H, Yang CS, Conney AH.   Inhibitory effect of topical application of a green tea polyphenol fraction on tumor initiation and promotion in mouse skin. Carcinogenesis (Lond.) 1992; 13:947-954

48. Wang ZY, Huang MT, Ferraro T, Wong CQ, Lou YR, Reuhl K, Latropoulos M, Yang CS, Conney AH.   Inhibitory effect of green tea in drinking water on tumorigenesis by ultraviolet light and 12-*O*-tetradecanoylphorbol-13-acetate in the skin of SKH-1 mice. Cancer Res 1992; 52:1162-1170

49. Katiyar S, Agarwal R, Wood GS. Inhibition of 12-*O*-tetradecanoyl-phorbol-13-acetate-caused tumor promotion in 7,12-dimethylbenz(a)anthracene-initiated SENCAR mouse skin by a polyphenolic fraction isolated from green tea. Cancer Res 1992; 52:6890-6897

50. Katiyar SK, Agarwal R, Mukhtar H. Protection against malignant conversion of chemically induced benign skin papillomas to squamous cell carcinomas in SENCAR

mice by a polyphenolic fraction isolated from green tea. Cancer Res 1993; 53:5409-5412

51. Wang ZY, Huang MT, Lou YR, Xie JG, Reuhl KR, Newmark HL, Ho CT, Yang CS, Conney AH. Inhibitory effects of black tea, green tea, decaffeinated black tea, and decaffeinated green tea on ultraviolet B light-induced skin carcinogenesis in 7,12-dimethylbenz[a]anthracene-initiated SKH-1 mice. Cancer Res 1994; 54:3428-3435

52. Balentine DA. Manufacturing and chemistry of tea. In: CT Ho, MT Huang, CY Lee (eds.), Phenolic Compounds in Food and their Effects on Health I: Analysis, Occurrence, and Chemistry, pp. 102-117, American Chemical Society, Washington, DC, 1992

53. Wang ZY, Wang LD, Lee MJ, Ho CT, Huang MT, Conney AH, Yang CS. Inhibition of N-nitrosomethylbenzylamine-induced esophageal tumorigenesis in rats by green and black tea. Carcinogenesis (Lond.) 1995; 16:2143-2148

54. Huang MT, Xie JG, Wange ZY, Ho CT, Lou YR, Wang CX, Hard GC, Conney AH. Effects of tea, decaffeinated tea, and caffeine on UVB light-induced complete carcinogenesis in SKH-1 mice: demonstration of caffeine as a biologically important constituent of tea. Cancer Res 1997; 57:2623-2629

55. Graham HN. Green tea composition, consumption, and polyphenol chemistry. Prev Med 1992; 21:334-350

56. Lea MA, Xiao Q, Sadhukhan AK, Cottle S, Wang ZY, Yang CS. Inhibitory effects of tea extracts and (-)-epigallocatechin gallate on DNA synthesis and proliferation of hepatoma and erythroleukemia cells. Cancer Lett 1993; 68:231-236

57. Yang GY, Liao J, Kim K, Yurkow EJ, Yang CS. Inhibition of growth and induction of apoptosis in human cancer cell lines by tea polyphenols. Carcinogenesis, in press

58. Shiraki M, Hara Y, Osawa T, Kumon H, Nakayama T, Kawakishi S. Antioxidative and antimutagenic effects of theaflavins from black tea. Mutat Res 1994; 323:29-34

59. Yu R, Jiao JJ, Duh JL, Gudehithlu K, Tan TH, Kong AN. Activation of mitogen-activated protein kinases by green tea polyphenols: potential signaling pathways in the regulation of antioxidant-responsive element-mediated phase II enzyme gene expression. Carcinogenesis 1997; 18:451-456

60. Jankun J, Selman SH, Swiercz R, Skrzypczak-Jankun E. Why drinking green tea could prevent cancer. Nature 1997; 387:561

61. Yang CS. Inhibition of carcinogenesis by tea. Nature 1997; 389:134-135

62. Dong Z, Ma WY, Huang C, Yang CS. Inhibition of tumor promoter-induced AP-1 activation and cell transformation by tea polyphenols, (-)-epigallocatechin gallate and theaflavins. Cancer Res 1997; 57:4414-4419

7

MECHANISMS BY WHICH GARLIC AND ALLYL SULFUR COMPOUNDS SUPPRESS CARCINOGEN BIOACTIVATION
Garlic and Carcinogenesis

John A. Milner

Nutrition Department
Graduate Program in Nutrition
The Pennsylvania State University
University Park, PA 16802

GARLIC: ITS HISTORICAL USAGE AND CURRENT PERSPECTIVES

For centuries garlic has been revered as a plant with medicinal properties. During this past 20 years these beliefs have been reinforced by exciting evidence documenting that garlic and its allyl sulfur components can alter a host of physiological processes that potentially foster health (Fenwick and Hanley, 1985b, Milner, 1996, Orekhov and Grunwald, 1997). Garlic's ability to reduce hyperlipidemia, hypertension, sterol synthesis and thrombus formation make it a strong candidate for lowering the risk of heart disease and stroke (Gebhardt, 1993, Orekhov and Grunwald, 1997, Abramovitz et al., 1999). In addition to antimicrobial properties (Adetumbi and Lau, 1983, Yoshida et al., 1999, Cellini et al., 1996, Dion et al., 1997), considerable evidence points to the ability of garlic and related components to serve as protectors of immunocompetence (Jeong and Lee, 1998, Morioka et al., 1993) and possibly mental function (Nishiyama et al., 1997). Garlic is a plant within

Nutrition and Cancer Prevention, edited under the auspices of AICR
Kluwer Academic / Plenum Publishers, New York, 2000.

69

the genus *Allium*. It along with onions, leeks and chives represent the major allium foods that are consumed by human beings. While it is possible that other allium foods possess similar health attributes, including a reduction in cancer risk, few comparative studies have been undertaken.

Although only a few epidemiological studies have examined garlic as a modifier of cancer risk those that have reveal an inverse relationship. Populations with the highest garlic intakes generally have the lowest risk of developing some forms of cancer (Cipriani et al., 1991, You et al., 1989, Arab, 2000). Notable among these are data from Shandong Province in the People's Republic of China (Mei et al., 1982) where stomach cancer mortality risk was found to be about 13 times lower in individuals consuming approximately 20 g garlic per day than occurred in people consuming about 1 g per day. Evidence that these benefits are not limited to a region of the world, or possibly a lifestyle, comes from comparable evidence of lower risks in residents of China, Italy, Germany and the United States who consume the highest amounts of garlic (Arab, 2000). Relatively modest intakes may offer protection as suggested by the reduction in colon cancer risk observed in women in the Iowa Women's Health Study who consumed garlic intermittently (Steinmetz et al., 1994). While these and other epidemiological data are tantalizing, not all studies support the anticarcinogenicity of garlic and related foods (Arab, 2000).

Laboratory based studies with model cancers provide some of the most compelling evidence that garlic and related sulfur components can alter cancer risk. Experimentally garlic and its associated components have been reported to have widespread protection against breast, colon, skin, uterine, esophagus and lung cancers (Wargovich et al., 1988, Sumiyoshi and Wargovich, 1990, Hussain et al., 1990, Liu et al., 1992, Ip et al., 1992, Amagase and Milner, 1993, Shukla et al., 1999, Song and Milner, 1999). While it remains to be firmly established, it appears that several mechanisms, which are briefly reviewed below, may account for this protection.

CANCER RISK: NITROSAMINE FORMATION AND METABOLISM

N-Nitroso compounds (NOCs) are potent carcinogens in a variety of biological models and presumably humans (Brown, 1999). Human exposure takes place following the ingestion or inhalation of preformed NOCs or after endogenous formation from naturally occurring precursors (Lijinsky, 1999). An acid environment and the presence of microorganisms can enhance the endogenous formation of nitrosamines. Both of these modifiers of nitrosamine formation can be influenced by the composition of the diet.

Several dietary factors are recognized to modify endogenous formation of nitrosamines (Shenoy and Choughuley, 1992, Kolb et al., 1997,

Dion et al., 1997, Atanasova-Goranova et al., 1997, Vermeer et al., 1999). These dietary components can either serve as catalysts or inhibitors of nitrosation. Garlic and some allyl sulfur compounds are capable of reducing the spontaneous formation of nitrosamines (Shenoy and Choughuley, 1992, Dion et al., 1997). Williams (1983) proposed that several sulfur compounds might foster the formation of nitrosothiols thereby reducing nitrosamine formation. Studies by Dion et al. (1997) provide evidence that not all sulfur compounds in garlic are equally effective in blocking the spontaneous formation of nitrosamines. Their studies reveal that water extracts of garlic, deodorized garlic powder, and onions were effect in reducing the spontaneous formation of N-nitrosomorpholine (NMOR), a known liver carcinogen. Interestingly, the inability of extracts of leeks to block NMOR formation suggest that all allium foods are not equal in their anticancer benefits. The ability of S-allyl cysteine (SAC) and its non-allyl analog S-propyl cysteine to effectively block NMOR formation suggest the cysteine residue is particularly important in this protection. This conclusion is supported by the relative inability of oil-soluble sulfur compounds such as diallyl disulfide (DADS), dipropyl disulfide, and diallyl sulfide to block spontaneous NMOR formation (Dion et al., 1997). Garlic preparations are known to vary in their content of specific allyl sulfur compounds. Thus, it is probable that these preparations are not equivalent in their ability to block nitrosamine formation.

Some of the most compelling evidence that garlic consumption alters nitrosamine formation in humans comes from studies by Mei et al. (1989). These investigators found that providing 5 g garlic per day was able to completely block the spontaneous formation of nitrosoproline resulting from ingestion of nitrate and proline supplements. While nitrosoproline is non-mutagenic and non-carcinogenic, its formation is thought to reflect the capacity to form other nitrosamines (Ohshima and Bartsch, 1999). The ability of garlic to reduce DNA adducts arising from the experimental feeding of nitrosamine precursors (Lin et al., 1994) provides additional evidence that this block in formation is physiologically important. Overall, of the plausible mechanisms by which garlic and at least some of its allyl sulfur compounds lowers cancer risk is by reducing exposure to NOCs.

The anticancer benefits attributed to garlic are not limited to its ability to retard NOC formation. Several studies reveal that allyl sulfur compounds also retard the bioactivation of carcinogens. For example, Dion et al. (1997) reported that water-soluble SAC and lipid-soluble DADS were both effective in reducing the mutagenicity of NMOR in *Salmonella typhimurium* TA100. While DADS was found to be cytotoxic to *Salmonella,* this property did not explain the observed reduction in mutagenicity. A block in mutagenicity following aqueous garlic extract exposure is also evident following treatment with ionizing radiation, peroxides, adriamycin, and N-methyl-N'-nitro-nitrosoguanidine (Knasmuller et al., 1989).

The ability of garlic to block nitrosamine metabolism is not restricted to procaryotic cells since similar protective effects are observed in experimental animals exposed to preformed nitrosamines (Hong et al., 1992, Lin et al., 1994, Haber-Mignard et al. 1996). DNA aklylation, a primary step in nitrosamine carcinogenesis, is markedly suppressed by ingestion of garlic (Lin et al., 1994). While this block in nitrosamine bioactivation may reflect several enzymatic changes, substantial evidence suggests a key alteration in cytochrome P450 2E1 (Chen et al., 1994, Jeong and Lee, 1998). Jin and Baillie (1997) provided evidence that autocatalytic destruction of CYP2E1 may account for some of the chemoprotective effects of diallyl sulfide, and possible other allyl sulfur compounds. Overall, considerable evidence suggests that part of the anticancer properties associated with garlic and allyl sulfur compounds revolve around their ability to retard the bioactivation of these potentially carcinogenic nitrosamines. The importance of the loss of P450 2E1 activity extends far beyond the cancer arena since Dion (1997) found garlic and associated water- and lipid-soluble allyl sulfur components retarded the metabolism of the muscle relaxing drug chlorzoxazone. It remains to be determined how much of the interindividual differences in the expression of cytochrome P450 enzymes, including 2E1, are due to specific dietary constituents and to what extent these influence drug effectiveness and/or disease risk.

Finally, garlic has also been observed to be effective in reducing tumors caused by treatment with a methylnitrosurea (MNU), a direct acting carcinogen (Lin et al., 1994). Addition of water-soluble S-allyl cysteine (57 μmol/kg diet) caused a 18% reduction in O6-methylguanine adducts while isomolar diallyl disulfide, oil soluble, resulted in a 23% reduction in adducts caused by MNU (Schaffer, et al. 1996). While the mechanism(s) by which garlic brings about this reduction in carcinogenesis remains to be determined, it may relate to a change in mammary gland terminal end bud formation and/or a change in rates of DNA repair.

GARLIC AND OTHER CANCER CAUSING AGENTS

Evidence that garlic and associated allyl sulfur constituents can alter carcinogenesis comes from many studies showing that they can retard the mutagenicity of a host of different compounds including nitrosomorpholine, benzo(a)pyrene, N-methyl N'-nitro-N-nitrosoguanidine, vinyl carbamate, N-nitrosodimethylamine and aflatoxin B1. Similarly, increasing evidence reveals that garlic and several allyl sulfur compounds can block the bioactivation and carcinogenicity of chemically diverse compounds (Table 1). This protection is not limited to a specific tissue but occurs widely since protection is observed in breast, esophagus, colon, lung and skin. The diversity of cancer causing compounds that are influenced suggests more than one mechanism may be involved. However, since many require metabolic activation there is a strong possibility that phase I and II enzymes are involved. Generally, garlic or associated components have not been observed to cause much, if any, change in cytochrome P-450 1A1, 1A2, 2B1, or 3A4 activities (Manson et al., 1997, Pan et al., 1993, Wang et al., 1999). Singh et al. (1998) provided evidence that the efficacy of various organosulfides to suppress benzo(a)pyrene tumorigenesis was correlated with their ability to suppress NAD(P)H:quinone oxidoreductase, an enzyme involved with the removal of quinones associated with this carcinogen. As mentioned below, changes in bioactivation resulting from a block in cyclooxygenase and lipoxygenase may partially account for the reduction in tumors following treatment with some carcinogens. Changes in glutathione concentration and the activity of specific glutathione-S-transferase, both factors involved in phase II detoxification, may be important in the protection provided by garlic. Both have been found to increase in liver and mammary tissue following consumption of processed garlic powder by the rat (Hatono et al., 1996, Manson et al., 1997, Singh and Singh, 1997). Hu et al. (1997) provided evidence that the induction of glutathione (GSH) S-transferase pi (mGSTP1-1) may be particularly important for the prevention of some chemically induced tumors.

Table 1. Carcinogens Known to be Influenced by Garlic or Associated Allyl Sulfur Compounds[1]

Compound	Site	Host
1,2-Dimethylhydrazine	colon	rat
3-Methylcholanthrene	cervix	mouse
4-(Methylnitrosamino)-1-(3-pyridyl)-1-butanone	nasal	rat
7,12 Dimethylbenz(a)anthracene	mammary	rat
7,12 Dimethylbenz(a)anthracene	skin	mouse
7,12-Dimethylbenz[a]anthracene	buccal pouch	hamster
7,12-Dimethylbenz[a]anthracene	forestomach	hamster
Aflatoxin B1	liver	toad
Aflatoxin B1	liver	rat
N-Methyl-N-nitrosourea	mammary	rat
Azoxymethane	colon	rat
Benzo(a)pyrene	forestomach	mouse
Benzo(a)pyrene	lung	mouse
Benzo(a)pyrene	skin	mouse
Benzo[a]pyrene	bone marrow	mouse.
Methylnitronitrosoguanidine	gastric	rat
N-nitrosodiethylamine	nasal	rat
N-nitrosodiethylamine	colon	rat
N-nitrosodimethylamine	nasal	rat
N-nitrosodimethylamine	liver	rat
N-nitrosodimethylamine	skin	mouse
N-nitrosomethylbenzylamine	esophagus	rat
Vinyl carbamate	skin	mouse

[1] The response to garlic and allyl sulfur components is highly dependent on the quantity provided as well as the amount of carcinogen examined.

VARIATION IN RESPONSE TO GARLIC SOURCE

The incidence of mammary, skin and buccal cavity tumors caused by 7,12-dimethylbenz(a)anthracene (DMBA) treatment is markedly reduced by the ingestion of garlic and/or by either its water- or lipid-soluble allyl sulfur constituents (Liu et al., 1992, Singh and Shukla,1998, Balasenthil et al., 1999). Such evidence suggests that several sources of garlic may be effective in retarding DMBA carcinogenesis and presumably other chemically induced tumors. Previous studies from our laboratory (Amagase and Milner, 1993) provide evidence that several sources of garlic are likely effective in retarding chemically induced tumors. These studies revealed that feeding locally purchased garlic or a high sulfur garlic powder were similar in their ability to retarding DNA adducts caused by DMBA. Interestingly, this response was also similar to the reduction caused by deodorized garlic. Overall, these and several other studies suggest that several, and certainly not one, sulfur-containing components of processed garlic can retard chemically induced tumors in model systems. Since a reduction in mammary tumors is highly correlated with a decrease in DMBA induced adducts bound to mammary cell DNA (Liu et al., 1992), these findings indicate that quantity rather than source of garlic may not be most important in determining the degree of protection. Subtle differences may become apparent as the quantity of the garlic preparation provided is reduced. It must be emphasized that several dietary components including total fat, selenium, methionine, and vitamin A can markedly influence the overall anticancer effects of garlic or its allyl sulfur constituents (Amagase and Milner, 1996, Ip et al., 1996, Schaffer and Milner, 1997).

Both water- and lipid-soluble allyl sulfur compounds have been recognized to suppress carcinogen bioactivation. Table 2 provides a list of those compounds that have been most extensively examined.

Table 2. Sulfur Compounds in Garlic with Observed Anticancer Properties

Diallyl sulfide	S-allyl cysteine
Diallyl disulfide	Ajoene
Diallyl trisulfide	Allixin

Few studies have simultaneously compared the water- and oil-soluble for their relative efficacy. Nevertheless, what is available do not indicate significant differences in efficacy (Schaffer et al., 1996, Schaffer et al., 1997). Tsai et al. (1996) found that diallyl disulfide, dipropyl disulfide, diallyl sulfide, allyl methyl sulfide, allyl mercaptan and cysteine were all effective in retarding the mutagenicity of boiled pork juice. In many studies diallyl disulfide is more effective than diallyl sulfide and replacing the allyl group by a propyl moiety reduces its ability to retard the cancer process (Hu et al., 1997, Sundaram and Milner, 1995).

Variation in garlic's overall efficacy may also be modified by preparation and handling procedures. This belief is emphasized by recent studies revealing that heating of unpeeled garlic in a microwave or convection oven virtually eliminates its anticancer properties (Song and Milner, 1999). These studies suggest that alliinase is critical for the formation of compounds that have anticancer benefits. Allowing peeled and crushed garlic to stand for about 15 minutes appears to minimize the loss of anticancer protection caused by normal heating (Song and Milner, 1999).

INTERACTIONS WITH OTHER DIETARY CONSTITUENTS

Several dietary constituents can markedly influence the response to supplemental garlic (Amagase and Milner, 1992, Schaffer et al., 1997). Two important variables are the quantity of selenium and unsaturated fatty acids provided by the diet. Amagase et al. (1996) and Ip et al. (1996) reported that selenium supplied either as a component of the diet or as a constituent of the garlic supplement, respectively, enhanced the protection against DMBA carcinogenesis over that provided by garlic alone. Again a depression in DMBA bioactivation, as evident by a reduction in DNA adducts, may account for this combined benefit of garlic and selenium. More recently, Schaffer and et al. (1997) reported that selenium enhanced the ability of both SAC and DADS to retard DMBA induced DNA adducts in rat mammary tissue. Dietary fatty acid supply can also dramatically influence the bioactivation of DMBA to metabolites capable of binding to rat mammary cell DNA. A significant portion of the enhancement in mammary DNA adducts caused by increasing dietary corn oil consumption can be attributed to linoleic acid intake (Schaffer and Milner 1997). While exaggerated oleic acid consumption also increased DMBA induced DNA adducts, the response was far less than that caused by linoleic acid. Interestingly, fortification of the diet with palmitic acid was not accompanied by a change in DMBA bioactivation (Schaffer and Milner, 1997). Thus, it can not be assumed that all fat sources will equally influence garlic's anticancer properties.

The ability of fatty acids to alter DMBA bioactivation may provide some clues to a mechanism by which garlic and its associated allyl sulfur compounds retard chemically induced tumors. As indicated previously, it does not appear that changes in cytochrome P450 enzymes can account for the protection provided by supplemental garlic. During the past few years, increased attention has focused on the possible involvement of cyclooxygenase in the bioactivation of some carcinogens. Smith et al. (1991) reported that prostaglandin H synthase could metabolize the bay region diol of benzo(a)pyrene to electrophilic diol epoxides that were capable of binding to DNA. Likewise, Liu et al. (1995) reported that 2-aminofluorene metabolism might involve this enzyme. Most recently, our laboratory has reported that DMBA bioactivation appears to depend on cyclooxygenase activity (Schaffer and Milner, 1997). Ali (1996) provided evidence that garlic can inhibit cyclooxygenase. Studies by McGrath and Milner (1999) provided evidence that both water and lipid soluble allyl sulfur compounds could retard the ability of cyclooxygenase to bioactivate DMBA. A close examination of the rate of formation of adducts in *in vitro* DMBA bioactivation studies suggests the involvement of possibly another enzyme. A logical enzyme to consider is lipoxygenase since it has also been found to bioactivate several carcinogens (Roy and Kulkarni, 1999, Rioux and Castonguay, 1998) including benz(a)pyrene (Hughes, et al. 1989, Joseph, et al. 1994), a carcinogen similar to DMBA. McGrath and Milner (1999) recently reported that lipoxygenase could bioactivate DMBA. The activation caused by lipoxygenase was about 10 times greater than that caused by cyclooxygenase (Figure 2). While limited, there is some data indicating that garlic and associated sulfur components can inhibit lipoxygenase activity (Belman et al., 1989).

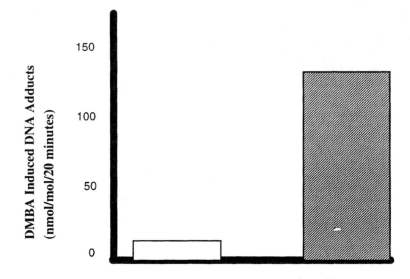

Figure 2. Influence of Cyclooxygenase and Lipoxygenase on the bioactivation of 7,12-dimethylbenz(a)anthrancene. The reaction mixtures contained either 40 units cyclooxygenase (COX) (Oxford Biomedical Research, Inc.) or 40 units 12/15 lipoxygenase (Sigma Chemical Co), 50 uM DMBA-3,4-diol, and 1 mg/mL calf thymus DNA. Reactions were initiated by addition of 100 uM linoleic acid and terminated after 20 min. Values are the mean of three reactions. Lipoxygenase was significantly more effective in bioactivating DMBA than was cyclooxygenase. A P1 nuclease enriched 32P-postlabeling method (Schaffer and Milner, 1996) was used for detection of DMBA induced DNA adducts. Presented in part McGrath and Milner, 1999).

Finally, evidence for the involvement of lipoxygenase in the bioactivation of DMBA comes from data from Song and Milner (1998). They reported that feeding the known lipoxygenase inhibitor, nordihydroguaiaretic acid (NDGA), was accompanied by a marked reduction in DMBA induced DNA adducts in rat mammary tissue. Collectively, these studies pose interesting questions about the role of both cyclooxygenase and lipoxygenase in not only forming prostaglandins and therefore modulating tumor cell proliferation and immunocompetence, but also their involvement in the bioactivation of carcinogens. Clearly, additional attention is need to clarify what role if any these enzymes have in determining the biological response to dietary garlic or its allyl sulfur components.

SUMMARY

Overall, a host of studies provides compelling evidence that garlic and its organic allyl sulfur components are effective inhibitors of the cancer process. These studies reveal that the benefits of garlic are not limited to a specific species, to a particular tissue, or to a specific carcinogen. Several mechanisms are likely to account for this protection. Notable among these is a depression in nitrosamine formation and a reduction in carcinogen bioactivation. The benefits provided by garlic must be viewed as part of the entire diet, since several dietary constituents can influence the degree of protection. More than one compound is responsible for the anticancer properties associated with garlic. Future research should focus on how genetic variability and daily environmental factors influence the anticancer benefits attributed to garlic and its allyl sulfur components.

ACKNOWLEDGMENTS

Supported in part by USDA National Research Initiative Competitive Grant Program and the American Institute for Cancer Research.

REFERENCES

1. Abramovitz D, Gavri S, Harats D, Levkovitz H, Mirelman D, Miron T, Eilat-Adar S, Rabinkov A, Wilchek M, Eldar M, Vered Z. Allicin-induced decrease in formation of fatty streaks (atherosclerosis) in mice fed a cholesterol-rich diet. Coron Artery Dis 1999; 10(7): 515-9.
2. Adetumbi MA, Lau BH. Allium sativum (garlic)--a natural antibiotic. Med Hypotheses 1983; 12(3): 227-37.
3. Ali M. Mechanism by which garlic (Allium sativum) inhibits cyclooxygenase activity. Effect of raw versus boiled garlic extract on the synthesis of prostanoids. Prostaglandins Leukot Essent Fatty Acids 1995; 53(6):3 97-400.

4. Amagase H, Milner JA. Impact of various sources of garlic and their constituents on 7,12-dimethylbenz(a)anthracene binding to mammary cell DNA. Carcinogenesis 1993;14:1627-31.
5. Amagase H, Schaffer EM, Milner, JA. Dietary components modify garlic's ability to suppress 7,12-dimethylbenz(a)anthracene induced mammary DNA adducts. 1996; J Nutr 126: 817-824.
6. Arab, K. Garlic and Cancer: A Critical Review of the Epidemiological Literature. 2000. Plenum Press
7. Atanasova-Goranova VK, Dimova PI, Pevicharova GT. Effect of food products on endogenous generation of N-nitrosamines in rats. Br J Nutr 1997; 78(2): 335-45.
8. Balasenthil S, Arivazhagan S, Ramachandran CR, Nagini S. Effects of garlic on 7,12-dimethylbenz[a]anthracene-induced hamster buccal pouch carcinogenesis. Cancer Detect Prev 1999; 23(6): 534-538.
9. Belman S, Solomon J, Segal A, Block E, Barany G. Inhibition of soybean lipoxygenase and mouse skin tumor promotion by onion and garlic components. J Biochem Toxicol 1989; 4(3): 151-60.
10. Block E. The chemistry of garlic and onion. Sci American 1985; 252: 114-9.
11. Brown JL. N-Nitrosamines. Occup Med 1999; 14(4): 839-848.
12. Cellini L, Di Campli E, Masulli M, Di Bartolomeo S, Allocati N. Inhibition of Helicobacter pylori by garlic extract (Allium sativum). FEMS Immunol Med Microbiol 1996; 13(4): 273-7.
13. Chen L, Lee M, Hong JY, Huang W, Wang E, Yang CS. Relationship between cytochrome P450 2E1 and acetone catabolism in rats as studied with diallyl sulfide as an inhibitor. Biochem Pharmacol 1994; 48(12): 2199-205.
14. Cipriani F, Buiatti E, Palli D. Gastric cancer in Italy.Ital J Gastroenterol 1991; 23(7):429-35
15. Clydesdale FM. A proposal for the establishment of scientific criteria for health claims for functional foods. Nutr Rev 1997; 55(12):413-22.
16. Dion ME, Agler M, Milner JA. S-allyl cysteine inhibits nitrosomorpholine formation and bioactivation. Nutr Cancer 1997; 28(1): 1-6.
17. Dion, M.. The Influence of Garlic and Associated Constituents on Nitrosamine Formation and Bioactivation. Master of Science Thesis. 1997. The Pennsylvania State University.
18. Fenwick, GR, Hanley AB. The genus Allium. Part 2. Crit Rev Food Sci Nutr 1985a; 22(4): 273-7.
19. Fenwick GR, Hanley AB. The genus Allium--Part 3. Crit Rev Food Sci Nutr 1985b; 23(1):1-73.
20. Ferguson LR. Natural and man-made mutagens and carcinogens in the human diet. Mutat Res 1999; 443(1-2):1-10.
21. Gebhardt R. Multiple inhibitory effects of garlic extracts on cholesterol biosynthesis in hepatocytes. Lipids 1993; 28(7):613-9.
22. Haber-Mignard D, Suschetet M, Berges R, Astorg P, Siess MH. Inhibition of aflatoxin B1- and N-nitrosodiethylamine-induced liver preneoplastic foci in rats fed naturally occurring allyl sulfides. Nutr Cancer; 1996; 25(1): 61-70.
23. Hatono S, Jimenez A, Wargovich MJ. Chemopreventive effect of S-allylcysteine and its relationship to the detoxification enzyme glutathione S-transferase. Carcinogenesis 1996; 17(5): 1041-4.
24. Hong JY, Wang ZY, Smith TJ, Zhou S, Shi S, Pan J, Yang CS.. Inhibitory effects of diallyl sulfide on the metabolism and tumorigenicity of the tobacco-specific carcinogen 4-(methylnitrosamino)-1-(3-pyridyl)-1-butanone (NNK) in A/J mouse lung. Carcinogenesis 1992; 13(5): 901-4.
25. Hu X, Benson PJ, Srivastava SK, Xia H, Bleicher RJ, Zaren HA, Awasthi S, Awasthi YC, Singh SV. Induction of glutathione S-transferase pi as a bioassay for the evaluation of potency of inhibitors of benzo(a)pyrene-induced cancer in a murine model. Int J Cancer 1997; 73(6): 897-902

26. Hughes MF, Chamulitrat W, Mason RP Eling TE. Epoxidation of 7,8-dihydroxy-7,8-dihydrobenzo[a]pyrene via a hydroperoxide-dependent mechanism catalyzed by lipoxygenases. Carcinogenesis 1989; 10: 2075-80.
27. Hussain SP, Jannu LN, Rao   AR.   Chemopreventive action of garlic on methylcholanthrene-induced carcinogenesis in the uterine cervix of mice. Cancer Lett 1990; 49: 175-180.
28. Ip C, Lisk DJ, Stoewsand GS. Mammary cancer prevention by regular garlic and selenium-enriched garlic. Nutr Cancer 1992; 7: 279-86.
29. Ip C, Lisk DJ, Thompson HJ. Selenium-enriched garlic inhibits the early stage but not the late stage of mammary carcinogenesis. Carcinogenesis 1996; 17(9): 1979-82.
30. Jeong HG, Lee YW   1998.   Protective effects of diallyl sulfide on N-nitrosodimethylamine-induced immunosuppression in mice. Cancer Lett 1998; 134(1): 73-9.
31. Jin L, Baillie TA 1997. Metabolism of the chemoprotective agent diallyl sulfide to glutathione conjugates in rats. Chem Res Toxicol 1997; 10(3): 318-27.
32. Joseph P, Srinivasan SN, Byczkowski JZ, Kulkarni AP.   Bioactivation of benzo(a)pyrene-7,8-dihydrodiol catalyzed by lipoxygenase purified from human term placenta and conceptal tissues. Reprod Toxicol 1994; 8: 307-13
33. Knasmuller S, de Martin R, Domjan G, Szakmary A. Studies on the antimutagenic activities of garlic extract. Environ Mol Mutagen 1989; 13(4): 357-65.
34. Kolb E, Haug M, Janzowski C, Vetter A, Eisenbrand. Potential nitrosamine formation and its prevention during biological denitrification of red beet juice. Food Chem Toxicol 1997; 35(2): 219-24.
35. Lawson LD, Wang ZJ, Hughes BG. Identification and HPLC quantitation of the sulfides and dialk(en)yl thiosulfinates in commercial garlic products. Planta Med 1991; 57(4): 363-70.
36. Lijinsky W. N-Nitroso compounds in the diet. Mutat Res 1999; 443(1-2):129-38.
37. Lin X-Y, Liu, JZ, Milner JA.. Dietary garlic suppresses DNA adducts caused by N-nitroso compounds. Carcinogenesis 1994; 15: 349-52.
38. Lipkin M, Reddy B, Newmark H, Lamprecht SA. Dietary factors in human colorectal cancer.Annu Rev Nutr 1999;19:545-86.
39. Liu JZ, Lin RI, Milner JA. Inhibition of 7,12-dimethylbenz(a)- anthracene induced mammary tumors and DNA adducts by garlic powder. Carcinogenesis 1992; 13: 1847-51.
40. Liu Y, Levy GN, Weber WW 1995. Activation of 2-aminofluorene by prostaglandin endoperoxide H synthase-2.Biochem Biophys Res Commun 215(1):346-54.
41. Manson MM, Ball HW, Barrett MC, Clark HL, Judah DJ, Williamson G, Neal GE. Mechanism of action of dietary chemoprotective agents in rat liver: induction of phase I and II drug metabolizing enzymes and aflatoxin B1 metabolism. Carcinogenesis 1997; 18(9):1729-38.
42. McGrath BC, Milner JA. Diallyl disulfide, S-allyl sulfide and conjugated linoleic acid   retard   12/15-lipoxygenase-mediated   bioactivation   of   7,12-dimethylbenz(a)anthracene (DMBA) in vitro. FASEB J. 1999; 13(4): A540.
43. Mei X, Lin X, Liu J, Lin XY, Song PJ, Hu JF, Liang XJ. The blocking effect of garlic on the formation of N-nitrosoproline in humans. Acta Nutr Sin 1989; 11:141-5.
44. Mei, X, Wang ML, Pan XY. Garlic and gastric cancer 1. The influence of garlic on the level of nitrate and nitrite in gastric juice. Acta Nutr Sin 1982; 4: 53-6.
45. Milner JA. Functional foods and health promotion. J Nutr 1999; 129(7 Suppl): 1395S-7S.
46. Milner JA. Garlic: its anticarcinogenic and antitumorigenic properties.Nutr Rev 1996; 54(11 Pt 2):S82-6.
47. Morioka N, Sze LL, Morton DL, Irie RF. A protein fraction from aged garlic extract enhances cytotoxicity and proliferation of human lymphocytes mediated by interleukin-2 and concanavalin A. Cancer Immunol Immunother 1993; 37(5): 316-22.

48. Nishiyama N, Moriguchi T, Saito H. Beneficial effects of aged garlic extract on learning and memory impairment in the senescence accelerated mouse. Exp Gerontol 1997; 32(1-2): 149-60.

49. Ohshima H, Bartsch H. Quantitative estimation of endogenous N-nitrosation in humans by monitoring N-nitrosoproline in urine. Methods Enzymol 1999; 301:40-9.

50. Orekhov AN, Grunwald J. Effects of garlic on atherosclerosis. Nutrition 1997; 13(7-8): 656-63.

51. Pan J, Hong JY, Li D, Schuetz EG, Guzelian PS, Huang W, Yang CS. Regulation of cytochrome P450 2B1/2 genes by diallyl sulfone, disulfiram, and other organosulfur compounds in primary cultures of rat hepatocytes. Biochem Pharmacol 1993; 45(11): 2323-9.

52. Rioux N, Castonguay A. Inhibitors of lipoxygenase: a new class of cancer chemopreventive agents. Carcinogenesis 1998; 19(8): 1393-400.

53. Roy P, Kulkarni AP. Co-oxidation of acrylonitrile by soybean lipoxygenase and partially purified human lung lipoxygenase. Xenobiotica 119; 29(5): 511-31

54. Salman H, Bergman M, Bessler H, Punsky I, Djaldetti M. Effect of a garlic derivative (alliin) on peripheral blood cell immune responses. Int J Immunopharmacol 1999; 21(9): 589-97.

55. Schaffer EM, Liu JZ, Green J, Dangler CA, Milner JA. Garlic and associated allyl sulfur components inhibit N-methyl-N-nitrosourea induced rat mammary carcinogenesis. Cancer Lett 1996. 102(1-2): 199-204.

56. Schaffer EM, Liu JZ, Milner JA. Garlic powder and allyl sulfur compounds enhance the ability of dietary selenite to inhibit 7,12-dimethylbenz[a]anthracene-induced mammary DNA adducts. Nutr Cancer 1997; 27(2): 162-8.

57. Schaffer EM, Milner JA. Cyclooxygenase-mediated formation of 7,12-dimethylbenz(a)anthracene (DMBA)-induced mammary DNA adducts. FASEB J. 1997; 11(3): A440.

58. Schaffer EM, Milner JA. Impact of dietary fatty acids on 7,12-dimethylbenz[a]anthracene-induced mammary DNA adducts. Cancer Lett 1996; 106(2): 177-83.

59. Shenoy NR, Choughuley AS. Inhibitory effect of diet related sulphydryl compounds on the formation of carcinogenic nitrosamines. Cancer Lett 1992; 65(3): 227-32.

60. Shukla Y, Singh A, Srivastava B. Inhibition of carcinogen-induced activity of gamma-glutamyl transpeptidase by certain dietary constituents in mouse skin. Biomed Environ Sci 1999; 12(2): 110-5.

61. Singh A, Shukla Y. Antitumor activity of diallyl sulfide in two-stage mouse skin model of carcinogenesis. Biomed Environ Sci 1998; 11(3): 258-63.

62. Singh A, Singh SP. Modulatory potential of smokeless tobacco on the garlic, mace or black mustard-altered hepatic detoxication system enzymes, sulfhydryl content and lipid peroxidation in murine system. Cancer Lett 1997; 118(1): 109-14.

63. Singh SV, Pan SS, Srivastava SK, Xia H, Hu X, Zaren HA, Orchard JL. Differential induction of NAD(P)H: quinone oxidoreductase by anti-carcinogenic organosulfides from garli. 1998; 244(3): 917-20.

64. Smith, BJ, Curtis JF, Eling TE. Bioactivation of xenobiotics by prostaglandin H synthase. Chem-Biol Interactions 1991; 79: 245-64.

65. Song K, Milner JA Heating garlic inhibits its ability to suppress 7, 12-dimethylbenz(a)anthracene-induced DNA adduct formation in rat mammary tissue. J Nutr 1999, 129(3): 657-61.

66. Steinmetz KA. Kushi LH, Bostick RM, Folsom AR, Potter JD. Vegetables, fruit, and colon cancer in the Iowa Women's Health Study. Amer J Epid 1994; 139: 1-15.

67. Sumiyoshi H, Wargovich MJ. Chemoprevention of 1,2-dimethylhydrazine-induced colon cancer in mice by natural occurring organosulfur compounds. Cancer Res 1990; 50: 5084-7.

68. Sundaran S, Milner JA. Diallyl disulfide inhibits the proliferation of human tumor cells in culture. *Biochem Biophy. Acta* 1995; 1315: 15-20,.

69. Tamaki T, Sonoki S. Volatile sulfur compounds in human expiration after eating raw or heat-treated garlic. J Nutr Sci Vitaminol (Tokyo) 1999; 45(2): 213-22.

70. Vermeer IT, Moonen EJ, Dallinga JW, Kleinjans JC, van Maanen. Effect of ascorbic acid and green tea on endogenous formation of N -nitrosodimethylamine and N-nitrosopiperidine in humans. Mutat Res 1999; 428(1-2): 353-61.

71. Wang BH, Zuzel KA, Rahman K, Billington D. Treatment with aged garlic extract protects against bromobenzene toxicity to precision cut rat liver slices. Toxicology 1999; 132(2-3): 215-25.

72. Wargovich MJ, Woods C, Eng VW, Stephens LC, Gray K. Chemoprevention of N-nitrosomethylbenzylamine-induced esophageal cancer in rats by the naturally occurring thioether, diallyl sulfide. Cancer Res. 1988; 48: 6872-5.

73. Weisburger JH. Mechanisms of action of antioxidants as exemplified in vegetables, tomatoes and tea. Food Chem Toxicol 1999; 37(9-10):943-8.

74. Williams D H. S-Nitrosation and the reactions of S-Nitroso compounds. Chem Soc Rev 1983; 15:171-196.

75. Winn LM, Wells PG. Evidence for embryonic prostaglandin H synthase-catalyzed bioactivation and reactive oxygen species-mediated oxidation of cellular macromolecules in phenytoin and benzo[a]pyrene teratogenesis. Free Radic Biol Med; 1997; 22(4): 607-21.

76. Yoshida H, Katsuzaki H, Ohta R, Ishikawa K, Fukuda H, Fujino T, Suzuki A. An organosulfur compound isolated from oil-macerated garlic extract, and its antimicrobial effect.Biosci Biotechnol Biochem 1999; 63(3): 588-90.

77. You WC, Blot WJ, Chang YS, Ershow A, Yang ZT, An Q, Henderson BE, Fraumeni JF Jr, Wang TG. Allium vegetables and reduced risk of stomach cancer. J Natl Cancer Inst 1989;81:162-4.

8

ANTIPROLIFERATIVE EFFECTS OF GARLIC-DERIVED AND OTHER ALLIUM RELATED COMPOUNDS

John T. Pinto[1,2,3], Sameer Lapsia[1], Amy Shah[1],
Harsha Santiago[1], and Grace Kim[1]

[1]Nutrition Research Laboratory
[2]The Clinical Nutrition Research Unit, Memorial Sloan-Kettering Cancer Center
[3]Weill Medical College of Cornell University New York, New York, USA

INTRODUCTION

An extensive and expanding information base that incorporates data from epidemiologic, animal, and laboratory investigations documents the relation between garlic consumption and decreased risk of developing cancer at various organ sites (1-3). Garlic and other allium-related plants contain alliin, an allylsulfinothiolated derivative of cysteine, that is transformed exogenously into a number of mono-, di-, and triallylsulfinyl analogues when the bulb is crushed, minced, or damaged (5). These bioactive compounds interact with a number of molecular targets whose functions range from control of cell cycle to expression of crucial antioxidant and detoxification enzymes (6-8). Modulation of each of these processes may underlie garlic's putative anticancer potential.

Nutrition and Cancer Prevention, edited under the auspices of AICR   **83**
Kluwer Academic / Plenum Publishers, New York, 2000.

In addition to thioallyl derivatives, garlic contains a number of other phytochemicals, synthesized constitutively or as part of a "stress response" by the plant, that demonstrate anticarcinogenic activity. These compounds include vinyl dithiins, allixins, saponins (β-cholorogenin), and gluco-arginine (N^{α}-fructosyl arginine) (9-14). Each of these compounds exhibits its own intrinsic capacity to affect growth of cancer cells and has the potential of acting alone or in combination with one or more of its co-constituents in garlic.

In view of the number of potentially bioactive components isolated from garlic, investigations that use aqueous or ethanolic extracts of crushed garlic prohibit accurate identification of which constituent reacts with a particular molecular target and which constituent(s) is(are) responsible for garlic's therapeutic properties. Although such studies reflect the type of effects that one might expect if garlic is consumed as a food, the majority of animal and laboratory investigations that focus on mechanism employ a pharmacological approach which attempts to describe the antitumor potential of garlic by examining efficacy of isolated derivatives. Clearly, the constraints in using this latter approach are that synergistic mechanisms of various constituents acting at single sites or multiple constituents acting at various molecular locations cannot be evaluated under these conditions.

Potential mechanisms of cancer prevention and control that are central to the action of allium derivatives impact upon several recognized stages of cancer, namely, initiation, promotion, and progression (15). In view of the many studies that have examined the efficacy of allium compounds as anti-initiators of chemical carcinogenesis (16-25), this chapter will highlight the effects of garlic-derived constituents on the latter stages of the carcinogenic process. Within the past few years, studies have emerged that demonstrate that thioallyl derivatives can antagonize growth of transformed cells by altering their mitogenic programming, inhibiting signal transduction protein kinases, blocking calcium ion channel function, and modifying steroid hormone responsiveness in breast and prostate carcinoma cells. In most instances, particular attention in this review will be given to hypothesized mechanisms that are associated with the antiproliferative effects of isolated thioallyl derivatives on a variety of transformed cell lines as well as on normal cells grown in culture.

STRUCTURAL FEATURES OF ALLIUM DERIVATIVES AND ENDOGENOUS REACTIONS THAT MAY UNDERLIE THEIR ANTIPROLIFERATIVE ACTIVITY.

Investigations of the chemopreventive activity of allium foods have concentrated on specific lipid- and water-soluble thioallyl constituents (*Figure 1*). All of these thioallyl compounds are derived *in situ* from a transitory, precursor diallylthiosulfinate, allicin, which, in turn, is enzymatically synthesized from the non-odorous, parent compound, alliin (26,27). Because of its anti-microbial properties, high reactivity with protein sulfhydryl groups, and strong pro-oxidant behavior, allicin was considered by early investigators to contribute significantly to garlic's therapeutic qualities in prevention of a wide variety of human diseases (28). However, due to its instability and spontaneous reactivity with a variety of reducing agents, it is doubtful whether allicin per se actually reached intracellular target sites that would impact on control of cell proliferation (29). Since allicin can react with endogenous sulfhydryl moieties, namely glutathione, cysteine, CoASH, and thiol containing proteins, within gastrointestinal cells (5,9,30), little if any allicin actually reaches the portal blood after consumption (29,30). In addition, allicin's utility in clinical trials has been limited because of its highly odiferous quality.

Feeding humans extracts of fresh raw garlic containing large amounts of allicin or other allylpolysulfides can produce gastric irritation and mucosal damage (31). Nonspecific liver injury and pulmonary edema has occurred in rats fed large amounts of raw garlic (31). By contrast to allylpolysulfides, monosulfinic derivatives such as DAS at similar dose levels exhibit less toxicity than those produced by a corresponding disulfide derivative such as DADS. Consumption of food or proteins rich in the amino acid, cysteine, can abrogate both pro-oxidant and irritant properties of allylpolysulfides.

Recent studies on the antiproliferative activity of thioallyl derivatives have utilized a number of mono-, di-, and triallylsulfide derivatives. The molecular structures of these derivatives are represented by the major lipid-soluble constituents, diallylsulfide (DAS), diallyldisulfide (DADS), diallyltrisulfide (DATS), and ajoene (*Figure 1*). A characteristic feature of these derivatives is that all have in common the reactive thioallyl moiety. As an example of the intrinsic differences in efficacy of some of these derivatives, in studies using human prostate cancer cells (32), growth inhibition in culture was most effective with compounds that contained a disulfide moiety, as in DADS or an active diallylsulfide moiety as in DAS. With the exception of significant growth inhibition with penta-1,3-dienyl-S-cysteine, marginal to no effect was observed with compounds containing benzyl and phenyl monosulfinic substituent groups (32). Thus, allium compounds that lack an active thioallyl moiety appear to exhibit only marginal antiproliferative activity on cancer cell growth.

The potential for allylpolysulfides to act as pro-oxidants and cross-react immediately with endogenous antioxidants, such as cysteine and reduced glutathione (GSH) is of particular interest (33). In as much as the

$CH_2=CH-CH_2-S(O)CH_2 CH(NH_2) COOH$	**ALLIIN**
$CH_2=CH-CH_2-S(O)SCH_2 CH=CH_2$	**ALLICIN**
$CH_2=CH-CH_2-S(O)CH_2 CH=CH-S-S-CH_2-CH=CH_2$	**AJOENE**
$CH_2=CH-CH_2-S-CH_2-CH=CH_2$	**DIALLYLSULFIDE**
$CH_2=CH-CH_2-S-S-CH_2-CH=CH_2$	**DIALLYLDISULFIDE**
$CH_2=CH-CH_2-S-S-CH_2-CH=CH_2$	**DIALLYLTRISULFIDE**
$CH_2=CH-CH_2-S-S-CH_3$	**ALLYLMETHYLDISULFIDE**
$CH_2=CH-CH_2-S-S-S-CH_3$	**ALLYLMETHYLTRISULFIDE**
$CH_2=CH-CH_2-S-CH_2-CH(NH_2) COOH$	**S-ALLYLCYSTEINE**
$CH_2=CH-CH_2-S-S-CH_2-CH(NH_2)COOH$	**S-ALLYLMERCAPTOCYSTEINE**
$CH_2=CH-CH_2-SH$	**ALLYLMERCAPTAN**
$CH_2=CH-CH_2-S-SH$	**ALLYLHYDRODISULFIDE**

Figure 1. Lipid- and water-soluble allium derivatives

intracellular concentration of GSH is in the range of 1-10 milliMolar (34), interactions of this type significantly alter the biological fate of the original garlic species and affect redox balance within cells. *Figure 2* illustrates possible molecular transformations of several di- and triallylsulfide derivatives with cysteine to form a water-soluble derivative, S-allylmercaptocysteine (SAMC) (9). Other viable compounds formed *in vivo* are ajocysteine and two highly reactive derivatives, allylmercaptan and allylhydrodisulfide (35). On the basis of available experimental evidence (5,12,29), it appears likely that the ability of allylpolysulfides derivatives to be transformed *in situ* into an allylmercaptan may be a prerequisite for garlic's potential anticancer effect. Objective evaluation of allium constituents as a chemopreventive strategy must be viewed in the light of their interactions with endogenous organosulfur components and other cellular metabolites as well as their capacity to affect the redox environment of cells (33).

Naturally-occurring, water-soluble derivatives of garlic have also been investigated for their anticancer potential. Two derivatives that are receiving particular attention are S-allylcysteine (SAC) and the aforementioned SAMC (*Figure 1*). These compounds are more suitable for study in cell culture systems than their lipid-soluble counterparts, DAS and

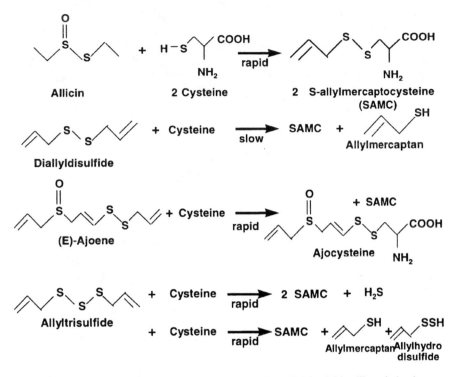

Figure 2. Formation of S-allylmercaptocysteine from lipid-soluble allium derivatives

DADS, since they obviate the need for non-aqueous solvent vehicles.

By contrast to polysulfide compounds, allylmonosulfinyl derivatives, such as DAS and SAC, do not exhibit the same type of reactivity with cysteine and GSH and appear to be more stable since significant levels are measurable in blood following their oral administration (29). It may be this difference in the reactivity of monosulfinic and allylpolysulfinic constituents with endogenous antioxidants that produces some of the differential responses observed when various garlic mixtures or extracts are applied to biological systems.

In addition to reacting with the free sulfhydryl groups of cysteine and GSH, allylpolysulfides can react with free sulfhydryl moieties in proteins, causing disulfide bond formation. Thiolation of proteins or formation of cysteinyl disulfide bonds with allylpolysulfide constituents has the potential of causing either loss or initiation of enzymatic activity as well as modifying structural integrity of membranes (36). In particular, a number of redox-sensitive enzymes and signal transduction proteins are capable of reacting with allylpolysulfide derivatives. Since many of these proteins require sulfhydryl integrity for maintaining enzymatic activity, interactions with di- and triallylsulfides that result in protein thiolation may, in part, be responsible for the antiproliferative effects observed with the use of various garlic constituents. Examples of these interactions will be discussed later in this chapter as possible mechanisms associated with cell cycle control and antipromotional potentials of allium derivatives.

EFFECTS OF ALLIUM DERIVATIVES ON TUMOR PROLIFERATION AND PROMOTION

Malignant cells enter the cell cycle and commit to DNA synthesis in response to activated proto-oncogenes, loss or inactivation of tumor suppressor genes, or alterations in programmed cell death (apoptotic pathway). In addition, a number of cytokines and growth factors as well as contacts between cells and interactions with cell matrix, provide positive and negative stimuli that govern the mechanisms of tumor cell proliferation, promotion, and growth arrest (37). Mutations in signal transduction proteins can effectively circumvent regulation exerted by extracellular stimuli, which, in turn, can result in uncontrolled cell growth. Recent studies suggest that allylsulfide derivatives inhibit growth of transplantable tumors and exert anti-promotional activity against a number of mammalian tumor cell lines (38-42). Growth arrest induced by allium compounds in transformed cells can be categorized as operating under four basic strategies a) antagonizing the mitogenic programming of the malignant cell, such as interfering with ornithine decarboxylase activity, modulating nuclear factor kappa B expression, or altering expression of the ras onco-protein; b) inhibiting activity of specific protein kinases; c) modifying trans-membraneous location of calcium by inhibiting calcium ATPase activity; and d) affecting hormonal responsiveness of transformed cells *(Figure 3)*. Each of these mechanisms will be considered in turn.

Antagonism of the Mitogenic Programming of Malignant Cells

Regulation of polyamine metabolism and ornithine decarboxylase activity

Polyamines (putrescine, spermidine and spermine) participate in DNA, RNA, and protein synthesis and play essential roles in cell growth and differentiation of both normal and neoplastic cells (43). Increased levels of polyamines, particularly putrescine and spermidine, are found in animal and human cancers. Growth factors, such as epidermal growth factor, stimulate

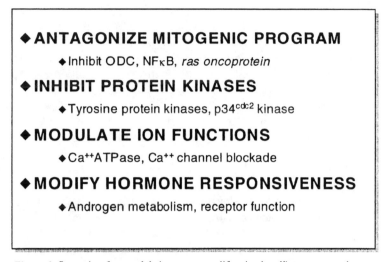

Figure 3. Strategies for modulating cancer proliferation by allium compounds

polyamine formation by increasing ornithine decarboxylase (ODC) activity and stimulate polyamine uptake from the extracellular environment by increasing the activity of a polyamine transporter (44-48). ODC and S-adenosylmethionine decarboxylase are the rate-limiting biosynthetic enzymes in polyamine synthesis (48). ODC catalyzes conversion of ornithine to putrescine and induction of this enzyme accompanies the stimulation of cell proliferation by growth factors, mitogens, and tumor promoters (43,47-50). Thus, as demonstrated in several types of tumor cells, the degree of enhancement of ODC activity correlates well with the growth rate of a neoplasm and its degree of malignancy (44).

Studies by Perchellet et al. (51) demonstrate that garlic oil blunts induction of ODC activity and reverses a prolonged decrease in glutathione peroxidase in mouse epidermal cells treated with phorbol ester. In comparable studies, Hu and Wargovich, (52) using a Wistar rat model for gastrointestinal cancer, showed that pretreatment of animals by gavage or intraperitoneal injection with DAS significantly reduces the N-methyl-N'-nitro-N-nitrosoguanidine induction of ODC. These studies illustrate that cellular injury by a number of mutagenic agents is associated with induction of ornithine decarboxylase and propose that specific allium derivatives may control the activity of this rate-limiting enzyme for polyamine synthesis.

Not all investigations using allium derivatives together with carcinogens, however, have demonstrated inhibitory effects on ODC. Takada et al. (53) evaluated the anticancer potential of organosulfur compounds from garlic and onions on diethylnitrosamine (DEN)-induced neoplasia in livers of male F344 rats. Their results revealed that dipropyl trisulfide from onion oil and allylmercaptan from garlic oil actually exerted an enhancing effect on hepatocarcinogenesis. In this study, allylmercaptan-treated liver tissue without prior DEN initiation caused a sequential increase in ODC activity after 4 hours with a maximum at 16 hours compared to results in livers of control animals. These investigators suggested that the highly reactive allylmercaptan may have promoted hepatocarcinogenesis by increasing cell proliferation in association with increased polyamine biosynthesis.

In a study to determine whether diallylsulfide (DAS) can diminish gamma-ray induced injury to colonic mucosa of laboratory animals, Baer and Wargovich (54) exposed DAS-treated and control female C57BL/6J mice to doses of whole body radiation. They found that, in control mice, the rate of incorporation of tritiated thymidine into DNA and the activity of ornithine decarboxylase were both elevated for more than 14 days but were markedly suppressed in DAS-treated animals. Analysis of the extent of nuclear aberrations revealed that pretreatment with DAS significantly reduced cellular damage in a dose related manner. However, in subsequent experiments, when animals were administered difluoromethylornithine, an ornithine decarboxylase inhibitor, prior to or following radiation treatment, the ability of DAS to decrease radiation-induced colonic nuclear damage was abolished. This observation suggests that DAS may protect against radiation-induced colonic injury via a polyamine-dependent pathway.

The aforementioned studies pertain to events that occur during early phases of cell insult and suggest that specific allium constituents and polyamines may interact as protective factors that stimulate DNA repair enzymes, stabilize DNA, and counteract oxidative stress, processes essential to cell survival. Cells exposed to a variety of allium derivatives demonstrate a marked increase in the intracellular ratio of GSH to GSSG, a major endogenous antioxidant (32,51,55). In addition, specific allium derivatives have been shown to affect sulfhydryl/disulfide exchange reactions that may involve both oxidized and reduced glutathione (56,57). Concomitantly, because of their anionic properties, polyamines can localize to and stabilize oxidant-prone membrane phospholipids and nucleic acids whereas their ability to bind with redox active cations efficiently prevents site specific generation of reactive oxygen species (58).

Although effects of allium derivatives on ODC activity and formation of polyamines in the early phases of carcinogenesis have been studied, little information is available about the later stages of carcinogenesis or about processes occurring in established tumor cells. In *in vitro* studies by Pinto et al. (32) of allium constituents on prostate cancer cell growth, concentrations of polyamines were measured at 3 and 5 days following a single treatment with SAMC. At 3 days, both putrescine and spermine concentrations were significantly decreased while spermidine concentration was significantly elevated. At 5 days post-treatment with a single dose of SAMC, polyamine levels returned to those of the controls. These and other findings (52-54) of decreased cell growth and altered polyamine levels suggest that SAMC may impede ODC, and perhaps S-adenosylmethionine decarboxylase, activity and thus antagonize the mitogenic program of transformed cells ultimately blocking synthesis of polyamines that are essential for cancer cell growth and proliferation (48).   A potential mechanism that requires further investigation is whether specific allylsulfides may modulate ODC, either by enhancing formation of intracellular GSH, which is known to inhibit ODC induction, or by reacting directly with ODC at its nucleophilic thiol moiety of cysteine 360, a target of ODC enzymic control by sulfhydryl binding reagents (57).

Modulation of nuclear factor kappa B (NFκB) expression

Flow cytometric analyses of DNA indicate that allium derivatives can prevent some human tumor cell lines from progressing through G_1/S phase while others are blocked in G_2/M.   In particular, erythroleukemic (HEL) (59), promyleoleukemic (HL60) (60) and colon carcinoma (HCT15, SW480, and HT29) cells (61,62) exposed to specific allium compounds exhibit marked decreases in the number of cells in G1 phase with a corresponding accumulation in G2/M phase. By contrast, human umbilical vein endothelial cells (HUVEC) and smooth-muscle cells appear to arrest in G1 (42).

The signaling cascade mechanisms associated with cell proliferation may involve reactive oxygen or nitrogen species as second messengers (63). Accordingly, the expression of transcription factors such as NFκB and AP-1, which contain easily oxidizable sulfhydryl groups, is increased during oxidative stress and thus is closely associated with malignancy and apoptosis (64). Other transcription and cell cycle regulators that undergo redox cycling or exhibit sulfhydryl moieties sensitive to oxidation are c-Fos/Jun complex, Ref-1, p53, and bcl-2 (65).   Redox regulation of transcriptional activators occurs through highly conserved cysteine residues in the DNA binding domains of these proteins (66).

Nuclear factor kappa B (NFκB) is a well characterized member of the Rel oncogene family that regulates genes encoding for proteins associated with immune function, inflammation, and cell proliferation (67). In addition, NFκB plays a crucial role in modulating gene expression during growth and development. Activation of this transcription factor can be attained by a variety of stimuli that include cytokines, mitogens, physical stresses such as ionizing radiation and oxidants, and chemical agents such as phorbol 12-myristate 13-acetate and okadaic acid, a phosphatase inhibitor. The predominant cytosolic form of NFκB exists as an inactive protein trimer consisting of p65, p50, and IκBα subunits. Oxidative stress activates NFκB by causing phosphorylation and dissociation of the inhibitory IκB subunit protein followed by a rapid translocation of the p50/p65 heterodimer to its nuclear binding domain. Once in the nucleus, the p50/p65 dimer activates transcription of a cadre of genes that includes those for cytokines, growth factors, acute-phase proteins, transcription factors, and cell cycle regulators (68). By contrast to the activating effects of oxidants, attenuation of NFκB induction can be achieved by antioxidants such as N-acetylcysteine, 2-mercaptoethanol, α-tocopherol, and chelators of transition metals (69). These relationships suggested to Geng et al. (70) that certain allylsulfide derivatives might be capable of blocking signal transduction pathways leading to expression of nuclear transcription factors. Accordingly, in Jurkat T (human lymphoma) cells subjected to oxidative stress by TNF-α and hydrogen peroxide, treatment of these cells with SAC did in fact block activation of NFκB as demonstrated by diminished antibody binding to the p50/p65 proteins. In similar fashion, Ide and Lau (71) demonstrated that pretreatment of endothelial cells with SAC inhibits lipid peroxide-induced activation of NFκB.

In view of the finding that oxidative stress activates NFκB and that activation of NFκB induces apoptosis in some cells (72), Dirsch et al. (60) sought to demonstrate that ajoene ((E,Z)-4,5,9-trithiadodeca-1,6,11-triene-9-oxide) was able to induce apoptosis in human promyelocytic leukemic cells (HL-60) by stimulating production of reactive oxygen species and activating nuclear translocation of NFκB. Conversely, pretreatment of leukemic cells with N-acetylcysteine blocked the ajoene-induced production of reactive oxygen species and prevented NFκB activation. Of particular interest was the finding that ajoene did not induce apoptosis in quiescent or proliferating mononuclear cells from healthy donors.

The contrasting effects observed with SAC and ajoene on NFκB activation exemplifies the diverse reactivity of monosulfinic and allylpolysulfinic derivatives and underscores the differential responses that are observed when various allium mixtures are applied to biological systems. Although NFκB is activated when cells are exposure to oxidative stress, excessive oxidation can affect attachment of the p50/p65 heterodimer to its DNA binding domain. Oxidation of NFκB subunits *in vitro* abolishes DNA-binding activity, whereas administration of reducing agents restores its binding domain (73).

The expression of these factors is sensitive to intracellular levels of reduced glutathione. More information is needed to define the dietary factors that impact on redox-sensitive effector systems in cells which, in turn, regulate cell growth, cell death, and transformation.

Alteration in ras oncoprotein expression

The *ras* family of proto-oncogenes plays a pivotal role in signal transduction and several members are mutated in about a third of all human cancers. Ras has four major isoforms, N-, H-, Ka- and Kb-, with each differing mainly in the post-translationally modified carboxy-terminus by the addition of a farnesyl and a palmitoyl moiety required before the ras protein can anchor to the plasma membrane. The distribution of the isoforms and the attachment of lipid moieties differ among various cancers which suggests that knowledge of the carboxy-terminus of ras may be of fundamental importance in understanding the carcinogenic process (74).

Studies by Singh et al. (75) have shown that DADS suppresses the growth of H-*ras* oncogene transformed tumors in nude mice by blunting the association of the p21^{H-ras} protein with the plasma membrane compartment. Measurements of the pool sizes of both the membrane bound p21^{H-ras} and the cytosolic p21^{H-ras} in tumors from DADS- and saline-treated mice revealed that DADS-treated mice have markedly higher cytosolic levels than controls whereas the converse was true in the saline-treated group. These studies suggested that the decreased association of p21^{H-ras} within tumor membranes of DADS-treated mice may be due to inhibition of hepatic 3-hydroxy-3-methylglutaryl coenzyme A (HMG-CoA) reductase, the rate limiting enzyme in the biosynthesis of isoprenoids, including farnesyl pyrophosphate within the cholesterol pathway (76).

The effect of allium constituents on cholesterol biosynthesis illustrates several important considerations. HMG-CoA reductase is a microsomal enzyme that catalyzes the rate-limiting step in the formation of farnesyl/isoprenoid units (77,78), the primary factor necessary to adjoin ras oncoproteins to membranes. Studies have demonstrated that HMG-CoA reductase is easily oxidized by compounds containing disulfide moieties which crosslink the enzyme into a totally inactive homodimer (79,80).

The biochemical effects of allium derivatives on expression and activation of the ras oncoprotein may also involve inhibition of farnesyl protein transferase, the enzyme necessary for post-translational modification (prenylation) of a cysteine residue located in the carboxyl-terminal tetrapeptide of the ras oncoprotein. As mentioned earlier, farnesylation is essential for membrane association and cell transforming activities of ras. Studies by Lee et al. (81) demonstrated that allicin, methyl allyl thiosulfinate, and allyl methyl thiosulfinate are more potent inhibitors of geranylgeranyl protein transferase (GGPT) than of the farnesyl protein transferase. In particular, methyl allyl thiosulfinate appears to be a competitive inhibitor of GGPP exhibiting a Ki of 15 microMolar.

Inhibition of prenylating enzymes has been demonstrated to blunt ras-dependent cell transformation and thus represents a potential therapeutic strategy for the treatment of certain human cancers. In light of the present studies on garlic, allylthiosulfinates are exceptionally promising dietary components whose structures might aid in design of novel antitumor agents.

Inhibition of Protein Kinases

A variety of protein kinases regulate cellular signaling events by catalyzing the transfer of the terminal phosphate moiety from ATP to specific tyrosine, serine, or threonine residues within target proteins (82). Isoforms of protein kinase C are activated at the inner surface of plasma membranes by endogenous cell signal messengers such as calcium and diacylglycerol, a product of receptor-mediated phosphatidylinositol hydrolysis as well as by certain tumor promoters such as phorbol 12-myristate. Thus, alterations in phospholipid metabolism are thought to be among the primary events involved in tumor promotion.

Studies by Nishino et al. (38) showed that an ethanolic extract from garlic inhibits, in a dose related manner, phorbol ester-induced stimulation of ^{32}Pi incorporation into phospholipids of HeLa Cells. These lipid and/or protein phosphorylation reactions may be relevant to studies involving protein kinases that interact with a variety of cytokine and transcription factors. In similar fashion, Lee et al. (42), using vascular smooth muscle and umbilical endothelial cells demonstrated that SAMC changes the extent of phosphorylation as well as the pattern of tyrosine phosphorylation in several proteins. Four proteins of 51.8, 45, 41 and 20 kDa displayed an increased level of tyrosine phosphorylation whereas five proteins of 58, 54, 47.8, 37, and 35 kDa exhibited a marked decrease in phosphorylation. Using immunoblotting techniques, these investigators identified three of the proteins from SAMC-treated smooth muscle cells that exhibited increased phosphotyrosine residues, namely, GTP-activating protein, tyrosine phosphatase-1B, and p34^{cdc2} . A change in the phosphorylated status of these proteins is thought to attenuate cell signaling mediated through the mitogen activated protein kinase (MAP kinase) pathway. The increased phosphorylation of these proteins correlates with the antiproliferative activity of allium constituents on normal smooth-muscle and endothelial cells (42). For example, in its phosphorylated state, p34^{cdc2} remains tethered to cyclin B, a mitotic phase protein kinase, keeping the complex inactive and thus maintaining cellular quiescence (83).

Important structural features of many of the protein kinases are their site-specific cysteine-rich regions in their catalytic and regulatory domains that are sensitive to oxidation (84). These cysteine regions may be sensitive to garlic-derived compounds through either direct interaction of the sulfhydryl moieties with specific allylpolysulfinic derivatives or indirect modification through the ability of certain allium derivatives to enhance endogenous production of glutathione.

Additional effects of allium derivatives on receptor complexes and the signal transduction system were demonstrated by Apitz-Castro et al. (85). Ajoene was observed to reversibly inhibit endogenous platelet aggregation *in vitro* as well as that induced by recognized agonists. These effects of ajoene were preceded by inhibition of several intra- and extracellular events, namely, agonist-induced exposure of fibrinogen receptors, activation of protein kinase C, and increase in cytoplasmic free calcium usually induced by receptor-dependent agonists such as collagen, ADP, platelet activating factor, and, low-dose thrombin.   In its entirety, these studies further illustrate and support the involvement of allium derivatives in modifying signal proteins in early events of cell proliferation.

Modulate Ion Functions by Inhibiting Calcium ATPase and/or Calcium Channels

Calcium in the presence of calmodulin participates in phosphorylation reactions of signal proteins and stimulates the activity of ODC (86). Changes in the thiol-sulfhydryl exchange mechanism are expected to modulate calcium ionic channel function by interfering with activity of Ca^{+2}ATPase. Such changes may also antagonize the mitogenic program of cancer cells by interfering with ODC and S-adenosylmethionine decarboxylase activities, ultimately blocking synthesis of polyamines that are essential for cell growth and differentiation.

Perturbations in the levels of intracellular calcium are associated with cell damage and fluctuations of thiol-disulfide metabolism associated with formation of reduced and oxidized glutathione correlates with alterations in cytosolic calcium homeostasis (87,88). A unifying theme in regulating cell function and controlling the cell cycle is to modulate protein kinases and calcium metabolism (89). Studies in human colon tumor (HCT-15) and skin (SK MEL-2) cells demonstrate that DADS induces a dose dependent rise in intracellular free calcium levels and that impairment of the extrusion mechanism of calcium, mediated through inactivation of calcium-dependent ATPases, may be involved (62). Similarly, in cultured lung carcinoma cells, Sakamoto et al. (90) showed that DATS administration caused a marked and progressive increase in intracellular calcium during the first four hours following treatment. When cells were re-cultured in fresh media in the absence of DATS, intracellular calcium levels returned to normal.

Corroboration of allium-induced impairment of intracellular calcium extrusion can be found in studies of vascular smooth muscle cells and cardiac tissue. Siegel et al. (91) found that an aqueous garlic extract and ajoene causes vasodilatation and hyperpolarization within vascular tissue because of closure of calcium channels. At the concentration of allium components used in the study, the hyperpolarizing and vasodilating influences were achieved at concentrations of ajoene in the extracellular space attainable by consumption of a single garlic clove. In studies to elucidate a possible role for calcium in the cardiotropic effects of garlic extract, Martin et al. (92) found that the negative inotropic effect of a garlic dialysate was related to the availability of the extracellular calcium concentration and that calcium channel blockers, such as nifedipine, verapamil, and diltiazem, induce a concentration-dependent synergism of the log concentration-effect of garlic dialysate on left atria. Changes in ion flux from closing calcium channels can trigger signal transduction mechanisms necessary for vasodilatory responses.

One of the more novel effects of allium compounds on platelet aggregation and calcium modulation that may also have relevance to cancer antiproliferation is the ability of garlic extracts and DAS to increase production of nitric oxide. Studies by Das et al. (93) showed that both water and ethanolic extracts of garlic are potent inhibitors of epinephrine- and ADP-stimulated platelet aggregation and that upregulation of the calcium-calmodulin dependent nitric oxide synthase may be responsible.

The role of nitric oxide as a signal transducer in vascular smooth muscle and other cell types is well established (94). For example, nitric oxide activates guanylate cyclase, and cyclic GMP is a second messenger of vascular smooth muscle relaxation. At high levels of production by macrophages, nitric oxide is quite toxic to most normal as well as tumor cells. It is generally accepted that the toxic species, peroxynitrite, is generated by the interaction of nitric oxide with molecular oxygen and inhibits a number important cellular processes including DNA formation and repair, mitochondrial respiration, and glycolysis (95). Although allium derivatives are capable of enhancing calcium-dependent nitric oxide synthase activity in platelets, treatment of lymph node-derived human prostate carcinoma (LNCaP) cells with SAC or SAMC, at concentrations that would have enhanced levels of intracellular calcium, did not elicit the same type of response (96).

Information from these studies suggests that allium constituents may affect cancer cells by interacting with factors that control cell cycle progression and affect signal transduction pathways. The possible targets may include among others alterations in synthesis and utilization of polyamines and glutathione, redox regulation of catalytic and regulatory domains of signal proteins, and changes in intracellular calcium homeostasis. Taken together, constituents from garlic are known to exert antiproliferative activity on normal and malignant cells and may block progression of tumor cells to more aggressive phenotypes.

Modification of Hormone Responsiveness and Effect on Steroid Hormone Metabolism

Through their inhibitory effect on HMG-CoA reductase activity and subsequent reduction of cholesterol biosynthesis, several allium derivatives also regulate steroid biosynthesis (97-100). Consistent findings from studies examining inhibition of chemical carcinogenesis by garlic-derived compounds indicate that covalent attachment of xenobiotic compounds to DNA is markedly depressed. The likely mechanism is selective suppression and/or induction of cytochrome P450 mixed function oxidases involved in phase I drug metabolism as well as activation of conjugating enzymes associated with phase II drug metabolism (101-103). Diallylsulfide (DAS) suppresses oxidative demethylation by competitively inhibiting cytochrome P450 2E1, an inducible isoenzyme that activates a number of known carcinogens, such as nitrosamines, hydrazines, and carbon tetrachloride (104). The effect of DAS on P450 enzymes appears to be specific rather than general in that the activities of other demethylating and hydoxylating cytochromes, namely P450 2B1, 1A1 and 1A2, are elevated by allium components (105).

In a fashion similar to that of environmental carcinogens, active estrogen and androgen metabolites enhance proliferation of breast and prostate cancers (106,107). Since the metabolism of these steroid hormones can occur through the same cytochrome P450 enzymes induced by allylsulfide derivatives (108-111), garlic consumption has the potential to alter the rates of metabolism of estrogen and testosterone (112,113). The balance of steroid hormone metabolites generated through the action of these P450 enzymes may be a critical mechanism whereby dietary constituents exert specific action in modulating the development of hormone-sensitive cancers(114-116).

Initial findings from our laboratory regarding allium constituents from garlic show antiproliferative effects on androgen-sensitive human prostate cancer cells. In preliminary studies (117), growth inhibition by the allium derivative, SAMC, was accompanied by a reduction in secretion of PSA by LNCaP cells. The reduction in PSA secretion induced by SAMC was even greater than the reduction in cell growth.

By contrast to its effect on inhibiting PSA secretion, SAMC actually increased activity of a newly identified marker for prostate cancer progression called prostate-specific membrane antigen (PSMA). We have identified PSMA as a unique transmembraneous folate hydrolase with exopeptidase activity that cleaves sequentially γ-glutamyl linkages from polygammaglutamated folates with accumulation of folate (118). Unlike the reduction in PSA expression in LNCaP that is associated with testosterone deprivation, PSM-folate hydrolase expression increases under these conditions. It is important to note that the pattern observed here of decreased PSA secretion and increased PSMA expression is consistent with the known effects of androgen deprivation (119). These results are also compatible with an alteration in the cell's ability to utilize testosterone.

Having demonstrated that SAMC can inhibit proliferation of LNCaP cells and may induce cells to enhance catabolism of testosterone, we then determined whether testosterone supplementation to growth media can reverse the antiproliferative effect of SAMC. Compared to cells treated with SAMC (200 uM) in the absence of testosterone, SAMC treated-LNCaP cells grown in media supplemented with 100 nM testosterone show significant increase in cell growth at day 3 (p < 0.01). However, for reasons yet unknown, growth declines around day 6 to levels not significantly different from cells treated with SAMC alone (*Figure 4*).

Our preliminary observations (113) indicate that testosterone does not enhance growth of SAMC-treated LNCaP cells to levels comparable to that of saline-treated cells. Although these experiments require further extension and confirmation, they suggest the possibility that the early inhibition of cell growth by SAMC may be reversed by testosterone, suggesting a hormonal mechanism, but that later inhibition of cell growth may not be due to a hormonal mechanism but to other effects of SAMC, perhaps on signal transduction or other events.

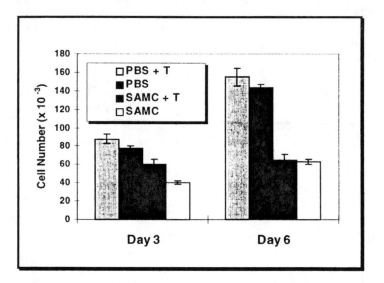

Figure 4. Effects of testosterone supplementation on growth of SAMC- and Saline-treated LNCaP cells.

Our findings demonstrate that SAMC exhibits differential effects on prostate specific biomarkers, namely reducing PSA secretion and enhancing PSM activity, and suggest the hypothesis that SAMC may inhibit the initial progression of androgen-responsive prostate cancer cells by altering testosterone metabolism.

CONCLUSION

Carcinogenesis is recognized as proceeding through a series of discrete phases termed initiation, promotion, conversion and progression that involve complex interactions between genetic and epigenetic factors. Advances in our knowledge of this process have led to the development of promising new approaches to prevention of cancer and have repeatedly confirmed the adage of the Statesman, Benjamin Franklin, that *"an ounce of prevention is worth a pound of cure" (Poor Richard's Almanack, 1732).* *Figure 5* outlines proposed mechanisms of cancer chemoprevention and control provided by allium derivatives.

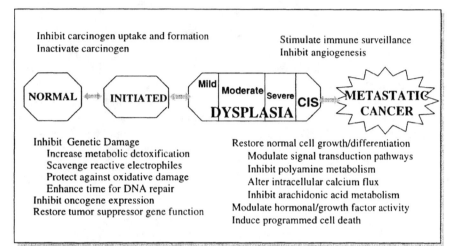

Figure 5. Proposed mechanisms of cancer chemoprevention by allium compounds.

At least 20 garlic-derived constituents have demonstrated chemopreventive and therapeutic activities. As inhibitors of carcinogenesis, compounds derived from garlic can be grouped into one or more of three possible functional categories (15):

a) compounds that impede the generation of a carcinogen from its precursor;

b) compounds that prevent a carcinogen from reacting with vulnerable cellular targets; and

c) compounds that delay or reverse expression of malignancy or demonstrate antiproliferative activity on tumor cells by modifying signal transduction mechanisms.

A number of the basic antiproliferative mechanisms of action of garlic and garlic-derived components have been described. Further research may be necessary to establish the most relevant of these mechanisms and to pave the way for human intervention trials with garlic derivatives involving not only cancer prevention but also control. One might argue that the use of cytotoxic drugs alone in the treatment of cancer has the goal of cell cycle retaliation while use of garlic or other diet-derived phytochemical that may induce apoptosis, change mitogenic programming, or maintain neoplastic cells in a quiescent phase has the goal of cell cycle reorganization.

ACKNOWLEDGMENTS

This work was supported in part by the Clinical Nutrition Research Unit grant (CA-29502) from the National Institutes of Health. Partial funding was also provided by grants from Wakunaga of America Co., Ltd., the Frank J. Scallon Medical Research Foundation, the Sunny and Abe Rosenberg Foundation, the Rosenfeld Heart Foundation, The Susan and Ronald Lynch Foundation and the NOW Company. Work on prostate cancer was performed in coordination with the Nutrition Research Laboratory and the George M. O'Brien Urology Research Center, Memorial Sloan-Kettering Cancer Center.

REFERENCES

1. Key TJA, Silcocks PB, Davey GK, Appleby PN, Bishop DT. A case-control study of diet and prostate cancer. Brit J Cancer 1997; 76: 678-687.
2. Dorant E, van den Brandt PA, Goldbohm RA, Hermus RJJ, Sturmans F. Garlic and its significance for the prevention of cancer in humans. A critical view. Br J Cancer 1993; 67: 424-429.
3. Milner JA. Garlic: Its anticarcinogenic and antitumorigenic properties. Nutr Rev 1996; 54: S82-S86.
4. Sumiyoshi H, Wargovich MJ. Garlic (Allium sativum): A review of its relationship to cancer. Asia Pacific J Pharmacol 1989; 4:133-140.
5. Block E. The chemistry of garlic and onions Sci. Amer 1985; 252: 114-119.
6. Pinto JT, Rivlin RS. Garlic and Other Allium Vegetables in Cancer Prevention. In "*Nutritional Oncology*" David Heber, George L. Blackburn, VLW Go, eds, New York, NY: Academic Press, 1999.
7. Agarwal KC. Therapeutic actions of garlic constituents. Med Res Rev 1996; 16: 111-124.
8. Yeh YY. Garlic phytochemicals in disease prevention and health promotion: An overview. New Drug Clin 1996; 45: 441-450.
9. Han J, Lawson L, Han G. A spectrophotometric method for quantitative determination of allicin and total garlic thiosulfinates. Anal Biochem 1995; 225: 157-160.
10. Weinberg DS, Manier ML, Richardson MD, Haibach FG. Identification and quantification of anticarcinogens in garlic extract and licorice root extract powder. J High Resolution Chromatography 1992; 15: 641-654.
11. Ide N, Lau BHS, Ryu K, Matsuura H, Itakura Y. Antioxidant effects of fructosyl arginine, a maillard reaction product in aged garlic extract. J Nutr Biochem 1999; 10: 372-376.
12. Yu TH, Wu CM, Liou YC. Volatile compounds from garlic. J Agric Food Chem 1989; 27: 725-730.

13. Yamasaki T, Teel RW, Lau BHS. Effect of allixin, aphytoalexin produced by garlic, on mutagenesis, DNA-binding and metabolism of aflatoxin B1. Cancer Lett 1991 59: 89-94.

14. Itakura Y, Ichikawa M, Mori Y, Okino R, Morita T How to distinguish garlic from the other allium vegetables? Recent Advances on the Nutritional Benefits Accompanying the Use of Garlic as a Supplement. Sponsored by The University of Pennsylvania and the National Cancer Institute. November 15-17, New Port Beach, CA, 1998.

15. Wattenberg LW. Chemoprevention of cancer. Cancer Res 1985; 45: 1-8.

16. Sparnins VL, Barany G, Wattenberg LW. Effects of organosulfur compounds from garlic and onion on benzo[a]pyrene-induced neoplasia and glutathione S-transferase activity in the mouse. Carcinogenesis 1988; 9:131-134.

17. Sparnins VL, Mott AW, Barany G, Wattenberg LE. Effects of allyl methyl trisulfide on glutathione S-transferase activity and BP-induced neoplasia in the mouse. Nutr Cancer 1986; 8: 211-215.

18. Hayes MA, Rushmore TH, Goldberg MT. Inhibition of hepatocarcinogenic responses to 1,2-dimethylhydrazine to diallyl sulfide, a component of garlic oil. Carcinogenesis 1987; 8:1155-1157.

19. Hatono S, Jimenez A, Wargovich MJ. Chemopreventive effect of S-allylcysteine and its relationship to the detoxification of enzyme glutathione S transferase. Carcinogenesis 1996; 17: 1041-1044.

20. Dwivedi C, Rohlfs S, Jarvis D, Engineer FN. Chemoprevention of chemically induced skin tumor development by diallyl sulfide and diallyl disulfide. Pharmaceutical Res 1992; 9: 1668-1670.

21. Sigounas G, Hooker JL, Li W, Anagnostou A, Steiner M. S-allylmercaptocysteine inhibits cell proliferation and reduces the viability of erythroleukemia, breast, and prostate cancer cell lines. Nutr Cancer 1997; 27: 186-191.

22. Sumiyoshi H, Wargovich MJ. Chemoprevention of 1,2-dimethylhydrazine-induced colon cancer in mice by naturally occurring organosulfur compounds. Cancer Res 1990; 50: 5084-5087.

23. Cheng JY, Meng CL, Tzeng CC, Lin JC. Optimal dose of garlic to inhibit dimethylhydrazine-induced colon cancer. World J Surg 1995; 19: 621-625.

24. Wattenberg LW, Sparnins VL, Barany G. Inhibition of N-nitrosodiethylamine carcinogenesis in mice by naturally occurring organosulfur compounds and monoterpenes. Cancer Res 1989; 49:2689-2692.

25. Lin X-Y, Liu J-Z, Milner JA. Dietary garlic suppresses DNA adducts caused by N-nitroso compounds. Carcinogenesis 1994; 15: 349-352.

26. Cavallito CJ, Buck JS, Suter CM. Allicin, the antibacterial principle of allium sativum. II. Determination of the chemical structure. J Am Chem Soc 1944; 66: 1952-1954.

27. Wills ED. Enzyme inhibition by allicin, the active principle of garlic. Biochem J 1956; 63: 514-520.

28. Stoll A, Seebeck E. Chemical Investigations of alliin, the specific principle of garlic. Adv Enzymol 1951; 11: 377-400.

29. Freeman F, Kodera Y. Garlic chemistry: Stability of S-(2-propenyl) 2-propene-1-sulfinothioate (allicin) in blood, solvents, and simulated physiological fluids. J Agric Food Chem 1995; 43: 2332-2338.

30. Koch HP, Lawson LD, Reuter HD, Hahn G, Siegers C-P. The Science and Therapeutic Application of Allium Sativum L. and Related Species. Baltimore, MD: Williams & Wilkins, 1996. pp 59-65.

31. Nakagawa S, Masamoto K, Sumiyoshi H, Kunihiro K, Fuwa T. Effect of raw garlic juice and aged garlic extract on growth of young rats and their organs after peroral administration. J Toxicol Sci 1980; 5: 91-112.

32. Pinto JT, Qiao CH, Xing J, Rivlin RS, Protomastro ML, Weissler ML, Tao Y, Thaler H, Heston WDW. Effects of garlic thioallyl derivatives on growth, glutathione concentration, and polyamine formation of human prostate carcinoma cells in culture. Am J Clin Nutr 1997; 66: 398-405.

33. Weisberger AS, Pensky J. Tumor inhibition by a sulfhydryl-blocking agent related to an active principle of garlic (Allium sativum). Cancer Res 1958; 18: 1301-1308.

34. Meister A, Anderson ME. Glutathione. Annu Rev Biochem 1983; 52: 711-760.

35. Pierson S. Garlic product organosulfur chemistry, pharmacology and toxicology: an overview for pharmacists. Pharm/alert Continuing Education 1994; 2: 1-9.

36. Harington JS. The sulfhydryl group and carcinogenesis. Adv Cancer Res. 1967; 10:247-309.

37. Roussel MF. Key effectors of signal transduction and G1 progression. Adv Cancer Res 1998; 74:1-25.

38. Nishino H, Iwashima A, Itakura Y, Matsuura H, Fuwa, T. Antitumor-promoting activity of garlic extracts. Oncology 1989; 46: 277-280.

39. Sundaram SG, Milner JA. Diallyl disulfide suppresses the growth of human colon tumor cell xenografts in athymic nude mice. J Nutr 1996; 126: 1355-1361.

40. Takeyama H, Hoon DSB, Saxton RE, Morton DL, Irie RF. Growth inhibition and modulation of cell markers of melanoma by S-allyl cysteine. Oncology 1993; 50: 63-69.

41. Welch C, Wuarin L, Sidell N. Antiproliferative effect of the garlic compound S-allyl cysteine on human neuroblastoma cells in vitro. Cancer Lett 1992; 63: 211-219.

42. Lee ES, Steiner M, Lin R. Thioallyl compounds: Potent inhibitors of cell proliferation. Biochim Biophys Acta 1994; 1221: 73-77.

43. Janne J, Poso H, Raina A. Polyamines in rapid growth and cancer. Biochim Biophys Acta 1978; 473:241-293.

44. Heby O. Role of polyamines in control of cell proliferation and differentiation. Differentiation 1981; 19:1-20.

45. Pohjanpelto P. Putrescine transport is greatly increased in human fibroblasts initiated to proliferate. J Cell Biol 1976; 68: 512-520.

46. O'Brien TG. The induction of ornithine decarboxylase as an early, possibly obligatory, event in mouse skin carcinogenesis. Cancer Res 1976; 36: 2644-2653.

47. DiPasquale A, White D, McGuire, JR. Epidermal growth factor stimulates putrescine transport and ornithine decarboxylase activity in cultivated human fibroblasts. Exp Cell Res 1978; 116: 317-323.

48. Pegg AE. Recent advances in the biochemistry of polyamines in eukaryotes. Biochem J 1986; 234:249-262.

49. Womble JR, Russell DH. Catecholamine-stimulated B2 receptors coupled to ornithine decarboxylase induction and to cellular hypertrophy and proliferation. Adv Polyamine Res 1983; 4: 549-562.

50. Russell DH. Ornithine decarboxylase as a biological and pharmacological tool. Pharmacology 1980; 20:117-129.

51. Perchellet JP, Perchellet EM, Abney NL, Zirnstein JA, Belman S. Effects of garlic and onion oils on glutathione peroxidase activity, the ratio of reduced and oxidized glutathione and ornithine decarboxylase induction in isolated mouse epidermal cells treated with tumor promoters. Cancer Biochem Biophys 1986; 8: 299-312.

52. Hu PJ, Wargovich MJ. Effect of diallyl sulfide on MNNG-induced nuclear aberrations and ornithine decarboxylase activity in the glandular stomach mucosa of the Wistar rat. Cancer Lett 1989; 47:153-8.

53. Takada N, Kitano M, Chen T, Yano Y, Otani S, Fukushima S Enhancing effects of organosulfur compounds from garlic and onions on hepatocarcinogenesis in rats: association with increased cell proliferation and elevated ornithine decarboxylase activity. Jpn J Cancer Res 1994; 85:1067-72.

54. Baer AR, Wargovich MJ. Role of ornithine decarboxylase in diallyl sulfide inhibition of colonic radiation injury in the mouse. Cancer Res 1989; 49:5073-5076.

55. Gudi VA, Singh SV. Effect of diallyl sulfide, a naturally occurring anti-carcinogen, on glutathione-dependent detoxification enzymes of female CD-1 mouse tissues. Biochem Pharmac 1991; 42:1261-1265.

56. Scharfenberg K, Ryll T, Wagner R, Wagner KG. Injuries to cultivated BJA-B cells by ajoene, a garlic-derived natural compound: cell viability, glutathione metabolism, and pools of acidic amino acids. J Cell Physiol 1994; 158:55-60.

57. Coleman CS, Stanley BA, Pegg AE. Effect of mutations at active site residues on the activity of ornithine decarboxylase and its inhibition by active site-directed irreversible inhibitors. J Biol Chem 1993; 268: 24572-24579.

58. Tadolini B. Polyamine inhibition of lipoperoxidation. Biochem J 1988; 249: 33-36.

59. Sigounas G, Hooker JL, Li W, Anagnostou A, Steiner M. S-Allylmercaptocysteine, a stable thioallyl compound, induces apoptosis in erythroleukemia cell lines. Nutr Cancer 1997; 28:153-159.

60. Dirsch VM, Gerbes AL, Vollmar AM. Ajoene, a compound of garlic, induces apoptosis in human promyeloleukemic cells, accompanied by generation of reactive oxygen species and activation of nuclear factor κB. Molec Pharmacol 1998; 53: 402-407.

61. Knowles LM, Milner JA. Garlic constituents alter cell cycle progression and proliferation. FASEB J 1997; 11:A422.

62 Sundaram SG, Milner JA. Diallyl disulfide inhibits the proliferation of human tumor cells in culture. Biochim Biophys Acta 1996; 1315: 15-20.

63. Hockenberry DM, Oltvai AN, Yin XN, Milliman CL, Korsmeyer SJ. Bcl-2 functions in an antioxidant pathway to prevent apoptosis. Cell 1993; 75: 241-251.

64. Meyer M, Schreck R, Baeuerle PA. H_2O_2 and antioxidants have opposite effects on activation of NF-κB and AP-1 in intact cells: AP-1 as secondary antioxidant responsive factor. EMBO J 1993; 12:2005-2015.

65. Powis G, Gashaska JR, Baker A. "Redox signaling and the control of cell growth and death." In *Antioxidants in disease mechanisms and therapy*. Helmut Sies, Volume Editor, Advances in Pharmacology, New York, NY: Academic Press 1997; 38:329-359.

66. Sun Y, Oberley LW. Redox regulation of transcriptional activators. Free Radical Biol Med 1996 21:335-348.

67. Sen CK, Packer L. Antioxidant and redox regulation of gene transcription. FASEB J 1996; 10: 709-720.

68. Siebenlist U, Franzoso G, Brown K. Structure, regulation and function of NFκB. Annu Rev Cell Biol 1994; 10: 405-455.

69. Schenk H, Klein M, Erdbrugger W, Droge W, Schulze-Osthoff K. Distinct effects of thioredoxin and antioxidants on the activation of transcription factors NF-kappa B and AP-1. Proc Natl Acad Sci. USA. 1994; 91:1672-1676.

70. Geng Z, Rong Y, Lau BHS. S allyl cysteine inhibits activation of nuclear factor kappa B in human T cells. Free Radical Biology Med 1997; 23: 345-350.

71. Ide N, Lau BHS. Garlic compounds minimize intracellular oxidative stress and inhibit NFκB action.. Abstract presented at the Recent Advances on the Nutritional Benefits Accompanying the Use of Garlic as a Supplement. Sponsored by The University of Pennsylvania and the National Cancer Institute. November 15-17. Newport Beach, CA. 1998.

72. Grimm S, Bauer, MKA, Baeuerle PA, Schulze-Osthoff K. Bcl-2 down regulates the activity of transcription factor NF-kappa B induced upon apoptosis. J Cell Biol 1996; 134: 13-23.

73. Matthews JR, Wakasugi N, Virelizier JL, Yodoi J, Hay RT. Thioredoxin regulates the DNA binding activity of NF-kappa B by reduction of a disulphide bond involving cysteine-62. Nucleic Acids Res 1992; 20: 3821-3830 .

74. Campbell SL, Khosravi-Far R, Rossman KL, Clark GJ, Der CJ. Increasing complexity of Ras signaling. Oncogene 1998; 17:1395-1413.
75. Singh SV, Mohan RR, Agarwal R, Benson PJ, Hu X, Rudy MA, Xia H, Katoh A, Srivastava SD, Mukhtar H, Gupta V, Zaren HA. Novel anti-carcinogenic activity of an organosulfide from garlic: Inhibition of H-*ras* oncogene transformed tumor growth in vivo by diallyl disulfide is associated with inhibition of p21^{H-ras} processing. Biochem Biophys Res Commun 1996; 225: 660-665.
76. Goldstein JL, Brown MS. Regulation of the mevalonate pathway. Nature 1990; 343:425-430.
77. Schaber MD, O'Hara MB, Garsky VM, Mosser SD, Bergstrom JD, Moores SL, Marshall MS, Friedman PA, Dixon RAF, Gibbs JB. Polyisoprenylation of *ras* in vitro by a farnesyl-protein transferase. J Biol Chem 1990; 265: 14,701-14,704.
78. Fukada Y, Takao T, Ohguro H, Yoshizawa T, Akino T, Shimonishi Y. Farnesylated γ-subunit of photoreceptor G protein indispensable for GTP-binding. Nature 1990; 346: 658-660.
79. Cappel RE, Gilbert HF. Thiol/disulfide exchange between 3-hydroxyl-3-methylglutaryl-CoA reductase and glutathione. A thermodynamically facile dithiol oxidation. J Biol Chem 1988; 263:12,204-12,212.
80. Gilbert HF, Stewart MD. Inactivation of hydroxymethylglutaryl-CoA reductase from yeast by coenzyme A disulfide. J Biol Chem 1981; 256:1782-1785.
81. Lee S, Park S, Oh JW, Yang C. Natural inhibitors for protein prenyltransferase. Planta Med 1998; 64:303-308.
82. Stabel S, Parker PJ. Protein kinase C Pharmacol Ther 1991; 51: 71-95.
83. Kikuchi K, Naito K, Noguchi J, Shimada A, Kaneko H, Yamashita M, Tojo H, Toyoda Y. Inactivation of p34cdc2 kinase by the accumulation of its phosphorylated forms in porcine oocytes matured and aged in vitro. Zygote 1999; 7:173-179.
84. Gopalakrishna R, Gundimeda U, Chen ZH. Cancer-preventive selenocompounds induce a specific redox modification of cysteine-rich regions in Ca(2+)-dependent isoenzymes of protein kinase C. Arch Biochem Biophys 1997; 348:25-36.
85. Apitz-Castro R, Jain MK, Bartoli F, Ledezma E, Ruiz MC, Salas R Evidence for direct coupling of primary agonist-receptor interaction to the exposure of functional IIb-IIIa complexes in human blood platelets. Results from studies with the antiplatelet compound ajoene. Biochim Biophys Acta 1991; 1094:269-280.
86. Veldhuis JD, Hammond JM. Role of calcium in the modulation of ornithine decarboxylase activity in isolated pig granulosa cells in vitro. Biochem J 1981; 196:795-801.
87. Akerman KEO. Ca^{+2}-Transport and cell activation. Med Biol 1982; 60: 168-182.
88. Gilbert HF. Molecular and cellular aspects of thiol-disulfide exchange. Adv Enzymology 1990; 63: 169-172.
89. Rasmussen H. The calcium messenger system. N Engl J Med 1986; 314: 1164-1170.
90. Sakamoto K, Lawson, LD, Milner JA. Allyl sulfides from garlic suppress the in vitro proliferation of human A549 lung tumor cells Nutr Cancer 1997; 29:152-156.
91. Siegel G, Walter A, Schnalke F, Schmidt A, Buddecke E, Loirand G, Stock G. Potassium channel activation, hyperpolarization, and vascular relaxation. Z Kardiol 1991; 80 Suppl 7:9-24.
92. Martin N, Bardisa L, Pantoja C, Barra E, Demetrio C, Valenzuela J, Barrios M, Sepulveda MJ. Involvement of calcium in the cardiac depressant actions of a garlic dialysate. J Ethnopharmacol 1997; 55:113-118.
93. Das I, Khan NS, Sooranna SR. Potent activation of nitric oxide synthase by garlic: a basis for its therapeutic applications. Curr Med Res Opin 1995; 13: 257-263.
94. Moncada S, Higgs A. The L-arginine-nitric oxide pathway. N Engl J Med 1993; 329: 2002-2112.
95. Dawson VL, Dawson TM, Bartley DA, Uhl GR, Snyder SH. Mechanisms of nitric oxide-mediated neurotoxicity in primary brain cultures. J Neurosci 1993; 13: 2651-2661.

96. Santiago H, Pinto JT, unpublished observation, 1999.
97. Bordia A, Bansal HC, Arora SK, Singh SV. Effect of essential oils of garlic and onion on alimentary hyperlipemia. Atherosclerosis 1975; 21: 15-19.
98. Chang MLW, Johnson, MA. Effect of garlic on carbohydrate metabolism and lipid synthesis in rats. J Nutr 1980; 110: 931-936.
99. Adamu I, Joseph PK, Augusti KT. Hypolipidemic action of onion and garlic unsaturated oils in sucrose fed rats over a two-month period. Experientia 1982; 38: 899-901.
100. Sodimu O, Joseph PK, Augusti KT. Certain biochemical effects of garlic oil on rats maintained on high fat-high cholesterol diet. Experientia 1984; 40: 78-80.
101. Brady JF, Li D, Ishizaki H, Yang CS. Effect of diallyl sulfide on rat liver microsomal nitrosamine metabolism and other monooxygenase activities. Cancer Res 1988; 48, 5937-5940.
102. Reicks MM, Crankshaw DL. Modulation of rat hepatic cytochrome P450 activity by garlic organosulfur compounds. Nutr Cancer 1996; 25: 241-248.
103. Wargovich MJ, Woods C, Eng VWS, Stephens LC, Gray K. Chemoprevention of N-nitrosomethylbenzylamine-induced esophageal cancer in rats by naturally occurring thioether, diallyl sulfide. Cancer Res 1988; 48: 6872-6875.
104. Brady JF, Ishizaki H, Fukuto JM, Lin MC, Fadel A, Gapac JM, Yang CS. Inhibition of cytochrome P450 IIE1 by diallyl sulfide and its metabolites. Chem Res Toxicol 1991; 4: 642-647.
105. Pan J, Hong J-Y, Ma B-L, Ning SM, Paranawithana SR, Yang CS. Transcriptional activation of P-450 2B1/2 genes in rat liver by diallyl sulfone, a compound derived from garlic. Arch Biochem Biophys 1993; 302:337-342.
106. Wilding G. The importance of steroid hormones in prostate cancer. Cancer Surv 1992; 14: 113-130.
107. Schneider J, Kinne D, Fracchia A. Abnormal oxidative metabolism of estradiol in women with breast cancer. Proc Natl Acad Sci USA 1982; 79: 3047-3051.
108. Guengerich FP. Human cytochrome P450 enzymes. Life Sci. 1992; 50: 1471-1478.
109. Nelson DR, Koymans L, Kamataki T, Stegeman JJ, Feyereisen R, Waxman DJ, Waterman MR, Gotoh O, Coon MJ, Estabrook RW, Gunsalus IC, Nebert DW. P450 superfamily: Update on new sequences, gene mapping, accession numbers and nomenclature. Pharmacogenetics 1996; 6: 1-42.
110. Musey PI, Collins DC, Bradlow HL, Gould KG, Preedy JR. Effect of diet on oxidation of 17 ß-estradiol in vivo. J Clin Endocrinol Metab 1987; 65: 792-795.
111. Relling MV, Lin JS, Ayers GD, Evans WE. Racial and gender differences in N-acetyltransferase, xanthine oxidase, and CYP1A2 activities. Clin Pharmacol Ther 1992; 52: 643-658.
112. Sepkovic DW, Qiao C, Pinto J, Bradlow HL. Phase II metabolism of various estrogens after treatment with aged garlic extract. Proceedings of the American Association for Cancer Research, April 27-30; Washington, D.C., 1996.
113. Pinto JT, Qiao CH, Xing J, Suffoletto BP, Rivlin RS, Heston, WDW. Garlic constituents modify expression of biomarkers for human prostatic carcinoma cells. FASEB J 1997; 11: 439A.
114. Nebert DW. Elevated estrogen 16α-hydroxylase activity: Is this a genotoxic or nongenotoxic biomarker in human breast cancer risk? [editorial; comment] J Natl Cancer Inst 1993; 85:1888-1891.
115. Swaneck GE, Fishman J. Covalent binding of the endogenous estrogen 16 alpha-hydroxyestrone to estradiol receptor in human breast cancer cells: Characterization and intranuclear localization. Proc Natl Acad Sci USA 1988; 85: 7831-7835.
116. Li G, Qiao CH, Lin RI, Pinto JT, Osborne MP, Tiwari RK. Antiproliferative effects of garlic constituents on cultured human breast cancer cells. Oncol. Rep 1995; 2: 787-791.

117. Pinto J, Qiao C, Xing J, Suffoletto B, Rivlin RS, and Heston W. Garlic constituents modify expression of biomarkers for human prostatic carcinoma cells. FASEB J 1997; 11:439A.
118. Pinto JT, Suffoletto BP, Berzin, TM, Qiao CH, Lin S, Tong WP, May F, Mukherjee B, Heston WDW. Prostate Specific Membrane Antigen: A novel folate hydrolase in human prostatic carcinoma cells. Clin Cancer Res 1996; 2:1445-1451.
119. Wright GL Jr, Grob BM, Haley C, Grossman K, Newhall K, Petrylak H, Troyer J, Konchuba A, Schellhammer PF, Moriarity R. Upregulation of prostate specific membrane antigen after androgen deprivation therapy. Urology 1996; 48: 326-334.

9

CONSIDERING THE MECHANISMS OF CANCER PREVENTION BY SELENIUM

Gerald F. Combs, Jr., Ph.D.
Division of Nutritional Sciences
Cornell University, Ithaca, NY

INTRODUCTION

Selenium (Se) was recognized as having nutritional importance fairly late in the development of nutrition knowledge (Schwarz and Foltz, 1957) and, for many years, the nature of its role in nutrition remained clouded by the lack of information about its biochemical mechanisms of action. First, it was regarded only as a factor that could somehow "spare" vitamin E in animal diets; and then it became clear that it was specifically required for the synthesis of a number of proteins, including some with antioxidant like functions (glutathione peroxidases [GPX], thioredoxin reductase), as well as others (iodothyronine 5'-deiodinases [DI]) with important metabolic significance of a different type, all of which contained Se in the form of the unusual amino acid, selenocysteine (SeCys). In fact, information about SeCys-proteins continues to emerge and, with it, understanding of the nutritional and health importance of the trace element continues to expand.

Only 12 years after the proposal that Se was an essential nutrient, Shamberger and Frost (1969) suggested that the element may also be related to cancer risk. Their case was based on their observation that U.S. local cancer mortality rates were inversely associated with the geographic distribution of Se in American forage crops. That suggestion provoked what has grown to be a large body of research that collectively has established that Se can reduce experimental carcinogenesis in animal models (see recent reviews by El-Bayoumey, 1991; Krämer et al, 1996; Combs and Gray, 1998; Ip, 1998) while also reducing cancer risk in humans (Blot et al, 1993; Li et al, 1993; An, 1995; Clark et al, 1996; Yu et al, 1997). Thus, Se is now seen as an essential nutrient that can also serve as a modifier of cancer risk. While its nutritional roles seem to be explained on the basis of the known or presumed functions of a number of specific SeCys proteins, understanding its anti-carcinogenic role is still the subject of speculation and continuing investigation.

This symposium undertook to discuss important recent findings concerning the mechanisms of anti-carcinogenic actions of Se. The present paper was offered by way of providing background and context for those discussions. To that end, five questions would appear to be relevant:

1. Is anti-carcinogenesis and nutritional or supra-nutritional role of Se?
2. What are the most active forms of Se?
3. What are the mechanisms of anti-tumorigenic action of Se-compounds?
4. Might Se deficiency increase cancer risk?
5. What is the optimal level of Se intake?

Is anti-carcinogenesis and nutritional or supra-nutritional role of Se?

Any discussion of Se as an effector of cancer risk must begin with a consideration of dose and form of the element. Unlike other trace elements, the various biological effects of Se are properties of its various covalent compounds rather than intrinsic properties of the element *per se*. In other words, discussions of biological effects of Se must be at least footnoted with indications of the particular Se-compounds in question. With this in mind, it can be stated that the anti-tumorigenic effects observed for various forms of supplemental Se have been consistently associated with supra-nutritional levels of the element. For experimental animals, this means levels >1 mg Se/kg diet or ca. 0.7 mg Se/l drinking water; these levels are at least 5-10 times those required to prevent clinical signs of Se deficiency or to support maximal expression of the known SeCys-enzymes. On a unit body weight basis, they are also much greater than those intakes of most people, which appear seldom to be greater than 2 mcg Se/kg/day or 200 mg/person/day.

A case in point is the study conducted by our group (Clark et al, 1996,

1998) which demonstrated that the use of a daily oral dose of supplemental Se was associated with very substantial (up to two-thirds) reductions in risks to carcinomas, particularly those of the colon-rectum and prostate. That our (American) subjects entered the trial with baseline plasma Se concentrations of 114 ± 23 ng/ml, indicated that few, if any, had histories of low Se intakes. Maximal expressions of the two SeCys-proteins in plasma (GPX and selenoprotein P) would be comprise sufficient Se to yield aplasma Se concentration of ca. 80 ng/ml. On the basis of the data of Yang et al (1989), that level could be supported by dietary Se intakes at little as 30-40 mcg/day. The plasma Se levels of our cohort at baseline, as well as that of the placebo group (114 ng/ml) during the 13 yrs. of active follow-up, suggest an average daily Se intake of at least 85 mcg from dietary sources, a number exceeding the RDAs for both women (55 mcg) and men (70 mcg). It is significant, therefore, that the use of a 200 mcg Se daily supplement in this study was associated with reductions in cancer risk, although it did *not* increase plasma GPX activities nor alter plasma T_3:T_4 ratios (which might indicate effects on DI activities).

If Se-compounds can be anti-carcinogenic at supra-nutritional levels of exposure, then it follows that such effects must involve mechanisms *other than* those attached to the known SeCys-enzymes. This is not to say that one or more of the SeCys-enzymes are not involved in cancer prevention; rather, it means that, in a population already consuming nutritionally adequate levels of the nutrient, any effects of further supplements must involve other mechanisms.

What are the most active forms of Se?

Until fairly recently, most studies with animal tumor models employed as the source of Se, the oxidized inorganic salt Na_2SeO_3 (sodium selenite). That form, as well as the further oxidized form selenate (Na_2SeO_4), are known to undergo thiol- or NADPH-dependent reductions ultimately to selenide (H_2Se) before being incorporated into SeCys in the synthesis of the specific SeCys-proteins or being methylated to a variety of excretion products (Fig. 1). An intermediate on the thiol-dependent pathway is the selenodiglutathione (GSSeSG), is potently anti-tumorigenic (Poirier and Milner, 1983). Thus, it is possible that relatively high doses of selenite may lead to the production of significant amounts of GSSeSG, which contributed to the reduced tumor yields observed in those animal studies.

There is no reason to expect that the subjects in our cohort had any exposure to inorganic Se. One would expect their diets to have provided Se mainly in the form of SeCys, selenomethionine (SeMet) and their methylated derivatives, and the supplement we used, a Se-enriched yeast, while poorly characterized, is thought to contain only organic forms of the element: SeMet, SeCys, Se-methylselenocysteine (MeSeCys), plus several other unidentified Se-compounds (Bird et al., 1997). These organic Se-compounds, in contrast to the oxidized inorganic forms, are already at a reduced valence state (Se^{-2}); thus, while they, too, are metabolized to H_2Se, the route is a fundamentally different one not involving reduction. Selenocysteine is converted directly to selenide by a β-lyase; while SeMet must first cycle through the general protein pool (as a mimic for its sulfur-analogue methionine, Met) before its Se

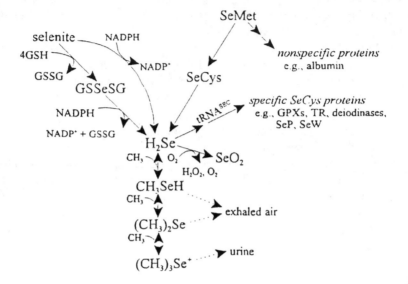

Figure 1. Selenium metabolism.

atom can be trans-selenated to form SeCys. The anti-tumorigenic activities of SeMet have generally been found to be less than selenite; but its efficacy can be expected to depend on the Met status of the host. For example, Ip (1988) found low-Met diets to reduce the chemopreventive efficacy of SeMet.

Results from Ip (1998) and Ganther (1999) have indicated that the anti-carcinogenic effects of Se are likely be discharged by one or more methylated Se-compounds that can be produced metabolically from H_2Se. Methylated forms of Se (methylselenol [CH_3SeH], dimethylselenide [$(CH_3)_2Se$] , trimethylselenonium [$(CH_3)_3Se^+$], collectively [$CH_3]_xSe$), have long been considered only as excretory forms of the element. However, it is clear that they can yield Se for the synthesis of SeCys-proteins through de-methylation to H_2Se; and Ip and Ganther (1990, 1991, 1992a, 1992b, 1993; Ip et al, 1991) have shown that the $(CH_3)_xSe$ and other Se-compounds that yield those forms metabolically can also function in anti-carcinogenesis.

Several alkyl and aryl selenocyanates have been synthesized and evaluated for anti-carcinogenicity in animal models. The more effective of these are benzylselenocyanate (El-Bayoumy, 1985; Reddy et al, 1987; Nayini et al, 1989; Ronai et al, 1995), p-methoxybenzylselenocyate (Reddy et al, 1997), *p*-xylylselenocyanate (El-Bayoumy, 1985; Reddy et al, 1987; Nayini et al, 1989; Ronai et al, 1995; Adler et al, 1996; Prokopczyck et al. 1996) and triphenylselenonium chloride (Ip et al, 1994; Lü et al, 1995). The metabolism of these Se-compounds appears limited, such that these tend not to be good sources of Se for the support of SeCys-enzyme expression. This suggests that these Se-compounds may be metabolized to anti-tumorigenic metabolites such as $(CH_3)_xSe$ and/or have inherent anti-tumorigenic properties.

Ip and Ganther (see review by Ip, 1998) have identified other anti-tumorigenic Se-compounds that serve as metabolic precursors to $(CH_3)_xSe$; these include Se-methylselenocysteine, which is a naturally occurring plant metabolite, and selenobetaine and selenobetaine methyl ester, which they synthesized. It would appear that the lipophilicities of these Se-compounds may allow each to provide Se at relatively sufficiently slow rates to support elevated steady-state levels of mono- and/or di-methylated components of the $(CH_3)_xSe$ pool without leading to quantitative urinary excretion of the dose as $(CH_3)_3Se^+$. The latter effect they proposed as the basis for the very poor anti-tumorigenicity of dimethyl selenoxide which appears to be metabolized very rapidly to $(CH_3)_2Se$ and lost either through respired air and or after further methylation to the urinary product $(CH_3)_3Se^+$. That the anti-tumorigenicity of these compounds does not depend on their metabolism to H_2Se (Ip and Ganther, 1992b) indicates that their cancer-preventive activities are not coupled to the nutritional role of Se discharged by the SeCys-proteins which depend on the metabolic availability of selenide.

If intermediates of Se metabolism, such as $(CH_3)_xSe$, are important in discharging anti-tumorigenic activities of various sources of Se that might be important in foods or considered as pharmaceuticals, then it would be extremely valuable to be able to measure those in subjects. The dogma in the field has been that "virtually all" Se in plasma is protein bound, those proteins being the SeCys-proteins selenoprotein P and GPX and also albumin which typically contains an appreciable amount of SeMet. However, we recently found that a small but measurable amount (2-5%) of Se in human plasma is non-covalently associated with proteins (Gray, Hyun and Combs, 1999). One might expect this low molecular weight fraction to contains such species as SeCys, SeMet, and $(CH_3)_xSe$; if so, then the development of methods to speciate its components may yield extremely useful means of monitoring efficacy as well as safety more effectively than is presently possible.

What are the mechanisms of anti-tumorigenic action of Se-compounds?

It is significant that, in our study (Clark et al, 1996, 1998), we observed reductions in cancer risk in Se-treated subjects after relatively short periods of intervention when compared to the time-lines proposed for most cancers. For example, we noted fewer cases of prostate cancer among Se-treated subjects in each calendar year and all but the first treatment year of the study. This suggests that Se-treatment must be effective at least in the latter stages of carcinogensis.

This does not exclude the possibility that Se-treatment may also affect other stages of carcinogenesis, as protective effects have been observed in different phases in different models. For example, it is reasonable to expect the GPXs and TR may play roles in inhibiting by free radical-initiated DNA damage and that deprivation of Se during initiation would enhance tumorigenesis. Accordingly, dietary selenite (>1 mg Se per kg) has been shown to reduce tumorigenesis in several models when it was given during the initiation phase, while other studies have shown Se-compounds to have significant post-initiation anti-tumorigenic effects (see review by Combs and Gray; 1998). Such results may indicate that the phase activity of Se may vary according to dose amount, if not also form. In humans given organic forms of the element, however, it is clear that the detectable protective effects must be late-stage ones.

The literature contains evidence for Se-supplements acting through several different but mutually exclusive mechanisms to prevent/delay tumorigenesis. These have been reviewed recently (Combs and Gray, 1998) and include effects that would be associated with tumor initiation (altered carcinogen metabolism; regulation of gene expression; favorable effects on hindgut microflora) as well as others associated with tumor progression (enhanced immune surveillance; enhanced apoptosis). Still the biochemical mechanisms for the involvement of Se-compounds at these levels are not clear.

Might Se deficiency increase cancer risk?

Because mutagenic oxidative stress is thought to be a major carcinogenic factor, it is logical to suggest that antioxidants, which scavenge reactive oxygen species (ROS) that can otherwise attack DNA bases, may be anti-carcinogenic. Therefore, because both the GPXs and TR are understood as playing important roles in cellular antioxidant protection, it is possible that these functions may contribute to anti-carcinogenic activities of Se-compounds. According to this hypothesis, through these enzymes Se would support the removal of DNA-damaging H_2O_2 and lipid hydroperoxides, thus blocking the generation of other ROS. In fact, skin tumorigenesis induced by ultraviolet (UV) irradiation (Burke et al, 1992; Pence et al, 1994; Diamond et al, 1996) or phorbol esters (Perchellet et al, 1987) was found to correlate inversely with skin GPX activity in Se-treated rats; and the restoration of GPX by selenite-treatment reduced N-nitrosobis(2-oxopropyl)amine-induced intrahepatic cholangiocarcinomas in Syrian golden hamsters (Kise et al, 1991). Both the carcinogenic and cytotoxic effects of UV-irradiation are diminished by treatment with selenite (Leccia et al, 1993; Pence et al, 1994; Moysan et al, 1995;Bertling et al, 1996; Diamond et al, 1996; Emonet et al, 1997) or SeMet (Burke et al, 1992) at Se-doses within the range (0.1-0.5 mg/kg diet) of maximization of selenoprotein expression.

Animal model studies, therefore, indicate that sub-optimal status with respect to Se (i.e., regular intakes that limit SeCys-enzyme expression) can, indeed, enhance tumorigenesis. As mentioned above, we have not observed such limiting status among apparently healthy Americans; but ample evidence from other parts of the world clearly show that Se-adequacy is not found in several other countries (e.g., most European countries, New Zealand, most of China, most of Australia, many parts of Russia, parts of Africa). For such populations, it is possible that sub-optimal Se intakes may contribute to cancer by way of compromised antioxidant protection.

What is the optimal level of Se intake?

If Se can be cancer-protective at supra-nutritional levels, then it is appropriate to ask what level of intake is necessary to realize that health benefit. That is, what is the optimal level of intake that will support not only adequate antioxidant defense but also minimal cancer risk. An appropriate data set upon which to base this sort of analysis would have informative measures of Se intake and Se status, as well as of cancer risk. Available data from human studies are few; at the moment, the best and perhaps only data of this nature come from our intervention trial (Clark et al, 1996, 1998, 1999). These show that Se-treatment to be effective in reducing risk to total carcinomas (Fig. 2) as well as to prostate cancers (Fig. 3) among subjects that entered the trial with plasma Se levels in the lower tertiles of the cohort. It should be pointed out that none of our subjects had plasma Se levels below 60 ng/ml and that very few had levels below 80 ng/ml; thus, as mentioned above, this cohort must be considered Se-adequate by current nutritional standards. Still, those subjects entering the trial with plasma Se levels less than 106 ng/ml showed not only the highest rates of cancer *but also* the strongest apparent protective effects of Se supplementation.

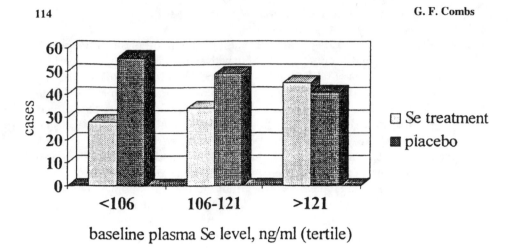

Figure 2. Effect of Se on total cancer risk by tertile of baseline plasma Se (from Clark et al., 1999).

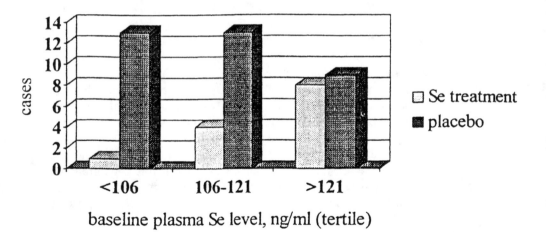

Figure 3. Effect of Se on prostate cancer risk by tertile of baseline plasma Se (from Clark et al., 1998).

Our data show, therefore, that persons with plasma Se levels above 121 ng/ml showed no cancer-protective benefits of taking the Se supplement. This might suggest that the plasma level of ca. 120 ng/ml may be associated with optimal cancer protection, and that strategies to reduce cancer risk might only need to raise Se status above that level.

CONCLUSION

Selenium appears to have two types of anti-carcinogenic roles: that of an essential nutrient providing the catalytic centers of antioxidant enzymes; and that as a source of metabolites that directly affect tumorigenesis. According to this view, Se is seen as potentially affecting a number of anti-carcinogenic activities depending on the form and level of the Se-dose. To the extent that these effects involve enhancements in the expression of selenoproteins (e.g., in Se-supplementation of Se-deficient populations), they would appear to be most relevant to the support of antioxidant defense and the inhibition of tumor initiation. To the extent that they involve supra-nutritional Se exposures (which is generally the case for the American population), they would appear to be mediated by Se-metabolites produced from relatively high doses of the many forms of the element. Current evidence suggests that the latter effects involve $(CH_3)_x Se$ acting in post-initiation stages of carcinogenesis.

REFERENCES

1.   Adler, V., Rincus, M. R., Posner, S., Upadhyay, P., El-Bayoumy., K., and Z. Ronai. Effects of chemopreventive selenium compounds on Jun-N-kinase activities. Carcinogenesis 17:1849-1854, 1996.
2.   An, P. Selenium and endemic cancer in China. In: Environmental bioinorganic chemistry of selenium, edited by P. M. Whanger, G. F. Combs, Jr., and J. Y. Yeh. Beijing: Chin. Acad. Sci. 1995; p. 91-149.
3.   Bertling, C. J., Lin, F., and A. W. Girotti. Role of hydrogen peroxide in the cytosolic effects of UCA/B radiation on mammalian cells. Photochem. Photobiol. 64:137-142, 1996.
4.   Bird, S. M., Uden, P.C., Tyson, J. F., Block, E., and E. Denoyer. Speciation of selenoamino acids and organoselenium compounds in selenium-enriched yeast using high-performace liquid chromatography-inductively coupled plasma mass spectrometry. J. Anal. Atom. Spectrom. 12:785-788, 1997.
5.   Blot, W. J., Li, J. Y., Taylor, P.R., Guo, W., Dawsey, S., Wang, G. Q., Yang. Nutrition intervention trials in Linxian, China: multiple vitamin/mineral supplementation, cancer incidence, and disease specific mortality among adults with esophagal dysplasia. J. Natl. Cancer Inst. 85: 1492-1498, 1993.
6.   Burke, K. E., Combs, Jr., G.F., Gross, E. G., Bhuyan, K. C., and H. Abu-Libdeh. The effects of topical and oral L-selenomethionine on pigmentation and skin cancer induced by ultraviolet irradiation. Nutr. Cancer 17:123-137, 1992.
7.   Clark, L. C., Combs, G. F., Jr., Turnbull, B. W., Slate, E., Alberts, D., Abele, D., Allison, R., Bradshaw. The nutritional prevention of cancer with selenium 1983-1993: a randomized clinical trial. J. Am. Med. Assoc. 276:1957-1963, 1996.
8.   Clark, L. C., Dalkin, B., Krongrad, A., Combs, G. F., Jr., Turnbull, B. W., Slate, E. H., Witherington, R., Herlong, J. H., Jansko, E., Carpenter, D., Borosso, C., Falk, S., and J. Rounder. Decreased incidence of prostate cancer with selenium supplementation: results of a double-blind cancer prevention trial. Br. J. Urol. 81:730-734, 1998.

9. Clark, L. C., Turnbull, B. W., Slate, E. H., Combs, G. F., Frischbach, L. Subgroup analysis of the nutritional prevention of cancer with selenium trial. Carcinoma of the skin: a randomized trial (unpublished research) 1999.

10. Combs, Jr., G. R. and W. P. Gray. Chemopreventive agents: selenium. Pharmacol. Therapeut. 79:179-192, 1998.

11. Diamond, A. M., Dale, P., Murray, J. L., and K. J. Grdina. The inhibition of radiation-induced mutagenesis by the combined effects of selenium and the aminothiol WR-1065. Mutat. Res. 356:147-154, 1996.

12. El-Bayoumy, K., The effects of organoselenium compounds on induction of mouse forestomach tumors by benzo(a)pyrene. Cancer Res. 45:3631-3635, 1985.

13. El-Bayoumy, K., The role of selenium in cancer prevention. In: Practice of oncology, 4th edition. Philadelphia: Lippincott 1991;p. 1-15. DeVita, V. T., Hellman, S., and S. S. Rosenberg (eds.).

14. Emonet, N., Leccia, M. R. Favier, A., Beani, J. C., and M. J. Richard. Thiols and selenium: protective effect of human skin fibroblasts exposed to UVA radiation. J. Photochem. Photobiol. B. 40:84-90, 1997.

15. Gray, W. P., Hyun, T., and G. F. Combs, Jr. Low molecular weight selenium in chick plasma. FASEB J. (in press), 1999.

16. Ip, C. Differential effect of dietary methionine on the biopotency of selenomethionine and selenite in cancer chemoprevention. J. Natl. Cancer Inst. 80:258-262, 1988.

17. Ip, C. Lessons from basic research in selenium and cancer prevention. J. Nutr. 128:1845-1854, 1998.

18. Ip, C., El-Bayoumy, K., Upadhyaya, P., Ganther, H., Vandanavikit, S., and H. Thompson. Comparative effect on inorganic and organic selenocyanate derivatives in mammary cancer prevention. Carcinogen. 15:187-192, 1994.

19. Ip, C., and H. Ganther. Activity of methylated forms of selenium in cancer prevention. Cancer Res. 50:1206-1211, 1990.

20. Ip, C. and H. Ganther. Combination of blocking agents and suppressing agents in cancer prevention. Carcinogenesis 12:365, 1991.

21. Ip, C. and H. E. Ganther. Comparison of selenium and sulfur analogs in cancer prevention. Carcinogenesis 13:1167-1170, 1992a.

22. Ip, C. and H. E. Ganther. Biological activities of trimethylselenonium as influenced by arsenite. J. Inorgan. Biochem. 46:215-222, 1992b.

23. Ip, C. and H. Ganther. Novel strategies in selenium cancer chemoprevention research. In: Selenium in biology and human health, edited by R. F. Burk. New York: Springer-Verlag 1993;p. 170-170.

24. Kise, Y., Yamamura, M., Kogata, M., Nakagawa, M., Uetsuji, S., Takada, H., Hioki, K., and M. Yamamoto. Inhibition by selenium of intrahepatic cholangiocarcioma induction in Syrian golden hamsters by N-nitrosobis(2-oxopropyl)amine. Nutr. Cancer 16: 153-164, 1991.

25. Kramer, K., Looks, M. P. Chrissafidou, A., Karsten, S., and J. Areads. Selen und tumarerkrankugen. Akt. Ernahr.-Med. 21:103-113. 1996.

26. Leccia, M. T., Richard, M. J., Beani, J. C., Faure, H., Monjo, A. M., Cadet, J., Amblard, P., and A. Favier. Protective effect of selenium and zinc on UV – A damage in human skin fibroblasts. Photochem. Photobiol. 58:548-553, 1993.

27. Li, J. Y., Taylor, P.R., Li, B., Blot, Wl J., Guo, W., Dawset, S., Wang, G. Q., Yang, C. S., Zheng, S. F., Gail, M., Li, G. Y., Liu, B. Q., Tangrea, I., Sun, Y. H., Liu, F., Fraumeni, F., Jr., and Y. H., Zhang. Nutrition intervention trials in Linxian, China. J. Nat. Cancer Inst. 85:1492-1498, 1993.

28. Lu, J., Jiang, C., Kaeck, M., Ganther, H. Ip, C., and H. Thompson. Cellular and metabolic effects of triphenyselenoium chloride in a mammary cell culturer model.

Carcinogenesis. 16:513-516, 1995.

29. Moysan, A., Morliere, P., Marquis, I., Richard, A., and L. Dubertret. Effects of selenium on UCA-induced lipid peroxidation in cultured human skin fibroblasts. Skin Pharmacol. 8:139-148, 1995.

30. Nayini, J., El-Bayoumy, K., Sugie, S., Cohen, L. A., and B. S. Reddy. Chemoprevention of experimental mammary carcinogenesis by the synthetic organoselenium compound, benzylselnocyanate, in rats. Carcinogenesis. 10:509-512, 1989.

31. Pence, B. C., Pelier, E., and D. M. Dunn. Effects of dietary selenium UCB-induced skin carcinogenesis and epidermal antioxidant status. J. Invest. Dermatol. 102:759-761, 1994.

32. Perchellet, J. P., Abney, N. L., Thomas, R. M., Guislan, Y. L., and E. M., Perchellet. Effects of combined treatments with selenium, glutathione and vitamin E on glutathione peroxidase activity, ornithine decarboxylase induction and complete and multistage carcinogenesis in mouse skin. Cancer Res. 47:477-485, 1987.

33. Poirier, K. A., and J. A. Milner, Factors influencing the antitumorigenic properties of selenium in mice. J. Nutr. 113:2147-2154, 1983.

34. Prokopczyk, B., Cox, J. E., Upadhyaya, P., Amin, S., Desai, D., Hoffmann, D., and K. El-Bayoumy. Effects of dietary 1, 4-phenylenebis(methylene)selenocyanate on 4-(methylnitrosamino)-1-(3-pyridyl)-1-butanone-induced DNA adduct formation in lung and liver of A/J mice and F344 rats. Carcinogenesis 17: 749-753, 1996.

35. Reddy, B. S., Sugie, S., Maruyama, H., El-Bayoumy, K., and P. Marra. Chemoprevention of colon carcinogenesis by dietary organselenium, benzylselenocyanate, in F344 rats. Cancer Res. 47:5901-5904, 1987.

36. Ronai, Z., Tillotson, J. K., Traganos, F., Darzynkiewice, Z., Conaway, C. C., Upadhyaya, P., and K. El-Bayoumy. Effects of organic and inorganic selenium compounds on rat mammary tumor cells. Int. J. Cancer 63:428-434, 1995.

37. Schwarz, K. C. M. Foltz. Selenium as an integral part of factor 3 agains dietary necrotic liver degeneration. J. Am. Chem. Soc. 79:3292-3293, 1957.

38. Shamberger, R. J. and D. V. Frost. Possible protective effect of selenium against human cancer. Can. Med. Assoc. J. 100:682-686, 1969.

39. Yang, G. Q., Yin, S., and R. Zhou. Studies of safe maximal daily dietary Se-intake in a seleniferous area in China. 1. Selenium intake and tissue selenium levels of the inhabitants. J. Trace Elem. Electrolytes Heatlh Dis. 3:77-86, 1989.

40. Yu, S. Y., Zhu, Y. J., and W. G. Li. Protective role of selenium against hepatitis B virus and primany level cancer in Qidong. Biol. Trace. Elem. Res. 56:117-124, 1997.

10

SELENIUM METABOLISM AND MECHANISMS OF CANCER PREVENTION

Howard E. Ganther

University of Wisconsin
Madison, Wisconsin, 53706

INTRODUCTION

It has been 50 years since the surprising discovery in 1949 that selenium (Se) had cancer preventing properties in animals given a chemical carcinogen (1). Numerous studies have confirmed the anticarcinogenic effects of supranutritional levels of Se in animals and more recently in humans given supplemental Se, as described by Combs (2). Proposed mechanisms of action for Se, as reviewed elsewhere in more detail (3), are based on (i) the formation of selenoproteins and (ii) the generation of low molecular weight Se metabolites by intermediary metabolism of Se in animals. A collaborative project (4,5) to investigate mechanisms and develop improved forms of Se for cancer prevention has provided considerable evidence that methylated metabolites of Se are important for Se anticarcinogenic action in animal model systems. The objective of this article is to summarize the findings that led to this concept and describe applications using methylated selenoamino acids that occur naturally in plants as a practical delivery mechanism for chemoprevention.

Nutrition and Cancer Prevention, edited under the auspices of AICR
Kluwer Academic / Plenum Publishers, New York, 2000.

SELENIUM METABOLISM

Methylation is a major fate of Se in animals (5). The garlic odor in breath of animals given inorganic Se salts was attributed to dimethyl selenide over 100 years ago (6). Animals synthesize selenoproteins from hydrogen selenide, a key intermediate in Se metabolism (Fig. 1). It is formed by reduction of inorganic salts such as sodium selenite, or by liberating Se from organoselenium compounds by scission of C-Se bonds. The metabolism of selenomethionine requires conversion to selenocysteine (transsulfuration pathway) followed by selenocysteine lyase to release inorganic Se. Hydrogen selenide is quite toxic but only miniscule amounts are formed to provide Se for selenoprotein synthesis. Animals deal with any excess by methylation, forming less toxic metabolites. Monomethylated forms are the major excretory products at normal Se intakes. Methylselenol (CH_3SeH) can be formed directly in one step from Se-methylselenocysteine (7), a major component of certain plants and selenized garlic (8). In this case the inorganic pool is largely bypassed, although sufficient demethylation to inorganic Se occurs to meet the needs for selenoprotein synthesis.

Hydrogen selenide is methylated by S-adenosylmethionine in three successive reactions, catalyzed by different enzymes. Steps 1 and 2 are catalyzed by an arsenite-sensitive microsomal enzyme called thiol S-methyltransferase (9; 10), forming dimethyl selenide; step 3 is catalyzed by thioether S-methyltransferase (10). The rate of methylation decreases with increasing degree of methylation, and the third step may become rate limiting. As a result, dimethyl selenide may escape and be excreted in the breath (10, 11). At normal levels of Se intake monomethylated forms are the major metabolites (11). When Se is fed to animals at chemopreventive levels, the urine contains much higher amounts of monomethylated forms of Se plus trimethylselenonium ion. At the highest Se intake, dimethyl selenide (breath) equals urinary monomethyl Se and exceeds urinary trimethylselenonium ion (11).

EFFICACY, BIOAVAILABILITY, AND TOXICITY

Selenomethionine or inorganic Se salts such as sodium selenite were used in most of the initial studies of cancer prevention because they were readily available (4). Cancer prevention activity in animals is lowest for selenomethionine, partly because it is incorporated into proteins in place of methionine. Selenite is more active and Se-methylselenocysteine is about twice as active as selenite (12). Other methylated forms of Se that bypass the inorganic pool also show good chemopreventive activity (12). These results suggested that activity might arise from some downstream metabolite of H_2Se. In that case, some of the potential toxic effects attributed to H_2Se, such as generation of superoxide radical (13), might be avoided by delivering the Se in pre-methylated forms, bypassing H_2Se.

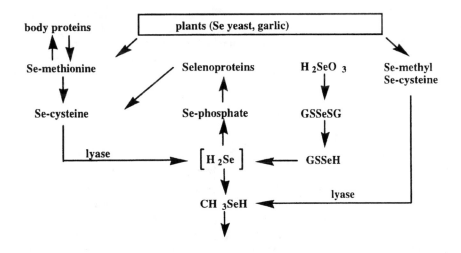

Figure 1. Selenium metabolism in animals (5). Plants supply Se to animals in the form of methylated selenoamino acids. Conversion to inorganic Se is necessary for synthesis of selenoproteins. Se-methylselenocysteine does not get incorporated into proteins and is directly converted to methyl selenol by cysteine conjugate β-lyase. At normal levels of Se intake the major urinary metabolites are monomethylated compounds (represented by methyl selenol). These can undergo further methylation (see text).

Dimethyl selenide and trimethylselenonium ion have low toxicity, partly because of the diminished reactivity of Se bound to two or three carbon atoms, and partly because these metabolites are readily excreted. Dimethyl selenide was not tested directly, but a non-volatile presursor, dimethyl selenoxide, was used to generate it. This compound had relatively low chemopreventive activity and was rapidly eliminated as dimethyl selenide (12). Trimethylselenonium chloride had little or no chemopreventive activity at dietary Se levels as high as 80 ppm, even though at 40 ppm Se it had

Table 1. Anticancer efficacy vs. bioavailability of selenium compounds

Compound	Dietary Se for 50% Tumor Inhibition	GSH Peroxidase (% of Control)
Se-Meselenocysteine	2 ppm	105 @ 0.5 ppm
$(CH_3)_3Se^+Cl^-$	No effect at 80 ppm	105 @ 40 ppm
$(C_6H_5)_3Se^+Cl^-$	10-20 ppm	1 @ 30 ppm

bioavailability sufficient for full synthesis of the selenoenzyme, glutathione peroxidase (14) (Table 1). In contrast, the novel organoselenium compound, triphenylselenonium chloride, had chemopreventive activity at 5 ppm Se but had no measurable bioavailability for synthesis of the selenoenzyme at 30 ppm Se (15); moreover, it produced no toxic effects at a level of 200 ppm Se. From these results it can be concluded that (i) selenoprotein synthesis can be independent of anticancer efficacy, and (ii) anticarcinogenic efficacy can be obtained independent of selenoprotein synthesis. In the case of triphenylselenonium chloride, there appears to be a rather distinct separation of anticancer efficacy from bioavailability and overt toxicity.

Additional evidence that cancer preventive activity could be independent of the inorganic Se pool was obtained using arsenite as a probe (16). A low level (5 ppm As) of arsenite alone had little cancer preventing activity. When this level of arsenite was fed together with a chemopreventive level of inorganic selenite, the chemopreventive activity was largely eliminated. However, when methylated forms of Se were used in combination with arsenite, chemopreventive activity was enhanced (16). Arsenite is known to antagonize many of the effects of inorganic selenium, and its failure to inhibit the chemopreventive activity of methylated forms of Se suggests that the formation of inorganic Se is not involved in the chemopreventive effects obtained with methylated Se compounds.

Chemopreventive efficacy for the final products of Se metabolism is shown diagramatically in Fig. 2. Activity is lower for H_2Se and reaches a peak at the monomethylated stage. Further methylation diminishes activity and increases excretability. This model predicts that with blockage (bars) of H_2Se methylation by inhibitors (arsenite) or genetic mutation, the absence of a functional methyl transferase activity would prevent the formation of monomethylated Se, thus giving lower chemopreventive activity with inorganic forms of Se. If Se is delivered at the monomethylated level from a suitable methylated precursor, however, there is no need for Step 1 methylation, and activity is as high or even higher because inactivation of monomethylSe by further methylation to dimethyl selenide would decrease if thiol S-methyltransferase is inhibited. In a human population where genetic polymorphisms are known to affect methylating abilities (17), individuals having low activity for enzymes catalyzing the initial stages of H_2Se methylation might respond poorly to chemopreventive forms of Se such as inorganic salts or selenomethionine that are metabolized through the H_2Se pool, but would likely show a response with Se compounds delivering Se in monomethylated forms.

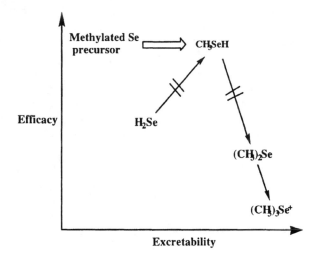

Figure 2. Profile of chemopreventive activity For Se metabolites. The bars indicate metabolic steps where interference with Se methylation might influence relative chemopreventive activities for inorganic forms of Se vs. methylated precursors (see text).

SE-METHYLSELENOCYSTEINE METABOLISM

Se-methylselenocysteine was one of the first naturally-occurring forms of Se to be identified in plants (18). It is present at high levels in certain species of *Astragalus* known as Se accumulators that tolerate high levels of Se. It is also the major form of Se in selenized garlic (8). The biosynthesis of Se-methylselenocysteine results from methylation of selenocysteine by a specific Se-methyltransferase recently identified in *Astragalus* that is inactive with cysteine but efficiently methylates selenocysteine, thus diverting selenocysteine to a form that cannot be incorporated into proteins (19).

Se-methylselenocysteine was readily metabolized to mono-, di-, and tri-methylated forms of Se in animals (11, 20) and scission by a lyase to methyl selenol was suggested (16). Cysteine conjugate β-lyase, found in kidney and other tissues, has no activity with S-methylcysteine but shows good activity with Se-methylselenocysteine and a number of other Se-alkylselenocysteine derivatives (21). Such activity makes it feasable to use Se-alkylselenocysteine derivatives as dietary chemopreventive agents that release the Se-alkyl moiety upon metabolism in vivo. Using this approach, the activity of Se-methyl-, Se-propyl-, and Se-allyl derivatives was compared at a level of 2 ppm dietary Se in the rat methylnitrosourea model (22). The Se-methyl and Se-propyl derivatives each gave about 50% reduction in tumor formation, whereas Se-allylselenocysteine gave almost 90% inhibition. These results show that the presence of a terminal double bond in the 3-carbon Se-allyl derivative confers greater activity compared to the saturated analogue or methyl derivative. Additional studies with Se-allylselenocysteine are in progress.

Since S-allylcysteine and related allyl sulfides are major forms of sulfur in garlic, it was anticipated that growth of garlic on a selenized medium might result in biosynthesis of Se-allylselenocysteine. Selenized garlic was shown to have very good chemopreventive activity, associated with a water-soluble component (23, 24). Chemical speciation studies have shown that Se-methylselenocysteine derivatives are the major forms of Se in selenized garlic, and Se-allyl derivatives were not detected (25). The chemopreventive activity of selenized garlic therefore is attributed to Se-methylselenocysteine. Se-garlic is a convenient means to deliver this form of Se using plant-based technology (23). The cancer preventing activity of Se-garlic was shown to be about twice that of selenized yeast in the rat models. This difference likely is related to Se-methylselenocysteine being the major form in Se-garlic whereas selenomethionine is the major form in Se-yeast (25).

CELLULAR MECHANISMS OF ACTION

Initial studies using inorganic sodium selenite showed inhibitory effects on growth, DNA synthesis, and many other cellular processes (4). These effects were more pronounced with transformed cells compared to normal cells, and greater in early stages of carcinogenesis (26). Apoptosis is an important mechanism for chemoprevention because the deletion of initiated cells prevents clonal expansion. Beginning with studies in Thompson's laboratory (27), many studies have shown the importance of apoptosis for Se chemoprevention (4). Apoptosis is one of several cellular processes showing very different action of monomethylated forms of Se vs. inorganic Se (4). Sinha and Medina observed altered cell cycle kinetics and found cdk2 kinase activity in mammary tumor cells was decreased by Se-methylselenocysteine, but not by inorganic selenite (29). Lu discusses apoptogenic mechanisms as well as his recent discovery of differential anti-angiogenesisis effects with monomethylated Se vs. inorganic Se in the following paper (28).

If monomethylated forms of Se such as methylselenol are critical chemopreventive metabolites, it would be expected that the direct addition of simple compounds generating methylselenol in vitro would be effective against transformed cells. With in vitro studies, systemic metabolism is not involved. Better control of experimental conditions is achieved, and the genetic makeup of cells can be varied. Direct addition of methylselenol is not feasible because of its facile oxidation, but alternative forms that are reducible to methylselenol can be used. Methylselenocyanate (CH_3SeCN) has substantial volatility and stench. Methylseleninic acid (CH_3SeO_2H) is more convenient to use because it ionizes at neutral pH in aqueous solutions to give the nearly odorless anion, and a number of studies are in progress using this compound. It has been shown to inhibit growth and DNA synthesis at low micromolar levels (30), and the recently described anti-angiogenic effects (28) are especially interesting. It has oxidizing properties comparable to selenite. A number of mechanisms based on formation of Se adducts with cysteine sulfhydryl groups of proteins or catalysis of reactions involving cysteine residues can be formulated. These mechanisms have been discussed at length in a recent review (3).

CYSTEINE CLUSTERS IN PROTEINS AS TARGETS

Clusters of cysteine residues occur in catalytic centers, regulatory sites, hormone binding domains, metal-binding sites, and in ion channel proteins. The stoichiometry of the reaction of oxidized forms of Se with sulfhydryl groups (up to four SH per Se) can be a basis for selectivity in protein modifications. Gopalakrishna's group has shown that the catalytic subunit of protein kinase C is inhibited by micromolar levels of selenite, whereas proteins lacking such clusters are unaffected (31).

Methylseleninic acid reacts with thiols in a 1:3 stoichiometric ratio, and modification of a protein cysteine cluster composed of three cysteine residues is depicted in Fig. 3. A methylselenenylsulfide derivative is formed with one cysteine, using reducing equivalents supplied by oxidation of two cysteine residues to an intramolecular disulfide bond.

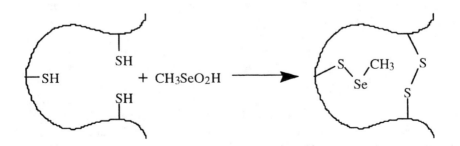

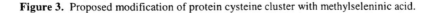

Figure 3. Proposed modification of protein cysteine cluster with methylseleninic acid.

A parallel type of modification was proposed for the reaction of methyl methanethiosulfonate with glucocorticoid receptor thiols, where the formation of a methylthio mixed disulfide and an intramolecular disulfide in the binding pocket for the steroid hormone inhibit steroid binding (32). Benzeneseleninic acid recently was shown to release zinc from tightly-bound zinc-sulfur clusters in metallothionein; the authors suggest that displacement by Se of zinc in zinc fingers of transcription factors or proteins involved in cell signaling could be a potential chemopreventive mechanism (33).

Formation of protein-Se adducts or catalysis of thiol/disulfide reactions may affect redox signaling (3). Figure 4 depicts a model where transcription factors, ion channel proteins, and other redox-regulated proteins could be poised in two states, ON/OFF, differing by the oxidation state of cysteine, and subject to time-limited activation. Se is proposed to catalyze reactions that return the activated state to the basal state by forming more reactive S-Se intermediates. The result is faster resetting of the basal state, and less time in the activated state.

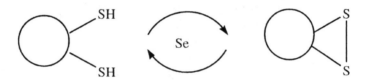

Figure 4. Se as a redox catalyst in modulation of redox-regulated proteins (3).

SELENOPROTEINS AND CANCER CHEMOPREVENTION

All of the known functions of Se as an essential nutrient involve selenoproteins. The presence of selenocysteine in proteins enables unique chemistry and high amplification mechanisms of action for Se. Although many believe that anticancer effects observed with Se at near nutritional levels must involve selenoproteins, the experimental animal models have not shown evidence that selenoproteins are increased by chemopreventive levels of Se. As discussed at greater length elsewhere, newly discovered selenoproteins such as thioredoxin reductase or novel selenoproteins having unidentified functions must be considered, along with classic Se-dependent peroxidases (3). Although chemopreventive activity is seen with Se compounds in which Se is unavailable for selenoprotein synthesis, selenoproteins hold promise for roles in cancer prevention, along with the better established roles for low molecular weight Se metabolites.

Lu has recently proposed an attractive model that integrates both concepts, with particular emphasis on the microvascular system (28). He proposes that Se interferes with angiogenesis, so that vascularization needed for growth and progression of small, early stage tumors is precluded. Such avascular masses of cells are suggested to develop a conditioned Se deficiency, so that synthesis of selenoproteins is impaired, even though Se supply elsewhere may be sufficient to allow the synthesis of normal levels of selenoproteins. His model predicts that higher Se intakes are required in order to drive sufficient Se into the avascular areas.

Based on physicochemical considerations of Se delivery, it might be speculated that some of the beneficial effects of methylated Se metabolites are exerted through provision of a bioavailable source of Se in the form of low molecular weight, readily diffusible forms of Se that can traverse avascular areas more readily than larger, more polar forms such as glutathione derivatives or inorganic Se. Production of methylated metabolites rises markedly with the attainment of chemopreventive levels of dietary Se (11). The greatest relative increase in any single metabolite was the 100-fold increase observed for dimethyl selenide. This volatile, neutral compound has sufficient lipophilic properties to move easily through membranes but also has appreciable water solubility. It is known that compounds such as dimethyl selenoxide, that generate mainly dimethyl selenide, provide sufficient Se for synthesis of selenoproteins (14). Moreover, anticarcinogenic activity of selenobetaine methyl ester, a compound undergoing direct and extensive metabolism to dimethyl selenide (34), is comparable to Se-methylselenocysteine and greater than that for inorganic selenite (35). The concept that methylation of Se might have implications for delivery of Se in vivo, where the degree of vascularization of tissues can influence the supply of nutrients, helps bridge the gap between in vivo studies suggesting efficacy even for extensively methylated forms of Se, and in vitro studies using cell cultures, where such compounds generally lack activity. Moreover, it is helpful in connecting the established efficacy of methylated Se metabolites with the tradional role of Se in selenoproteins. Multiple chemopreventive mechanisms, as in the integrated model of Lu, are likely to be involved.

It is concluded that animals have a long, comfortable relationship with methylated forms of Se. They consume methylated selenoamino acids in the diet, metabolize them to release methylated or inorganic forms, and readily methylate any excess inorganic Se for excretion. Through such metabolic processes, chemopreventive methylated Se metabolites are generated, with a peak in activity at the monomethylated stage. The appearance of dimethylselenide in breath may be a useful marker for attainment of maximal levels of Se methylation. There is evidence that Se selectively affects transformed cells compared to normal cells, and has greater effectiveness in early stages of carcinogenesis. Multiple chemopreventive actions are known, including growth inhibition, altered cell cycle kinetics, and induction of apoptosis independent of DNA damage and functional p53. Se-methylselenocysteine is a good precursor for generating active monomethylated Se metabolites in vivo. It is more active than selenomethionine, gives a lower body burden of Se, and is rapidly eliminated upon cessation of intake. It delivers a steady stream of monomethylated Se in one step, beyond the hydrogen selenide pool. It occurs naturally in plants and can be delivered through food sources or provided in synthetic form.

ACKNOWLEDGMENT

This contribution was supported by grant no. CA 45164 from the National Cancer Institute, NIH.

REFERENCES

1. Clayton, C.C., and Baumann, C.A. (1949) Diet and azo dye tumors: Effect of diet during period when the dye is not fed. *Cancer Res.*, 9, 575-592.
2. Combs, G. F. , Jr. Considering the mechanisms of cancer prevention by selenium. In *Nutrition and Cancer Prevention: New Insights Into the Role of Phytochemicals.* Kluwer Academic/Plenum, New York, 2000 [This volume].
3. Ganther, H. E. (1999) Selenium metabolism, selenoproteins, and mechanisms of cancer prevention: Complexities with thioredoxin reductase. *Carcinogenesis,* 20, 1657-1666.
4. Ip, C. (1998) Lessons from basic research in selenium and cancer prevention. *J. Nutr.,* 128, 1845-1854.
5. Ganther, H.E., and Lawrence, J.R. (1997) Chemical transformations of selenium in living organisms. Improved forms of selenium for cancer prevention. *Tetrahedron,* 53, 12229-12310.
6. Hoffmeister, F. (1894) Ueber Methylirung im Thierkörper. *Arch. Exp. Path. Pharmacol.,* 33, 198-215.
7. Andreadou, I, Water, B, Commandeur, J.N.M., Worthington, E.A, and Vermeulen, N.P.E. (1996) Comparative cytotoxicity of 14 novel selenocysteine Se-conjugates in rat renal proximal tubular cells. *Toxicol. Appl. Pharmacol.,* 141, 278-287.
8. Uden, P. C., Bird, S. M., Kotrebai, M., Nolibos, P., Tyson, J. F., Block, E., and Denoyer, E. (1998) Analytical selenoaminoacid studies by chromatography with interfaced atomic mass spectrometry and atomic emission spectral detection. *Fresenius J. Anal. Chem.,* 362, 447-456.
9. Hsieh, H. S., and Ganther, H. E. (1977) Biosynthesis of dimethyl selenide from sodium selenite in rat liver and kidney cell-free systems. *Biochim. Biophys. Acta,* 497, 205-217.
10. Mozier, N. M., McConnell, K. P., and Hoffman, J. L. (1988) S-adenosyl-L-methionine:thioether S-methyltransferase, a new enzyme in sulfur and selenium metabolism. *J. Biol. Chem.,* 263, 4527-4531.
11. Vadhanavikit, S., Ip, C., and Ganther, H. E. (1993) Metabolites of sodium selenite and methylated selenium compounds administered at cancer chemopreventive levels in the rat. *Xenobiotica,* 23, 731-745.
12. Ip, C., and Ganther, H. E. Novel strategies in selenium cancer chemoprevention research. In *Selenium in Biology and Health,* Burk, R., ed., Springer-Verlag, Berlin, 1994.

13. Spallholz, J. E. (1994) On the nature of selenium toxicity and carcinostatic activity. *Free Radical Biol. & Med.*, 17, 45-64.
14. Ip, C., and Ganther, H. E. Relationship between the chemical form of selenium and anticarcinogenic activity. In *Cancer Chemoprevention*. Wattenberg, L, Lipkin, M, Boone, C. W., and Kelloff, G, J., eds., CRC Press, Boca Raton, l992.
15. Ip, C., Lisk, D. J., and Ganther, H. E. (1998) Activities of structurally-related lipophilic selenium compounds as cancer chemopreventive agents. *Anticancer Res.*, 18, 4019-4026.
16. Ip, C., Hayes, C., Budnick, R. M., and Ganther, H. E. (1991) Chemical form of selenium, critical metabolites, and cancer prevention. *Cancer Res.*, 51, 595-600.
17. Weinshilboum, R. M., Otterness, D. M., and Szumlanski, C. L. (1999) Methylation pharmacogenetics: Catechol O-methyltransferase, thiopurine methyltransferase, and histamine N-methyltransferase. *Annu. Rev. Pharmacol. Toxicol.* 39, 19-52.
18. Trelease, S. F., Di Somma, A. A., and Jacobs, A. L. (1960) Seleno-amino acid found in Astragalus bisulcatus. *Science,* 132, 618.
19. Neuhierl, B., Thanbichler, M., Lottspeich, F., and Böck, A. (1999) A family of S-methylmethionine-dependent thiol/selenol methyltransferases. *J. Biol. Chem.*, 274, 5407-5414.
20. Foster, S. J., Kraus, R.J., and Ganther, H. E. (1986) The metabolism of selenomethionine, Se-methylselenocysteine, their selenonium derivatives, and trimethylselenonium in the rat. *Arch. Biochem. Biophys.*, 251, 77-86.
21. Andreadou, I, Menge, W. M. P. B., Commandeur, J.N.M., Worthington, E.A, and Vermeulen, N.P.E. (1996) Synthesis of novel Se-substituted selenocysteine derivatives as potential kidney selective prodrugs of biologically active selenol compounds: Evaluation of kinetics of β-elimination reactions in rat renal cytosol. *J. Med. Chem.*, 39, 2040-2046.
22. Ip, C., Zhu, Z., Thompson, H. J., Lisk, D., and Ganther, H. E. (1999) Chemoprevention of mammary cancer with Se-allylselenocysteine and other selenoamino acids in the rat. *Anticancer Res.*, 19 (in press)
23. Ip, C, and Lisk, D. J. (1996) The attributes of selenium-enriched garlic in cancer prevention. *Adv. Exp. Med. Biol.*, 401, 179-187.
24. Lu, J., Pei, H., Ip, C., Lisk, D. J., Ganther, H., and Thompson, H. J. (1996) Effect of an aqueous extract of selenium-enriched garlic on in vitro markers and in vivo efficacy in cancer prevention. *Carcinogenesis,* 17, 1903-1907.
25. Ip, C., Birringer, M., Block, E., Kotrebai, M., Tyson, J. F., Uden, P. C., and Lisk, D. J. Chemical speciation influences comparative activity of selenium-enriched garlic and yeast in mammary cancer prevention. (submitted)
26. Medina, D., and Morrison, D.G. (1988) Current ideas on selenium as a chemopreventive agent. *Pathol. Immunopathol. Res.*, 7,187-199.
27. Wilson, A.C., Thompson, H.J., Schedin, P.J., Gibson, N.W., and Ganther, H.E. (1992) Effect of methylated forms of selenium on cell viability and the induction of DNA strand breakage. *Biochem. Pharmacol.*, 43, 1137-1141.
28. Lu, J. Apoptosis and angiogenesis in cancer prevention by selenium. In *Nutrition and Cancer Prevention: New Insights into the Role of Phytochemicals.* Kluwer Academic/Plenum, New York, 2000. [This volume]
29. Sinha, R, and Medina, D. (1997) Inhibition of cdk2 kinase activity by methylselenocysteine in synchronized mouse mammary epithelial tumor cells. *Carcinogenesis,* 18, 1541-1547.
30. Sinha, R., Ganther, H. E., and Medina, D. (1999) Methylseleninic acid, a novel selenium compound inhibits mouse mammary epithelial tumor cells in vitro. *Proc. Amer. Assoc. Cancer Res.*, 40, 360.
31. Gopalakrishna, R., Gundimeda, U., and Chen, S.-H. (1997) Cancer-preventive selenocompounds induce a specific redox modification of cysteine-rich regions in Ca^{2+}-dependent isozymes of protein kinase C. *Arch. Biochem. Biophys.*, 348, 25-36.

32. Simons, S. S., Jr., and Pratt, W. B. (1995) Glucocorticoid receptor thiols and steroid-binding activity. *Methods Enzymoll.*, 251, 406-422.

33. Jacob, C., Maret, W., and Vallee, B. L. (1999) Selenium redox biochemistry of zinc-sulfur coordination sites in proteins and enzymes. *Proc. Nat. Acad. Sci. (U. S.)*, 96, 1910-1914.

34. Foster, S. J., Kraus, R. J., and Ganther, H. E. (1986) Formation of dimethyl selenide and trimethylselenonium from selenobetaine in the rat. *Arch. Biochem. Biophys.*, 247, 12-19.

35. Ip, C., and Ganther, H. E. (1990) Activity of methylated forms of selenium in cancer prevention. *Cancer Res.*, 50, 1206-1211.

11

APOPTOSIS AND ANGIOGENESIS IN CANCER PREVENTION BY SELENIUM

Junxuan Lu, Ph.D.

Center for Cancer Causation and Prevention
AMC Cancer Research Center
Denver, CO 80214

INTRODUCTION

Epidemiological and laboratory findings have long implicated a potential anti-cancer activity of the trace element nutrient selenium (Se). Note that it is often for convenience reasons to describe such anti-cancer activity in terms of the element. A vast volume of data have been accumulated supporting the theme that cancer preventive activity is expressed as a function of the dose and chemical form in which the element resides, not elemental Se *per se* (1,2). The landmark cancer prevention trial by Clark, Combs and coworkers demonstrated for the first time that a supra-nutritional Se supplement (provided as selenized yeast) to a US skin cancer patient population otherwise adequate in Se nutrition might be an effective preventive agent for several major human epithelial cancers (3). With profound public health implications at stake, many serious issues demand a clear understanding of the mechanisms through which Se exerts anti-cancer activity. Some of these pressing questions, for example, include what form(s) and what doses of Se should be used? What populations should be given the intervention? How long should the intervention be given?

With respect to "mechanisms", a number of them have been investigated: antioxidant protection (via SeCys-glutathione peroxidases), altered carcinogen metabolism, enhanced immune surveillance, cell cycle effects, enhanced apoptosis (1,2) and more recently inhibition of neo-angiogenesis (4).   The mechanisms that are actually involved in cancer prevention by Se will likely depend on the dose and form of Se-compounds, the Se status of the individual and perhaps the type and etiology of malignancy to be prevented.   It is probable that Se supplementation of individuals with relatively low or frankly deficient Se intakes can be expected to support enhanced antioxidant protection due to increased expression of the SeCys-enzymes or enhanced immune surveillance (2). On the other hand, in animal models and in clinical studies, anti-tumorigenic activities have been associated with Se intakes that are more than sufficient to correct nutritional deficiency. That is, Se appears to be anti-tumorigenic at intakes that are substantially greater than those associated with maximal expression of the known SeCys-containing glutathione peroxidase enzymes (1,2). Therefore, a favored hypothesis that has enjoyed considerable experimental support is that cancer chemopreventive functions of Se are attributable to active Se-metabolite(s) produced in significant amounts at high Se intakes (1,2,5). Specifically methylselenol has been implicated as a candidate *in vivo* active Se metabolite (5-7).

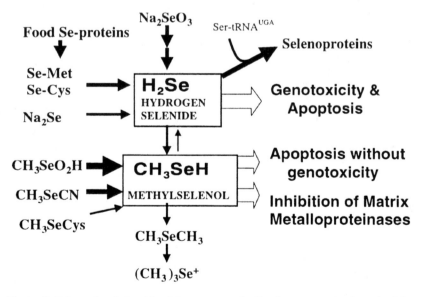

Figure 1. Schematic relationship of Se precursors feeding into two pools of proximal Se metabolites that exert distinct biochemical and cellular effects. The fate of Se amino acids derived from food Se-proteins was also indicated. The genotoxicity (or lack of) effect of the two Se pools was based on studies with mammary cancer epithelial cells and leukemia cells (ref. 15,16, 23-25). Abbreviations: Se-cys, selenocysteine; Se-Met, selenomethionine; CH_3SeCN, methylselenocyanate; CH_3SeCys, Se-methylseleno-cysteine; CH_3SeO_2H, methylseleninic acid.

In this chemopreventive context, we have used cell culture and animal models to seek a better understanding of how Se confer growth/fate regulation of transformed cells (15,16, 23-25) and more recently the role of angiogenesis in mammary cancer and its prevention by Se (4).

In this chapter, I will focus on the following questions: Does Se induce apoptotic death of cancerous cells? What pathways mediate such an effect? Does Se inhibit neo-angiogenesis and if so, how? The scope of discussion will be limited to those forms of Se that are related to *in vivo* Se metabolism (Figure 1) (8). Interested readers are referred to recent review articles concerning the cancer preventive activity of novel synthetic aromatic organo-selenium compounds (1, 9). I will review pertinent data that support two pools of proximal Se metabolites, namely hydrogen selenide and methylselenol, that induce apoptosis with distinct biochemical/cellular pathways and a specific inhibitory activity of methylselenol on endothelial matrix metalloproteinases (MMPs) which are required for the angiogenic process (Figure 1). In the discussion section, I will propose an integrated (albeit speculative) model of cancer prevention by Se based on the interaction of epithelial lesions and the vasculature that supports such lesions.

SELENIUM AND CELL DEATH/APOPTOSIS

Selenite-induced apoptosis is causally linked to genotoxicity

Treatment of fibroblasts and other cell lines with selenite, a commonly used reference Se compound, has been reported to lead to DNA single strand breaks (defined as genotoxicity) in the late 1980s and early 90s (10-12). Generation of reactive oxygen species (ROS) such as superoxide was demonstrated in *in vitro* models by the reaction of selenite with glutathione and other thiol compounds (13,14). These observations suggested that ROS and genotoxicity might be causally involved in the cytostatic and cytocidal effects of Se.

To test this hypothesis, we examined the sequence of events in the induction of apoptotic cell death (as evidenced by morphology and DNA apoptotic fragmentation) by sodium selenite using murine L1210 leukemia cells as our model (15). Cell death and DNA apoptotic fragmentation as well as double stranded breaks (DSBs) were preceded by the occurrence of DNA single strand breaks (SSBs) as measured using a filter elution assay (15,16). Much insight was gained by using inhibitors of key biochemical processes to probe the likely sequence of events (Table 1). Copper diisopropylsalicate (CuDIPS), a superoxide dismutase (SOD) mimetic compound that blocks the generation of hydrogen selenide from selenite (11), completely blocked the effect of selenite on DNA integrity and cell viability. Because the free radical quencher mannitol failed to modulate the treatment effect of selenite, hydroxy

Table 1. Modulation of selenite-induced DNA strand breaks and cell viability of L1210 murine leukemia cells (Modified based on ref. 15)

Treatment	DNA SSBs	DNA DSBs	Cell Viability,%
None	5.7 ± 0.7	5.0 ± 0.1	99
+ 50 μM CuDIPS[1]	4.8 ± 0.4	5.8 ± 0.6	98
+ 5 mM mannitol[2]	5.2 ± 0.4	4.8 ± 0.2	98
+ 0.25 mM ATA[2]	4.3 ± 0.4	3.4 ± 0.2	99
+ 39 μM ZnSO₄ [2]	6.0 ± 1.1	5.9 ± 0.1	99
10 μM selenite	93.4 ± 0.4	27.1 ± 1.6	72
+ 50 μM CuDIPS	5.6 ± 0.5	4.8 ± 0.2	97
+ 5 mM mannitol	89.0 ± 0.6	25.5 ± 0.9	65
+ 0.25 mM ATA	54.9 ± 0.9	3.7 ± 0.1	97
+ 39 μM ZnSO₄	62.4 ± 1.9	8.8 ± 0.6	95

Mean±sem (n=4).
[1]CuDIPS, copper diisopropylsalicylate, is a superoxide dismutase mimetic.
[2]ATA, aurintricarboxylic acid. ATA and zinc are inhibitors of Ca^{2+}/Mg^{2+}-dependent endonucleases. Mannitol is a hydroxy free radical quencher.

free radicals were not likely involved as mediators of DNA strand breaks and apoptosis. These data indicated that metabolism of selenite, not selenite *per se*, was required for the induction of DNA damage and subsequent apoptosis and implicated superoxide and/or hydrogen selenide as likely proximal mediators of the observed effects.   Co-treatment of L1210 cells with aurin tricarboxylic acid (ATA) and zinc, known inhibitors of Ca^{2+}/Mg^{2+}-dependent endonucleases responsible for nucleosomal apoptotic DNA fragmentation, prevented DNA DSBs and cell viability loss, attenuated but did not block the occurrence of DNA SSBs.

These data indicated that the occurrence of DNA SSBs preceded and was likely causal to Ca^{2+}/Mg^{2+}-dependent endonuclease activation and apoptotic fragmentation of the DNA. The likely sequence of events in apoptosis induction by selenite treatment is shown schematically in Figure 2. Results from other laboratories published recently have provided confirmation of growth inhibition and apoptosis induction by selenite and related Se forms through genotoxicity mediated by ROS (17-22).   The generality of this mechanism appears to extend to human leukemia (17), hepatoma (18), colon carcinoma (20,21), glioma (22) and mouse keratinocytes (19).

Methylselenol induces apoptosis without inducing DNA SSBs (23)

To further define the Se metabolite(s) responsible for induction of DNA damage and apoptosis, we took advantage of Se compounds that enter the Se metabolic pathways at different points (Figure 1). Selenite treatment of

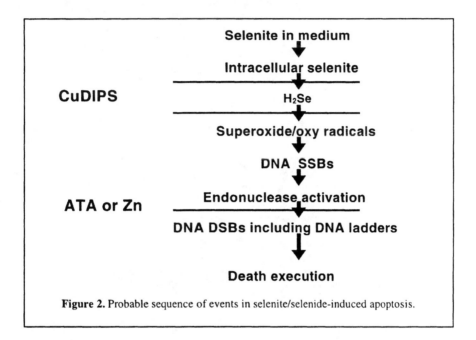

Figure 2. Probable sequence of events in selenite/selenide-induced apoptosis.

MOD mouse mammary cancer epithelial cells led to a rapid induction of DNA SSBs (Figure 3A) and DSBs (Figure 3B), and subsequent cell death by a composite of acute lysis and apoptosis (Figure 3C). Sodium selenide, which metabolizes to hydrogen selenide (H_2Se), recapitulated the effects of selenite treatment on DNA SSBs and DSBs and cellular morphological responses (23). In contrast, methylselenocyanate (MSeCN or CH_3SeCN) and methylselenocysteine (MSeC or CH_3SeCys) induced exclusively apoptosis of cancerous mammary epithelial cells (Figure 3D) without induction of DNA SSBs (Figure 3, A and B). *Therefore, hydrogen selenide is likely the proximal Se metabolite involved in the induction of DNA SSBs and apoptosis by Se compounds that feed into this Se pool. Methylselenol, on the other hand, is the proximal Se metabolite for induction of apoptosis without the genotoxicity elicited by hydrogen selenide* (Figure 1). It is striking that only a single methylation step separates the two forms of Se metabolites that are responsible for eliciting distinct biochemical and cellular responses.

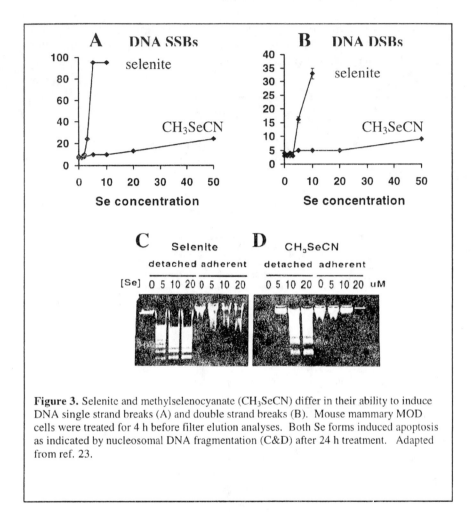

Figure 3. Selenite and methylselenocyanate (CH₃SeCN) differ in their ability to induce DNA single strand breaks (A) and double strand breaks (B). Mouse mammary MOD cells were treated for 4 h before filter elution analyses. Both Se forms induced apoptosis as indicated by nucleosomal DNA fragmentation (C&D) after 24 h treatment. Adapted from ref. 23.

How does methylselenol induce apoptosis?

Very little is known at the present concerning the underlying mechanisms triggering apoptosis by methylselenol. Some insights are suggested by additional differences, besides genotoxicity, in the biochemical and cellular consequences of treatment with the two types of Se compounds (Table 2). The methylselenol precursors MSeCN, MSeC and MSeA exert a moderate anti-proliferative effect as assessed by ^{3}H-thymidine incorporation into DNA and arrest cells in the G_1 phase of the cell cycle, whereas selenite rapidly blocks DNA synthesis and arrests cells in the S phase (24,25 and unpublished data). Consistent with G_1 arrest by methylselenol, MSeC has been shown to inhibit key cyclin dependent kinases (cdks) whereas selenite lacks such an effect (26). We have reported a differential induction of the *growth arrest and DNA damage inducible* (*gadd*) genes by selenite and MSeCN in mammary cancer cells (25), although no induction of *gadd* genes was detected in mammary tumors induced to regress by Se *in vivo* (unpublished data).

Table 2. Representative data illustrating the distinct response patterns of MOD cells to selenite (5 μM) and methylselenocyanate (CH₃SeCN, 5 μM)

Parameters	Selenite		CH₃SeCN	
	4 h	24 h	4 h	24 h
Cellular Se, ng/10[6] cells	24	36	4	4
Thymidine incorporation[1]	16	7	59	45
Adherent Cell number[1]	93	44	98	41
DNA single strand breaks[2]	12.5	5.3	1	0.7
DNA double strand breaks[2]	6.4	3.5	1	2.4
Membrane leakage[2]	3.8	7.4	1.3	3.3
Cell cycle disturbance	No	S-arrest	No	G_1 arrest
*gadd*153 gene expression	-	+++	+++	-
*gadd*34 gene expression	+	+++	++	+
*gadd*45 gene expression	+	+++	++	+
Morphological cell death	Acute lysis	Apoptosis	No change	Apoptosis

[1]untreated control=100
[2]untreated control = 1

In a recent review article, Ganther proposed several potential chemical reactions in which methylselenol may participate that can either directly modify protein activities or through regulation of gene expression (5). The relevance of these reactions remains to be established. Much work is needed to elucidate the underlying mechanism(s) through which methylselenol regulates cancer cell growth and survival.

SELENIUM AND ANGIOGENESIS REGULATION

It is now well recognized that angiogenesis, i.e., the growth of capillary vessels from existing ones, is obligatory for the growth, progression and metastasis of solid cancer (27,28). During solid cancer carcinogenesis, initiated cells undergo clonal expansion in an avascular state when the expanding lesions are small enough to take in nutrients and to expel metabolic wastes by diffusion. However diffusion is not sufficient to support continued growth of the lesion beyond a certain physical size (estimated ~2 mm diameter) as the expanding lesions consume nutrients at a rate proportional to their volume whereas the supply of nutrients is delivered at a rate proportional to their surface area (34,35). In order for avascular lesions to progress beyond the size limit imposed by simple diffusion, they must turn on the angiogenesis switch to form a neo-vasculature (29).   Because of the critical dependence of tumor growth and metastasis on angiogenesis, therapeutic strategies are being developed targeting various aspects of the angiogenic processes, many with promising results. We have recently initiated work to explore the hypothesis that Se may exert cancer chemopreventive activity, at least in part, through an anti-angiogenic mechanism (4).

Mammary cancer prevention by Se is associated with decreased microvessel density (4)

In a chemoprevention setting, Se (3 ppm) as either Se-garlic (Experiment 1) or selenite (Experiment 2) was fed for ~2 months to Sprague-Dawley rats that were given a single i.p. injection of methylnitrosourea (MNU) to initiate mammary carcinogenesis a week earlier. The microvessels in the mammary tumors were visualized with immunohistochemical staining for Factor VIII and the microvessel number (counts/0.5 mm^2, 10 fields) in "hotspot" stromal areas was counted.   Mammary carcinomas in the Se-fed rats was 34% (Expt 1) and 24% (Expt 2) lower than in those of rats fed the control diet (Table 3).

Table 3. Effects of a chemopreventive level of dietary Se as either Se-garlic (EXPT 1) or selenite (EXPT 2) on the microvessel density (counts/0.5 mm^2) of 1-methyl-1-nitrosourea-induced rat mammary carcinomas and non-involved mammary glands. Adapted from Ref. 4.

Dietary group		Large $\phi>9$	Medium $\phi5-9$	Small $\phi1-4$ cells	Total vessels
Experiment 1					
Carcinomas					
Control	n=9	5±1	10±1	**55±6**	**69±6**
Se-garlic	n=6	3±1	8±2	**35±6**	**46±6**
Mammary glands					
Control	n=6	1.8±0.5	2.7±0.4	4.2±0.8	8.7±0.7
Se-garlic	n=6	1.3±0.4	2.0±0.7	3.8±0.6	7.2±0.9
Experiment 2					
Carcinomas					
Control	n=8	0.9±0.4	4±2	**75±5**	**80±4**
Selenite	n=4	0.3±0.3	4±3	**57±2**	**61±3**

Mean ± sem. Bold face pairs are significantly different (p<0.05).

When categorized by the size of the microvessels, the observed reduction of microvessel density in the Se-fed groups was almost exclusively confined to the small microvessels (1-4 cells in diameter). The microvessel density of the uninvolved mammary glands was not decreased by Se-garlic treatment (Table 3). Similar results were obtained when established mammary carcinomas were treated acutely through bolus doses of Se (4). These results indicated a potential anti-angiogenic effect of chemopreventive intake of Se and that the effect was neoplasia-specific. Because growing and newly sprout microvessels are likely to be smaller, the observed reduction of small vessels by Se treatment indicated that mechanism(s) governing the genesis of new vessels might be inhibited.

Multiple mechanisms are likely for the anti-angiogenic activity (4)

Sustained angiogenesis depends on the concerted coordination and participation of the following processes (27-29). The angiogenic stimulus (angiogenic factors such as VEGF, FGF, hypoxia, etc.) must be maintained; the endothelial cells must secrete MMPs required to break down the extracellular and adjacent tissue matrix; the endothelial cells must be capable of movement/migration; and endothelial cells must proliferate to provide the necessary number of cells for the growing vessels. To define the potential contribution of these elements, we have examined the expression of VEGF, a primary angiogenic mediator, in Se-treated tumors and also the effects of direct Se exposure in cell culture on the proliferation and survival and MMPs of human umbilical vein endothelial cells (HUVEC). Preliminary results are summarized below.

(A) Selenium decreases expression of VEGF in some carcinomas. The expression level of VEGF in mammary carcinomas was measured by Western blot analyses (Figure 4A). Based on the limited number of samples analyzed, 2 out of 5 carcinomas in the Se-garlic group and 2 out of 4 carcinomas in the selenite group (4) showed a marked reduction in VEGF expression to almost non-detectable levels. These results indicated that VEGF down regulation might be involved in some, but not all, tumors. Similar to the chemoprevention setting, acute Se treatment of established mammary carcinomas showed a marked reduction of VEGF expression in some, but not all, treated carcinomas (4).

(B) Selenium induces apoptosis of endothelial cells. Treatment of HUVEC with MSeA in monolayer culture led to cell retraction and detachment from flask and such changes started to appear 12 h after treatment was initiated. Most affected cells displayed morphological apoptotic features as indicated by nuclear condensation and formation of apoptotic bodies. Re-plating these detached cells in fresh medium did not result in any cell attachment or growth. By 48 h of MSeA treatment, adherent cell number was reduced by as much as 80% at 2 μM (a level achievable in human blood) and

virtually no cell remained attached at 6 μM MSeA (Figure 4B). The cytocidal
effect of MSeA was ~4 fold more efficacious than selenite.

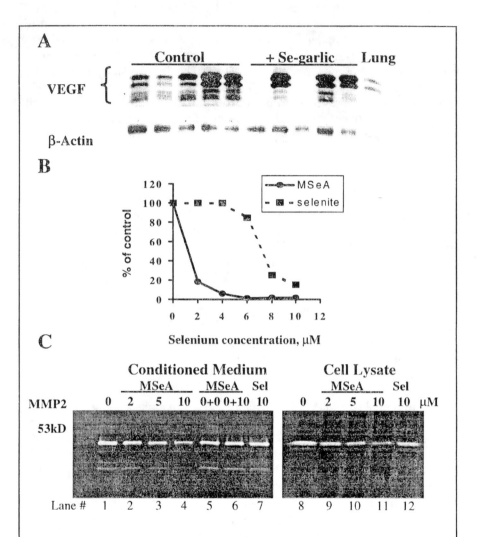

Figure 4. A. Representative Western blot analysis of expression of VEGF proteins in
MNU-induced rat mammary carcinomas after the rats were fed for 2 months a control diet
(0.1 ppm Se) or 3 ppm Se as Se-garlic. Actin was re-probed for correction of loading
differences. A lung sample was included as a positive control for VEGF proteins. **B**.
Effect of Se as selenite or methylseleninic acid (MSeA) on HUVEC cell number remaining
adherent after 48 h treatment. Apoptotic cells detached from culture vessels. **C**. Effect of
Se on HUVEC MMPs after 6 h treatment as detected by zymography on type I gelatin gels.
Lanes 5 & 6 were control conditioned medium incubated for 6 h with PBS or MSeA to
determine whether MSeA *per se* inactivated MMPs. Sel, sodium selenite. Adapted from
ref. 4.

This comparison indicated that the inhibitory effect did not result from a direct reaction of MSeA *per se* with the secreted MMPs and was therefore dependent on cell activation to generate methylselenol. This *(C)*

(C) Methylselenol specifically inhibits endothelial MMPs. Treatment with MSeA led to a Se concentration-dependent inhibition of the gelatinolytic activity in both the conditioned medium and the cell lysate (Figure 4C) of the 72kD gelatinase A/MMP-2 and a 53 kD MMP. Methylselenocyanate (MSeCN) treatment had a comparable inhibitory potency as MSeA (unpublished data). Incubating the conditioned medium from the untreated cells for 6 h at 37°C with 10 μM MSeA in a test tube did not inhibit MMPs (lanes 7 vs. 6). This comparison indicated that the inhibitory effect did not result from a direct reaction of MseA *per se* with the secreted MMPs and was therefore dependent on cell activation to generate methylselenol. This postulation was consistent with a time course experiment in which the inhibitory action of MSeA on MMPs followed a 10 min delay, probably a reflection of time needed for this active Se metabolite to reach a critical intracellular level (unpublished data).

In contrast to methylselenol precursors, treatment with 10 μM selenite for 6 h did not inhibit the MMPs (Figure 4C, lanes 7 vs. 1 and 12 vs. 8). Na_2Se had no inhibitory effect when provided at a concentration (~25 μM) that produced a similar extent of cell number reduction as MSeA (unpublished data). These results indicate that the proximal Se metabolite for MMP inhibition is methylselenol and that the MMP inhibitory effect is independent of apoptosis, which requires continued exposure of greater than 12 h. This discovery not only provides a specific mechanism for methylselenol to inhibit angiogenic sprouting (30,31), but also has mechanistic implications on processes, such as lesion progression and metastasis, that require MMPs for extracellular matrix degradation and remodeling (32,33).

CONCLUSIONS AND IMPLICATIONS

The data reviewed above support the apoptogenic activities of two pools of proximal Se metabolites, hydrogen selenide and methylselenol, that are mediated by distinct biochemical and cellular pathways. Compared to our understanding of the sequence of events in selenite/selenide induced growth arrest and apoptosis, much work is needed to elucidate the biochemical and molecular mechanisms underlying the apoptogenic activity of the methylselenol pool. Furthermore, the data support a methylselenol-specific inhibitory activity on endothelial MMPs. In addition to its involvement in angiogenesis regulation, methylselenol may therefore have a potential inhibitory activity on lesion progression and metastasis as they represent processes that require MMPs for extracellular matrix degradation and remodeling. The MMP inhibitory activity of methylselenol may underlie the increased *in vivo* efficacy of forms of Se that are precursors of this Se pool in comparison to selenite and other Se-amino acids (1). Considering the potential mutagenic side effects of genotoxicity on normal cells, Se compounds that feed into the hydrogen selenide pool may be less desirable for chemoprevention use by humans. Conversely, Se compounds that enter the methylselenol pool may be more desirable Se forms for human applications.

An Integrated Model for Cancer Prevention by Se

Much mechanistic research effort has so far focused on how Se affects the cancer epithelial cells. Because epithelial lesions do not exist in isolation *in vivo*, but instead intimately interact with the stroma and vasculature, cancer prevention mechanisms by Se should and must integrate the actions of Se on epithelial as well as non-epithelial targets. Figure 5 schematically illustrates a model based on this thesis. The angiogenesis aspect of the work reviewed here is consistent with a potential for Se to regulate non-epithelial targets.

It is probable that apoptogenic activity in the cancer epithelial cells may be triggered by Se through mechanisms reviewed above, if the Se metabolites (hydrogen selenide or methylselenol) can reach critical concentrations in the target cells. However, the physio-chemistry of Se delivery to transformed epithelial cells in *in vivo* lesions may be a major determinant of the actual mechanism(s) as well as the process(es) that are invoked to regulate the epithelial cell fate and growth. It is speculated that Se delivery to epithelial cells in the avascular lesions may follow a concentration gradient similar to oxygen tension that has been known to decline precipitously as the distance to the nearby microvessel increases, resulting in hypoxic state in the interior of such lesions (34,35) (Figure 5). Should such a declining gradient exist for Se, a "conditional Se deficiency" state may be created inside expanding avascular epithelial lesions even when the Se supply is sufficient to saturate selenoprotein activities in the serum or normal tissues. This model predicts that more Se is required to enrich the Se metabolite pools in the avascular lesions in order to elicit the anti-proliferative and apoptotic pathways in the transformed epithelial cells. This model may warrant a re-evaluation of the current paradigm that discounts the likelihood of involvement of selenoproteins for the chemopreventive activity of Se (1,2). For example, is it possible that Se intake much higher than that is required to saturate serum/tissue selenoproteins will be needed to optimize the activity of key selenoproteins such as thioredoxin reductase and Se-Gpx's in the epithelial lesions so as to re-regulate their transformation status/physiology?

This model also highlights the need for investigations that incorporate hypoxia as a feature of the solid lesions when evaluating the efficacy of Se to induce growth arrest and cell death responses. Hypoxia is known to affect cellular energy metabolism (34,35) and therefore it may affect the cellular redox status. It would be important to address whether a hypoxic state alters the apoptogenic efficacy of the different pools of Se metabolites. Hypoxia is also a known potent stimulus for the angiogenic switch. An inhibitory activity by Se on the ability of the epithelial lesions to produce angiogenic factors is an avenue through which Se may regulate angiogenesis and cancer. The observed effect of Se on VEGF expression is consistent with this thesis.

In contrast to the Se delivery physics in epithelial lesions, the endothelial cells in the vasculature are the first line of exposure to blood Se. Direct anti-proliferative and apoptogenic action on vascular endothelial cells as well as inhibitory activity on their MMPs by methylselenol may therefore present a likely and perhaps more significant avenue for Se to inhibit avascular lesion expansion/growth through blocking angiogenesis, provided that the Se actions are preferential against tumor/neo-angiogenesis. The angiogenic microenvironment during clonal expansion and lesion progression may provide a plausible biological basis for such desired selectivity. Sustained angiogenic stimulation provided by the transformed cells in the lesion sites will elicit concerted actions of MMPs, motility and cell division for angiogenic sprouting. It is possible and probable that angiogenically-stimulated endothelial cells, not the quiescent ones in the normal vessels/tissues, may be preferentially targeted for action by blood Se.

It is my hope that the model presented here can serve as a new paradigm to stimulate Se research in both the non-epithelial and the epithelial targets. With such an integrated approach, a more comprehensive mechanistic understanding may be achieved on how Se exerts its cancer preventive activity.

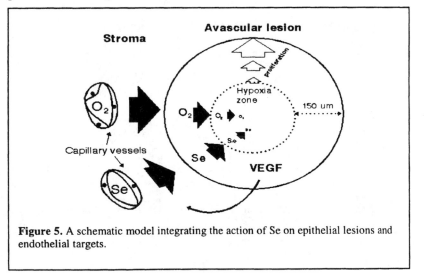

Figure 5. A schematic model integrating the action of Se on epithelial lesions and endothelial targets.

ACKNOWLEDGMENTS

Data cited in this presentation represented team efforts of many individuals including Henry Thompson, Cheng Jiang, Mark Kaeck, Weiqin Jiang, Zaisen Wang, Hongying Pei, Gretchen Garcia and Adrian Wilson at AMC and our collaborators Howard Ganther and Clement Ip. Work in the Lu laboratory was supported by grants from American Institute for Cancer Research 97AO83 and Department of Defense BC980909.

REFERENCES

1. Ip C. Lessons from basic research in selenium and cancer prevention. J Nutr. 1998; 128:1845-1854.
2. Combs GF Jr and Gray WP. Chemopreventive agents: selenium. Pharmacol Ther. 1998; 79:179-192.
3. Clark LC, Combs GF Jr, Turnbull BW, et. al. Effects of selenium supplementation for cancer prevention in patients with carcinoma of the skin. A randomized controlled trial. Nutritional Prevention of Cancer Study Group. JAMA. 1996; 276: 1957-1963.
4. Jiang C, Jiang W, Ip C, Ganther H and Lu JX. Selenium-induced inhibition of angiogenesis in mammary cancer at chemopreventive levels of intake. Mol. Carcinogenesis. 1999. In press.
5. Ganther HE. Selenium metabolism, selenoproteins, and mechanisms of cancer prevention: complexities with thioredoxin reductase. Carcinogenesis, 1999. 20:1657-1666. Review.
6. Ip C and Ganther HE. Activity of methylated forms of selenium in cancer prevention. Cancer Res 1990; 50:1206-1211.
7. Ip C, Hayes C, Budnick RM, and Ganther HE. Chemical form of selenium, critical metabolites, and cancer prevention. Cancer Res 1991; 51:595-600.
8. Ganther HE. Pathways of selenium metabolism including respiratory excretory products. J Am. Coll. Toxicol. 1986; 5:1-5.
9. El-Bayoumy K, Upadhyaya P, Chae YH, Sohn OS, Rao CV, Fiala E, Reddy BS. Chemoprevention of cancer by organoselenium compounds. J Cell Biochem Suppl. 1995; 22:92-100. Review.
10. Snyder RD. Effects of sodium selenite on DNA and carcinogen-induced DNA repair in human diploid fibroblasts. Cancer Lett. 1987; 34:73-81.
11. Garberg P, Stahl A, Warholm M, Hogberg J. Studies of the role of DNA fragmentation in selenium toxicity. Biochem Pharmacol. 1988; 37:3401-3406.
12. Wilson AC, Thompson HJ, Schedin PJ, Gibson NW, Ganther HE. Effect of methylated forms of selenium on cell viability and the induction of DNA strand breakage. Biochem Pharmacol. 1992; 43:1137-41.
13. Seko Y, Saito Y, Kitahara J. and Imura N. Active oxygen generation by the reaction of selenite with reduced glutathione in vitro. In: Proceedings of the 4th International Symposium on Selenium in Biology and Medicine (Ed. Wendel A). Springer, Heidelburg, Germany. 1989. pp 70-73.
14. Yan L and Spallholz JE. Generation of reactive oxygen species from the reaction of selenium compounds with thiols and mammary tumor cells. Biochem Pharmacol. 1993; 45:429-37.
15. Lu J, Kaeck M, Jiang C, Wilson AC, Thompson HJ. Selenite induction of DNA

strand breaks and apoptosis in mouse leukemic L1210 cells.   Biochem Pharmacol. 1994; 47:1531-1535.

16. Lu J, Kaeck MR, Jiang C, Garcia G, Thompson HJ. A filter elution assay for the simultaneous detection of DNA double and single strand breaks.   Anal Biochem. 1996; 235:227-233.

17. Cho DY, Jung U, Chung AS.   Induction of apoptosis by selenite and selenodiglutathione in HL-60 cells: correlation with cytotoxicity. Biochem Mol Biol Int. 1999; 47:781-793.

18. Shen HM, Yang CF, Ong CN. Sodium selenite-induced oxidative stress and apoptosis in human hepatoma HepG2 cells. Int J Cancer. 1999; 81:820-828.

19. Stewart MS, Spallholz JE, Neldner KH, Pence BC. Selenium compounds have disparate abilities to impose oxidative stress and induce apoptosis. Free Radic Biol Med. 1999; 26:42-48.

20. Davis RL, Spallholz JE, Pence BC. Inhibition of selenite-induced cytotoxicity and apoptosis in human colonic carcinoma (HT-29) cells by copper. Nutr Cancer. 1998; 32:181-189.

21. Stewart MS, Davis RL, Walsh LP, Pence BC. Induction of differentiation and apoptosis by sodium selenite in human colonic carcinoma cells (HT29). Cancer Lett. 1997; 117:35-40.

22. Zhu Z, Kimura M, Itokawa Y, Aoki T, Takahashi JA, Nakatsu S, Oda Y, Kikuchi H. Apoptosis induced by selenium in human glioma cell lines. Biol Trace Elem Res. 1996; 54:123-134.

23. Lu J, Jiang C, Kaeck M, Ganther H, Vadhanavikit S, Ip C and Thompson HJ. Dissociation of the genotoxic and growth inhibitory effects of selenium. Biochem Pharmacol 1995; 50: 213-219.

24. Lu J, Pei H, Ip C, Lisk D, Ganther H and Thompson HJ. Effect of an aqueous extract of selenium enriched garlic on in vitro markers and in vivo efficacy in cancer prevention. Carcinogenesis, 1996; 17:1903-1907.

25. Kaeck M, Lu J, Strange R, Ip C, Ganther HE, Thompson HJ. Differential induction of growth arrest inducible genes by selenium compounds.   Biochem Pharmacol 1997; 53:921-926.

26. Sinha R, Medina D. Inhibition of cdk2 kinase activity by methylselenocysteine in synchronized mouse mammary epithelial tumor cells.   Carcinogenesis. 1997; 18:1541-1547.

27. Folkman J. Tumor angiogenesis: therapeutic implications. N Engl J Med. 1971; 285:1182-1186.

28. Folkman J. New perspectives in clinical oncology from angiogenesis research. Eur J Cancer. 1996; 32A:2534-2539.

29. Hanahan D, Folkman J. Patterns and emerging mechanisms of the angiogenic switch during tumorigenesis. Cell. 1996; 86:353-364.

30. Itoh T, Tanioka M, Yoshida H, Yoshioka T, Nishimoto H, Itohara S.   Reduced angiogenesis and tumor progression in gelatinase A-deficient mice.   Cancer Res. 1998; 58:1048-1051.

31. Hiraoka N, Allen E, Apel IJ, Gyetko MR, Weiss SJ. Matrix metalloproteinases regulate neovascularization by acting as pericellular fibrinolysins.   Cell. 1998; 95:365-377.

32. Deryugina EI, Bourdon MA, Reisfeld RA, Strongin A. Remodeling of collagen matrix by human tumor cells requires activation and cell surface association of matrix metalloproteinase-2. Cancer Res. 1998; 58:3743-3750.

33. Zetter BR. Angiogenesis and tumor metastasis. Annu Rev Med. 1998; 49:407-424.

34. Sutherland RM. Cell and environment interactions in tumor microregions: the multicell spheroid model. Science. 1988; 240:177-184.

35. Brown JM, Giaccia AJ. The unique physiology of solid tumors: opportunities (and problems) for cancer therapy.   Cancer Res. 1998; 58:1408-1416.

RESVERATROL INHIBITS THE EXPRESSION OF CYCLOOXYGENASE-2 IN MAMMARY EPITHELIAL CELLS[*]

Kotha Subbaramaiah and Andrew J. Dannenberg

Department of Medicine, New York Presbyterian Hospital
Cornell and Anne Fisher Nutrition Center
Strang Cancer Prevention Center
New York, New York 10021

INTRODUCTION

Cyclooxygenases (COX) catalyze the synthesis of prostaglandins (PGs) from arachidonic acid. There are two isoforms of COX, designated COX-1 and COX-2. COX-1 is a housekeeping gene that is expressed constitutively in most tissues (1). In contrast, COX-2 is undetectable in most normal tissues but is induced by mitogenic and inflammatory stimuli (2-4).

There is growing evidence that COX-2 is important in carcinogenesis. For example, COX-2 is overexpressed in transformed cells (2,5,6) and in malignant tissues (7-10) whereas levels of COX-1 remain essentially unchanged. Moreover, a null mutation for COX-2 in $APC^{\Delta716}$ knockout mice, a murine model of familial adenomatous polyposis, markedly reduces the number and size of intestinal tumors (11). Furthermore, treatment with a selective inhibitor of COX-2 caused nearly complete suppression of azoxymethane-induced colon cancer (12). These studies suggest that targeted inhibition of

Nutrition and Cancer Prevention, edited under the auspices of AICR
Kluwer Academic / Plenum Publishers, New York, 2000.

COX-2 is a promising approach to prevent cancer. Although chemopreventive strategies have focused on specific inhibitors of COX-2 enzyme activity, an equally important strategy may be to identify compounds that suppress amounts of COX-2 (13-15).

Resveratrol, a phytoalexin found in grapes and other foods, has anti-inflammatory and anti-cancer effects (Fig. 1)(16).

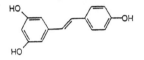

Figure 1. Structure of resveratrol.

It inhibits the development of preneoplastic lesions in carcinogen-treated mouse mammary glands, for example; and it blocks tumorigenesis in a two-stage model of skin cancer that was promoted by treatment with phorbol ester (PMA) (16). The anti-inflammatory properties of resveratrol were demonstrated by suppression of carrageenan-induced pedal edema, an effect attributed to suppression of PG synthesis (16). In this study, we have extended upon prior observations concerning the effects of resveratrol on PG synthesis by determining if resveratrol inhibits the induction of COX-2 by PMA. Our data show that resveratrol suppresses the activation of COX-2 gene expression by inhibiting the PKC signal transduction pathway. These data provide a mechanistic basis for the chemopreventive and anti-inflammatory properties of resveratrol.

MATERIALS AND METHODS

Materials

MEM medium, PKC assay kits and LipofectAMINE were from Life Technologies, Inc. (Grand Island, NY). Keratinocyte basal medium (KBM) was from Clonetics Corp. (San Diego, CA). Phorbol 12-myristate 13-acetate, sodium arachidonate, <u>trans</u>-resveratrol, epidermal growth factor, hydrocortisone and o-nitrophenyl-β-D-galactopyranoside were from Sigma Chemical Co. (St. Louis, MO). Enzyme immunoassay reagents for PGE_2 assays were from

Cayman Co. (Ann Arbor, MI). [^{32}P]-CTP was from DuPont-NEN (Boston, MA). Random-priming kits were from Boehringer Mannheim Biochemicals (Indianapolis, IN). Nitrocellulose membranes were from Schleicher & Schuell (Keene, NH). Reagents for the luciferase assay were from Analytical Luminescence (San Diego, CA). The 18S rRNA cDNA was from Ambion, Inc. (Austin, TX). Rabbit polyclonal anti-human COX-2 antiserum was from Oxford Biomedical Research, Inc. (Oxford, MI). Goat polyclonal anti-human COX-1 antiserum was from Santa Cruz Biotechnology, Inc. (Santa Cruz, CA). Western blotting detection reagents (ECL) were from Amersham (Arlington Heights, Ill.). Plasmid DNA was prepared using a kit from Promega Corp. (Madison, WI).

Tissue Culture

The 184B5/HER cell line has been described previously (17). Cells were maintained in MEM-KBM mixed in a ratio of 1:1 (basal medium) containing EGF (10 ng/ml), hydrocortisone (0.5 µg/ml), transferrin (10 µg/ml), gentamicin (5 µg/ml) and insulin (10 µg/ml). Cells were grown to 60% confluence, trypsinized with 0.05% trypsin-2 mM EDTA, and plated for experimental use. In all experiments, 184B5/HER cells were grown in basal medium for 24 h prior to treatment. Treatment with vehicle (0.2% DMSO), resveratrol or PMA was always carried out in basal medium.

PGE$_2$ Production

5 X 10^4 cells/well were plated in 6-well dishes and grown to 60% confluence. Levels of PGE$_2$ released by the cells were measured by enzyme immunoassay. Amounts of PGE$_2$ produced were normalized to protein concentrations.

Western blotting

Analysis was done with a rabbit polyclonal anti-COX-2 antiserum or a polyclonal anti-COX-1 antiserum as described in detail in Ref. 15.

Northern Blotting

Analysis was done with a radiolabeled human COX-2 cDNA as described in Ref. 15.

Nuclear Run-off Assay

2.5 X 10^5 cells were plated in four T150 dishes for each condition.

Cells were grown until approximately 60% confluent prior to experimental treatment. Nuclei were isolated and stored in liquid nitrogen. The transcription assay was performed as described previously (15).

Plasmids

The COX-2 promoter construct (-327/+59) was a gift of Dr. Tadashi Tanabe (National Cardiovascular Center Research Institute, Osaka, Japan) (18). The human COX-2 cDNA was generously provided by Dr. Stephen M. Prescott (University of Utah, Salt Lake City, UT). RSV-c-jun was a gift from Dr. Tom Curran (Roche Laboratories, Nutley, NJ). The AP-1 reporter plasmid (2xTRE-luciferase), composed of two copies of the consensus TRE ligated to luciferase, was kindly provided by Dr. Joan Heller Brown (University of California, La Jolla, CA). pSV-βgal was obtained from Promega Corp. (Madison, WI).

Transient Transfection Assays

184B5/HER cells were seeded at a density of 5×10^4 cells/well in 6-well dishes and grown to 50-60% confluence. Transfections and analyses were carried out as described previously (15).

Protein Kinase C Assay

The activity of PKC was measured according to directions from Life Technologies, Inc. Briefly, cells were plated in 10 cm dishes at 10^6 cells/dish and grown to 60% confluence. Cells were then treated with fresh basal medium containing vehicle (0.2% DMSO), PMA (50 ng/ml) or PMA (50 ng/ml) plus resveratrol (15 µM) for 30 min. Total PKC activity was measured in cell lysates. To determine cytosolic and membrane bound PKC activity, cell lysates were centrifuged at 100,000 x g for 30 min. The resulting supernatant contains cytosolic PKC; membrane bound PKC activity is present in the pellet. Subsequently, DEAE cellulose columns were used to partially purify PKC enzymes. Protein kinase C activity was then measured by incubating partially purified PKC with $[\gamma\text{-}^{32}P]ATP$ (3000-6000 Ci/mmol) and the substrate myelin basic protein for 20 min at room temperature. The activity of PKC is expressed as CPM incorporated/µg protein.

Statistics

Comparisons between groups were made by the Student's t test. A difference between groups of $P < 0.05$ was considered significant.

RESULTS

Resveratrol inhibits the induction of COX-2 by phorbol esters

The possibility that resveratrol inhibited PMA-mediated induction of PGE_2 synthesis was investigated. Cells were co-treated for 4.5 h with PMA and the indicated concentrations of resveratrol. The medium then was replaced, and the synthesis of PGs was measured in the absence of resveratrol over the next 30 min. PMA in this setting caused about a 2-fold increase in synthesis of PGE_2. This effect was suppressed by resveratrol in a dose-dependent manner (Fig. 2).

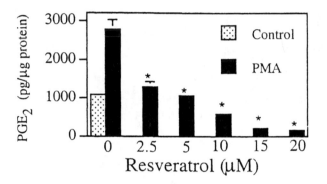

Figure 2. Resveratrol inhibits phorbol ester-mediated induction of PGE_2 synthesis. 184B5/HER cells were treated with vehicle (stippled column), PMA (50 ng/ml, black column) or PMA (50 ng/ml) and resveratrol for 4.5 h. The medium was then replaced with basal medium and 10 µM sodium arachidonate. Thirty min later, the medium was collected to measure the amount of production of PGE_2. Synthesis of PGE_2 was determined by enzyme immunoassay. Columns, means; bars, SD; n=6. *, P<0.001 compared with PMA.

Immunoblotting was performed to determine whether the above effects on production of PGE_2 could be related to differences in levels of COX. Figure 3 shows that PMA induced COX-2 in human mammary epithelial cells, an effect that was suppressed by resveratrol in a dose-dependent manner. Neither PMA nor resveratrol altered amounts of COX-1 (data not shown).

To further elucidate the mechanism responsible for the changes in amounts of COX-2 protein, steady-state levels of COX-2 mRNA were determined.

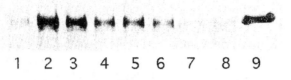

Figure 3. Resveratrol inhibits PMA-mediated induction of COX-2 in human mammary epithelial cells. Lysate protein was from 184B5/HER cells treated with vehicle (lane 1), PMA (50 ng/ml, lane 2) or PMA (50 ng/ml) and resveratrol (2.5, 5, 7.5, 10, 15, 30 μM; lanes 3-8) for 4.5 h. Lane 9 represents an ovine COX-2 standard. Cellular lysate protein (25 μg/lane) was loaded onto a 10% SDS-polyacrylamide gel, electrophoresed and subsequently transferred onto nitrocellulose. The blot was probed with antibody specific for COX-2.

Treatment with PMA resulted in a marked increase in levels of COX-2 mRNA, an effect that was suppressed by resveratrol in a concentration dependent manner (Fig. 4).

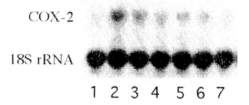

Figure 4. Resveratrol inhibits PMA-mediated induction of COX-2 mRNA. 184B5/HER cells were treated with vehicle (lane 1), PMA (50 ng/ml, lane 2) or PMA (50 ng/ml) and resveratrol (2.5, 5, 10, 15, 20 μM; lanes 3-7) for 3 h. Total cellular RNA was isolated; 10 μg of RNA was added to each lane. The Northern blot was hybridized with probes that recognized mRNAs for COX-2 and 18S rRNA. Results of densitometry in arbitrary units: lane 1, 18; lane 2, 225; lane 3, 135; lane 4, 72; lane 5, 45; lane 6, 42; lane 7, 9.

Nuclear run-offs were performed to determine if these differences in levels of mRNA reflected altered rates of COX-2 transcription. As shown in Fig. 5, we observed higher rates of synthesis of nascent COX-2 mRNA after treatment with PMA, consistent with the differences observed by Northern blotting. This effect was suppressed by resveratrol.

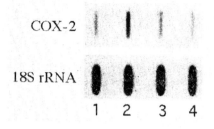

COX-2

18S rRNA

1   2   3   4

Figure 5. Phorbol ester-mediated induction of COX-2 transcription is inhibited by resveratrol. 184B5/HER cells were treated with vehicle (lane 1), PMA (50 ng/ml, lane 2) or PMA (50 ng/ml) and resveratrol (5 µM, lane 3; 10 µM, lane 4) for 3 h. Nuclear run-offs were performed. The COX-2 and 18S rRNA cDNAs were immobilized onto nitrocellulose membranes and hybridized with labeled nascent RNA transcripts. Results of densitometry in arbitrary units: lane 1, 19; lane 2, 44; lane 3, 29; lane 4, 16.

Determining the mechanism by which resveratrol inhibits PMA-mediated induction of COX-2

PMA regulates COX-2 gene expression by activating the PKC signal transduction pathway. A key feature of this mechanism is the translocation of PKC activity from cytosol to membrane. Hence, we determined whether resveratrol inhibited PMA-mediated activation of PKC or AP-1. Treatment of cells with PMA stimulated the translocation of PKC activity from cytosol to membrane, an effect that was blocked by resveratrol (Fig. 6).

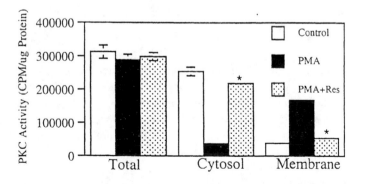

Figure 6. Resveratrol inhibits the redistribution of PKC activity mediated by phorbol ester. 184B5/HER cells were treated with vehicle (open column), PMA (50 ng/ml, black column) or PMA (50 ng/ml) and resveratrol (15 µM) (stippled column) for 30 min. Total, cytosolic and membrane PKC activities were determined. Columns, means; bars, SD. n=6, *, P<0.01 vs. PMA.

Additionally, transiently overexpressing c-Jun, a component of the AP-1
transcription factor complex, caused about a 4-fold increase in COX-2 promoter
activity. This effect was blocked by resveratrol (Fig. 7A). Resveratrol also
suppressed the activation of an AP-1 reporter plasmid by PMA (Fig. 7B).

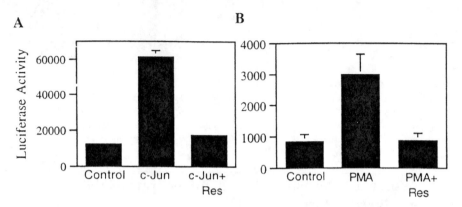

Figure 7. Resveratrol inhibits AP-1-mediated induction of COX-2 promoter activity. A,
184B5/HER cells were transfected with 0.9 μg of a human COX-2 promoter construct ligated to
luciferase (-327/+59) (control) or 0.9 μg of COX-2 promoter construct and 0.9 μg of expression
vector for c-jun. All cells received 0.2 μg of pSVβgal. The total amount of DNA in each reaction
was kept constant at 2 μg by using empty vector. Twenty four h later, cells were treated with
vehicle or resveratrol (15 μM) for 6 h. B, 184B5/HER cells were co-transfected with 1.8 μg of
2xTRE-luciferase and 0.2 μg of pSVβgal. Twenty four h after transfection, cells were treated with
vehicle, PMA (50 ng/ml) or PMA (50 ng/ml) and resveratrol (15 μM) for 6 h. Luciferase activity
represents data that have been normalized with β-galactosidase activity. Six wells were used for
each of the conditions. Columns, means; bars, SD.

DISCUSSION

There is considerable evidence that inhibitors of COX-2 are useful for
treating inflammation and preventing cancer (11,12,19). Compounds that
interfere with the signaling mechanisms that up-regulate COX-2 should also be
useful in this regard because they too decrease COX-2 activity (13,14). We
have shown in the present experiments that resveratrol suppressed PMA-
mediated induction of PG synthesis at least, in part, by inhibiting COX-2 gene
expression (15).

Tumor-promoting phorbol esters induce COX-2 gene expression by
activating the PKC pathway (20). A downstream target of activated PKC is the
AP-1 transcription factor complex. Resveratrol suppressed PMA-mediated
activation of COX-2 transcription by inhibiting the PKC signal transduction
pathway at multiple levels. It blocked both PMA-induced translocation of PKC

activity from cytosol to membrane (Fig. 6), and the increase in COX-2 promoter activity mediated by c-Jun (Fig. 7). These inhibitory effects can be explained, in part, by the antioxidant properties of resveratrol since other phenolic antioxidants inhibit both PMA-mediated activation of PKC and AP-1 (21,22). These results are significant because PKC activity is up-regulated in some cancers and is considered a potential target for anti-cancer therapy (23). Additionally, since AP-1 has been implicated in promoting carcinogenesis, these effects are likely to contribute to the anti-tumor activity of resveratrol.

Xie and Herschman showed that the AP-1 transcription factor complex is important for the activation of the murine COX-2 promoter via a cyclic AMP response element (CRE) (24). Thus, it is possible that resveratrol blocks PMA-mediated induction of COX-2 by suppressing AP-1-dependent transactivation via the CRE. The anti-AP-1 effect of resveratrol can potentially be explained if resveratrol induced Fra expression like other phenolic antioxidants (25). Heterodimers of c-Jun and Fra do not activate AP-1-mediated gene expression as effectively as c-Jun homodimers or c-Jun/c-Fos heterodimers (26). Alternatively, resveratrol could suppress PMA-mediated increases in AP-1 activity by inhibiting the induction or phosphorylation of c-Jun (27).

We reported previously that retinoids blocked PMA-mediated induction of COX-2 in oral epithelial cells (13). The same effect of retinoids was observed in the human mammary epithelial cells used in this study. However, whereas resveratrol and retinoids both block PMA-mediated induction of COX-2 transcription, they appear to do so via different mechanisms. Thus, in contrast to resveratrol, retinoids did not block the PMA-induced redistribution of PKC activity from cytosol to membrane (data not shown). Additionally, resveratrol and retinoids antagonize AP-1 activity via different mechanisms. Retinoids antagonize AP-1 activity via a receptor-dependent mechanism (28) whereas our data suggest that resveratrol blocks PMA-mediated stimulation of AP-1-activity by inhibiting the PKC signaling cascade. Thus, chemopreventive agents can inhibit AP-1-mediated induction of COX-2 by disrupting PKC signal transduction at different levels in the pathway. Finally, based on the finding that resveratrol inhibited COX-2, further studies are warranted to determine how effective this compound or its analogues will be in preventing or treating inflammation and cancer.

NOTES

*Data in this manuscript were previously reported in Ref. 15.

REFERENCES

1.   Funk,C.D., L.B. Funk, M.E. Kennedy, A.S. Pong. & G.A. FitzGerald. 1991. Human

platelet/erythroleukemia cell prostaglandin G/H synthase: cDNA cloning, expression, and gene chromosomal assignment. FASEB J. 5:2304-2312.

2.   Subbaramaiah,K., N. Telang, J.T. Ramonetti, R. Araki, B. DeVito, B.B. Weksler & A.J. Dannenberg. 1996. Transcription of cyclooxygenase-2 is enhanced in transformed mammary epithelial cells. Cancer Res. 56:4424-4429.

3.   DuBois,R.N., J. Award, J. Morrow, L.J. Roberts & P.R. Bishop. 1994. Regulation of eicosanoid production and mitogenesis in rat intestinal epithelial cells by transforming growth factor-α and phorbol ester. J. Clin. Invest. 93:493-498.

4.   Kelley,D.J., J.R. Mestre, K. Subbaramaiah, P.G. Sacks, S.P. Schantz, T. Tanabe, H. Inoue, J.T. Ramonetti & A.J. Dannenberg. 1997. Benzo[a]pyrene up-regulates cyclooxygenase-2 gene expression in oral epithelial cells. Carcinogenesis 18: 795-799.

5.   Kutchera,W., D.A. Jones, N. Matsunami, J. Groden, T.M. McIntyre, G.A. Zimmerman, R.L. White & S.M. Prescott. 1996. Prostaglandin H synthase-2 is expressed abnormally in human colon cancer: evidence for a transcriptional effect. Proc. Natl. Acad. Sci. USA 93:4816-4820.

6.   Sheng,G.G., J. Shao, H. Sheng, E.B. Hooton, P.C. Isakson, J.D. Morrow, R.J. Coffey, R.N. DuBois & R.D. Beauchamp. 1997. A selective cyclooxygenase-2 inhibitor suppresses the growth of H-ras-transformed rat intestinal epithelial cells. Gastroenterology 113: 1883-1891.

7.   Kargman,S.L., G.P. O'Neil, P.J. Vickers, J.F. Evans, J.A. Mancini & J.A. Jothy. 1995. Expression of prostaglandin G/H synthase-1 and -2 protein in human colon cancer. Cancer Res. 55: 2556-2559.

8.   Chan, G., J.O. Boyle, E.K. Yang, F. Zhang, P.G. Sacks, J.P. Shah, D. Edelstein, R.A. Soslow, A.T. Koki, B.M. Woerner, J.L. Masferrer & A.J. Dannenberg. 1999. Cyclooxygenase-2 gene expression is up-regulated in squamous cell carcinoma of the head and neck. Cancer Res. 59: 991-994.

9.   Ristimaki,A., N. Honkanen, H. Jankala, P. Sipponen & M. Harkonen. 1997. Expression of cyclooxygenase-2 in human gastric carcinoma. Cancer Res. 57: 1276-1280.

10. Tucker, O.N., A.J. Dannenberg, E.K. Yang, F. Zhang, L. Teng, J.M. Daly, R.A. Soslow, J.L. Masferrer, B.M. Woerner, A.T. Koki and T.J. Fahey. 1999. Cyclooxygenase-2 expression is up-regulated in human pancreatic cancer. Cancer Res. 59:987-990.

11. Oshima,M., J.E. Dinchuk, S.L. Kargman, H. Oshima, B. Hancock, E. Kwong, J.M. Trzaskos, J.F. Evans & M.M. Taketo. 1996. Suppression of intestinal polyposis in Apc$^{\Delta716}$ knockout mice by inhibition of cyclooxygenase 2 (Cox-2). Cell 87: 803-809.

12. Kawamori,T., C.V. Rao, K. Seibert & B.S. Reddy. 1998. Chemopreventive activity of celecoxib, a specific cyclooxygenase-2 inhibitor, against colon carcinogenesis. Cancer Res. 58: 409-412.

13. Mestre,J.R., K. Subbaramaiah, P.G. Sacks, S.P. Schantz, T. Tanabe, H. Inoue & A.J. Dannenberg. 1997. Retinoids suppress phorbol ester-mediated induction of cyclooyxgenase-2. Cancer Res. 57: 1081-1085.

14. Mestre,J.R., K. Subbaramaiah, P.G. Sacks, S.P. Schantz, T. Tanabe, H. Inoue & A.J. Dannenberg. 1997. Retinoids suppress epidermal growth factor-induced transcription of cyclooxygenase-2 in human oral squamous carcinoma cells. Cancer Res. 57: 2890-2895.

15. Subbaramaiah,K., W.J. Chung, P. Michaluart, N. Telang, T. Tanabe, H. Inoue, M. Jang, J.M. Pezzuto & A.J. Dannenberg. 1998. Resveratrol inhibits cyclooxygenase-2 transcription and activity in phorbol ester-treated human mammary epithelial cells. J. Biol. Chem. 273: 21875-21882.

16. Jang,M., L. Cai, G.O. Udeani, K.V. Slowing, C.F. Thomas, C.W.W. Beecher, H.H.S. Fong, N.R. Farnsworth, A.D. Kinghorn, R.G. Mehta, R.C. Moon & J.M. Pezzuto. 1997. Cancer chemopreventive activity of resveratrol, a natural product derived from grapes. Science 275: 218-220.

17. Zhai, Y-F., H. Beittenmiller, B. Wang, M.N. Gould, C. Oakley, W.J. Esselman & C.W.

Welsch. 1993. Increased expression of specific protein tyrosine phosphatases in human breast epithelial cells neoplastically transformed by the neu oncogene Cancer Res. 53: 2272-2278.

18. Inoue, H., C. Yokoyama, S. Hara, Y. Tone & T. Tanabe. 1995. Transcriptional regulation of human prostaglandin-endoperoxide synthase-2 gene by lipopolysaccharide and phorbol ester in vascular endothelial cells. J. Biol. Chem. 270: 24965-24971.

19. Masferrer,J.L., B.S. Zweifel, P.T. Manning, S.D. Hauser, K.M. Leahy, W.G. Smith, P.C. Isakson, & K. Seibert. 1994. Selective inhibition of cyclooxygenase-2 in vivo is antiinflammatory and nonulcerogenic. Proc. Natl. Acad. Sci. USA 91: 3228-3232.

20. Subbaramaiah, K., D. Zakim, B.B. Weksler & A.J. Dannenberg. 1997. Inhibition of cyclooxygenase: a novel approach to cancer prevention. Proc. Soc. Exp. Biol. Med. 216, 201-210.

21. Liu,J-Y., S-J. Lin & J-K. Lin. 1993. Inhibitory effects of curcumin on protein kinase C activity induced by 12-O-tetradecanoyl-phorbol-13-acetate in NIH 3T3 cells. Carcinogenesis 14: 857-861.

22. Huang, T-S., S-C. Lee & J-K. Lin. 1991. Suppression of c-Jun/AP-1 activation by an inhibitor of tumor promotion in mouse fibroblast cells. Proc. Natl. Acad. Sci. USA 88: 5292-5296.

23. Gordge, P.C., M.J. Hulme, R.A. Clegg & W.R. Miller. 1996. Elevation of protein kinase A and protein kinase C activities in malignant as compared with normal human breast tissue. Eur. J. Cancer 32A: 2120-2126.

24. Xie, W. & H.R. Herschman. 1995. v-src induces prostaglandin synthase-2 gene expression by activation of c-Jun N-terminal kinase and the c-Jun transcription factor. J. Biol. Chem. 270: 27622-27628.

25. Yoshioka, K., T. Deng, M. Cavigelli & M. Karin. 1995. Antitumor promotion by phenolic antioxidants: inhibition of AP-1 activity through induction of Fra expression. Proc. Natl. Acad. Sci. USA 92:4972-4976.

26. Suzuki, T., H. Okuno, T. Yoshida, T. Endo, H. Nishina & H. Iba. 1992. Difference in transcriptional regulatory function between c-Fos and Fra-2. Nucleic Acids Res. 19: 5537-42.

27. Karin, M. 1995. The regulation of AP-1 activity by mitogen-activated protein kinases. J. Biol. Chem. 270: 16483-16486.

28. Pfahl, M. 1993. Nuclear receptor/AP-1 interaction. Endocrine Rev. 14: 651-658.

13

THE WORLD OF RESVERATROL

George J. Soleas[1] , Eleftherios P. Diamandis[2,3] and
David M. Goldberg[2]

[1]Quality Assurance, Liquor Control Board of Ontario,
Toronto, Ontario, Canada; [2]Department of Laboratory
Medicine and Pathobiology, University of Toronto, Ontario,
Canada; [3]Department of Pathology and Laboratory Medicine,
Mount Sinai Hospital, Toronto, Ontario, Canada

INTRODUCTION

Since the discovery of *trans*-resveratrol (3,5,4'-trihydroxystilbene) as
a constituent of wine by Siemann and Creasy, first reported in 1992 (1), the
possibility that this compound, almost unique to red wine among constituents
of the human diet, may in large measure account for the putative health
benefits of this beverage beyond its mere content of vulgar ethanol, excited
the imagination of the scientific and medical communities, initiating a ferment
of research and enquiry that continues to this day. Indeed, ripples of these
activities from time to time flow into the pages of the lay press, so that
resveratrol has become a molecule impacting the consciousness of many well-
informed members of the lay public. In March, 1997 we published a major
review incorporating 183 references forming the bulk of the world literature
on resveratrol up to that time (2). Our *bottom line* was that the future of
resveratrol did not look particularly promising given the reality that, despite
its miraculous performances in the culture dish and the test tube, the intact

bodies of mice and men proved to be an inhospitable millieu robbing it of its presumed powers. To us, it seemed to be a compound *for whom the bell tolled*, but others did not share this gloomy prognosis. In fact, so much new work on this topic has been published in a mere two years-and-a-bit that a re-appraisal of the situation deserves a welcome and is mandated by the present Symposium. Resveratrol exists as *trans* and *cis* isomers. Very little is known about the latter. When the nature of resveratrol is not specified, the reader should assume that the text refers to the *trans* isomer.

Before plunging into the biological effects of resveratrol, some background concerning its chemical nature, natural occurrence and biosynthesis would appear to be desirable. These themes were in fact extensively described in our earlier review (2), but a brief synopsis of these themes is not out of place and should prove helpful. The statements made will not be referenced since the relevant primary literature is already cited (2). The only further preliminary task is to draw attention to two other short reviews that describe its functions in plant biology (3) and human health (4), respectively.

OCCURRENCE AND FUNCTION OF RESVERATROL IN THE PLANT KINGDOM

More that 30 stilbenes and stilbene glycosides occur naturally among members of the plant kingdom classified as spermatophytes. The essential structural skeleton comprises two aromatic rings joined by a methylene bridge. Resveratrol is a pivotal molecule in plant biology with homologies extending into the realm of mammalian fatty acid metabolism. Its main significance lies in its role as the parent molecule of a family of polymers given the name viniferin. These compounds are able to inhibit fungal infection, a property which has earned their inclusion in the class of plant antibiotics known as phytoalexins. Until 1992, there was no interest in resveratrol from the perspective of mammalian biochemistry or clinical science, but in that year Siemann and Creasy reported the presence of *trans*-resveratrol in wine and drew attention to the fact that it was also a constituent of oriental folk medicines reputed to benefit persons afflicted by a wide range of disorders.

Resveratrol does not enjoy a wide distribution in the plant world, and has been reported in few fruits and vegetables employed for human consumption (Table 1). One of the richest sources is the weed *Polygonum cuspidatum*, root extracts of which have played an important role in Japanese and Chinese folk-medicine. Its occurrence has been documented in a number of trees: these include eucalyptus and spruce. Cotyledons of groundnuts (*Arachis hypogaea*) synthesise an array of phytoalexin stilbenes, including resveratrol, concentrations of which are greatly increased in response to infection, wounding, and irradiation with ultraviolet (but not visible) light.

Most interest has centered upon resveratrol in grapevines (*Vitaceae*) because its function as a phytoalexin and its role as a marker of infection by various pathogens has been intensively investigated in this genus. The first reports describing the presence of resveratrol in grapevine tissues

Table 1. Natural Occurrence of Resveratrol Among Spermatophytes

Type	Species
Weeds	Polygonum cuspidatum
Trees	Eucalyptus Spruce Bauhimia racemosa Scottish pine (pinosylvin)
Plants	Veratrum formosanum Veratrum grandiflorum
Legumes	Pterolobium hexapetallum (non-edible)
Nuts	Arachis hypogaea
Vines	Vitaceae. Present in roots, Canes, leaves and berry skin

and its induction by fungal infection emphasized that ultraviolet irradiation, but not natural sunlight, could stimulate its synthesis as well as that of the viniferins. Whereas none of these phytoalexins are present in healthy vine leaves or berries, they are quite abundant in mature vine wood. Detailed investigations demonstrated a relationship between susceptibility to fungal infection (*Botrytis cinerea*), and the concentrations of stilbenes (resveratrol and viniferins) in the leaves and berries of different *Vitaceae*. Stilbene production in leaves and berries were positively correlated, and there was a negative correlation between stilbene production and susceptibility to *B. cinerea*. Without infection, only very low concentrations of both stilbenes could be detected in these parts of the vine. Resveratrol is not present in the berry flesh, but only in the skins, with very low concentrations found in the latter in the absence of induction. Resistant species produced five-times the maximum concentrations of resveratrol as susceptible species. The concentrations were greatest in the non-infected fruit close to necrotic lesions and appeared to help in limiting their spread. It appears that resveratrol production enables the vine to withstand *Botrytis* attack until climatic conditions (mild and humid) favourable to the pathogen tip the balance against the host. The stimulus to resveratrol production in healthy berries at some distance from infected areas must take the form of a chemical signal regulating stilbene synthase activity, generated by the pathogen or by the infected berries.

BIOSYNTHESIS AND GENE TRANSFER

Resveratrol and related stilbenes are strongly implicated as an important mechanism in host defense against infection and injury among those members of the plant community that can conjure up its existence. Since the gene specifying its synthesis enjoys a very restricted distribution, it is not surprising that crops subject to endemic fungal attack from which it is constitutively absent have become the target of genetic engineering in an attempt to correct this natural deficiency.

The immediate precursors of resveratrol are *p*-coumaroyl CoA and malonyl CoA in a molar ratio of 1-to-3. The latter is derived by elongation of acetyl CoA units and the former from phenylalanine which, in plants, can be synthesised from sugars via the shikimate pathway. The condensation of *p*-coumaroyl CoA with three molecules of malonyl CoA is accomplished through the activity of the stilbene synthase, resveratrol synthase, in most species of the *Vitaceae* and four moles of CO_2 are released for each mole of resveratrol synthesised (Figure 1).

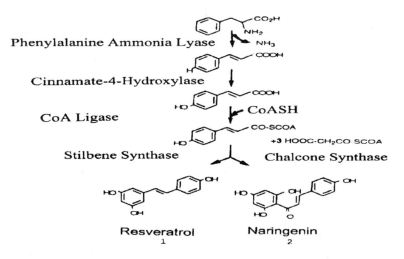

Figure 1. Biosynthetic pathway from phenylalanine to resveratrol.

The *Vitaceae* possess another enzyme, chalcone synthase, which catalyses a reaction involving one molecule of *p*-coumaroyl CoA and three of malonyl CoA, but in this instance only three molecules of CO_2 are generated; the other product is naringenin chalcone which, in a further series of reactions, gives rise to the flavonoid family.

Resveratrol synthase and chalcone synthase are different in this fundamental respect; the latter is expressed constitutively, such that its activity is substrate-driven and its products accumulate in proportion to the generation of precursor sugars during ripening and maturation of the berries, a process stimulated by UV light and possibly accounting for the ability of the latter to modulate its mRNA production. By contrast, the former is normally unexpressed and is inducible only by a range of provocations which include UV-irradiation, trauma and infection. Because of its potential to confer disease resistance upon plants incapable of performing its synthesis, resveratrol and stilbene synthase have been the targets of investigations to transfer the gene specifying its synthesis to disease-susceptible plants lacking this genetic information. The first step was the expression in *E. coli* of a full-length stilbene synthase cDNA prepared from grapevine mRNA yielding an enzymatically-active dimer exhibiting only stilbene synthase activity. Next, the gene from groundnut (*Arachis hypogaea*) that codes for stilbene synthase was transferred to tobacco plants (*Nicotiana tabacum*). Three years later, evidence was presented that the regenerated tobacco plants containing these genes were more resistant to *B. cinerea* infection than the wild type.

INFLAMMATION AND ATHEROSCLEROSIS

These disease processes involve mechanisms common to both, notably activation of polymorphonuclear leukocytes (PMN) with release of cytokines and synthesis of pro-inflammatory eicosanoids. Oxygen free radicals and immune responses also play important roles in their initiation and propagation. By contrast, lipid abnormalities predispose to atherosclerosis but not inflammation as such, while infectious agents are common precursors of inflammation. However, these distinctions are becoming increasingly blurred as our knowledge expands to reveal that in many respects atherosclerosis behaves as an inflammatory disease (5), and that micro-organisms may play a role in its etiology (6).

Resveratrol has been shown to modulate a number of metabolic and enzymatic pathways that are central to the inflammatory response, and has been reported to inhibit carrageenan-induced injury in the mouse (7). These authors attributed the observed protection to down-regulation of cyclo-oxygenase (COX) I, a constitutively expressed enzyme responsible for the biosynthesis of prostaglandins and thromboxanes. Subbaramaiah *et al* (8) subsequently described inhibition by resveratrol of the inducible enzyme

COX II that is increased following stimulation by mitogens such as phorbol ester. This inhibition operated at several levels: direct enzymatic activity, protein and mRNA synthesis, a cyclic AMP response element, protein kinase C, and AP-1-mediated gene expression. Their experiments were performed with human mammary epithelial cells and with resveratrol concentrations in the range 2.5-30 μM. Paradoxically, the same group of investigators were unable to detect resveratrol-induced changes in the COX I or COX II content of mouse skin cells stimulated by phorbol ester (9,10). However, the production of prostaglandin E_2 by an osteoblastic cell line was inhibited by resveratrol (11). It appears, therefore, that the alterations in COX gene expression by resveratrol are not identical in different experimental models of tissue damage, and that they may manifest tissue specificity dependent upon the response evoked by the compound on the expression of c-fos.

In actual fact, COX acts in conjunction with a peroxidase to comprise the Prostaglandin H Synthase (PGHS) multienzyme system. Employing a different *in vitro* model, Johnson and Maddipati found that resveratrol inhibits PGHS-1, but causes a 2-fold increase in the activity of PGHS-2 (12). Inhibition of the peroxidase activity of the former took place with an IC_{50} of 15 μM; the peroxidase activity of the latter was inhibited with an IC_{50} of 200 μM. These data are inconsistent with a number of contemporaneous reports. Resveratrol appears to inhibit the COX activity of PGHS-2 purified from sheep seminal vesicles although with a potency that is only 25-30% of the inhibitory capacity manifested by the resveratrol polymer α-viniferin (13,14). It also inhibits a COX-like enzyme, tentatively identified as a COX-2, from the invertebrate *Ciona intestinalis* (15).

Formation of fibrous tissue to replace necrotic cells is a fundamental and irreversible part of the chronic inflammatory process. In the liver, stellate cells subserve this function. Kawada *et al* demonstrated inhibition by resveratrol of rat hepatic stellate cell proliferation using an *in vitro* model (16). Simultaneously, the following functions were decreased: activity of mitogen-activated protein (MAP) kinase; concentration of the cell cycle protein, cyclin D1; production of nitric oxide and of the pro-inflammatory cytokine tumor necrosis factor α (TNF-α). These effects would be expected to reduce both acute and chronic inflammatory reactions in the liver, but the resveratrol concentrations used were quite high (10-100 μM). A possible protective effect of resveratrol against immunological hepatocyte damage assessed by release of the enzyme alanine aminotransferase into the medium has recently been demonstrated in experiments with cultured hepatocytes (17).

The inhibition by resveratrol of COX and PGSH *in vitro* leads to marked reduction of eicosanoid production in affected cells. This was first demonstrated for rat peritoneal polymorphonuclear leukocytes (18) in which the cyclo-oxygenase pathway (evaluated by the synthesis of HHT and thromboxane B_2) was blocked (IC_{50} around 0.5-1 μM), as was the 5-

lipoxygenase pathway (assessed by 5-HETE production, IC_{50} 2.72 µM). It was subsequently shown that resveratrol inhibited the 5-lipoxygenase and 15-lipoxygenase pathways in washed neutrophils from healthy human subjects with IC_{50} concentrations of 22.4 µM and 8.7 µM, respectively (19), in line with the earlier observations of Kimura and colleagues (20) who reported that resveratrol prevented the formation of an array of 5-lipoxygenase products in human leukocytes (IC_{50} values 1.37-8.90 µM).

The synthesis of eicosanoids by platelets is also blocked by resveratrol. A series of papers by Chinese investigators described its inhibition of thromboxane B_2 production from arachidonate in rabbit platelets (21-23). Similar inhibition of thromboxane B_2 synthesis in human platelets was reported, as well as a modest reduction in the activity of the platelet 12-lipoxygenase pathway leading to the production of pro-atherogenic hepoxillins (24).

Aggregation of platelets is a prelude to thrombus formation, the mechanism that precipitates coronary artery occlusion in the majority of patients who go on to develop acute myocardial infarction. This phenomenon is prevented by resveratrol in rabbit platelets (22,23) and in human platelets (24); in the latter, the IC_{50} is around 10 µM with ADP or thrombin as agonist. Bertelli and colleagues (25,26) reported an IC_{50} for *trans*-resveratrol with human platelets of 15 nmol/l and a slightly lower value for *cis*-resveratrol when collagen was employed as agonist. These are orders of magnitude less than IC_{50} values for various biological effects reported by virtually all other investigators. Moreover, no information was provided about the nature of the *cis*-resveratrol whose synthesis has never been reported, apart from the name of the institution from which it was obtained. Confirmation of the antiplatelet aggregation activity of resveratrol has recently been provided (27).

Contact between circulatory blood cells, especially polymorphonuclear leukocytes and monocytes, and the vascular endothelium is a necessary prelude to the entry of these cells into the underlying intimal layers where the latter can undergo transformation into macrophages that then take up lipids, particularly oxidized LDL, to become the 'foam cells' characteristic of the early atherosclerotic lesion known as the 'fatty streak'. This contact is facilitated by an array of adhesion molecules whose expression is up-regulated by endothelial damage and cytokine signalling typically observed in atherosclerosis (28,29). Resveratrol, in concentrations ranging from 100 nM to 1 µM blocked the expression of at least two of these adhesion molecules in TNFα-stimulated human umbilical vein endothelial cells (30), as shown in Figure 2. It also reduced the expression of the β_2 integrin MAC-1 on the surface of activated human polymorphonuclear leukocytes (31). Both of these functions could have important implications for the potential anti-atherosclerotic role of resveratrol.

The release of lysosomal enzymes from activated PMN leukocytes causes degranulation and contributes to inflammatory damage in adjacent tissues. Resveratrol prevents this secretion in cells stimulated by the calcium ionophore A23187, but the IC_{50} has been reported to be around 0.1-1 mM by

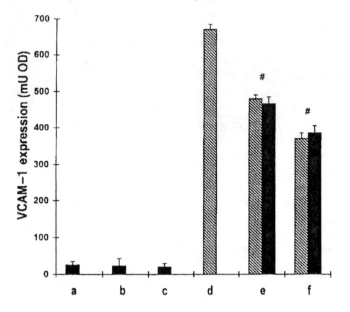

Figure 2: Inhibition by resveratrol of LPS-induced VCAM-1 expression of vascular endothelial cells. The letters represent the following conditions: a. unstimulated cells; b. same with 100 nM resveratrol; c. same with 1 μM resveratrol; d. cells stimulated with LPS; e. same with 100 nM resveratrol; f. same with 1 μM resveratrol; #, P<0.05 (From Ref. 30, with permission).

one group (20) and around 30 μM by other investigators (31). The liberation of β-hexosaminidase from cultured RBL-2H3 cells was also inhibited by resveratrol with an IC_{50} of 14 μM (32).

An important inflammatory pathway involves activation of the transcription factor NF-KB which promotes the synthesis of several cytokines, including TNFα, and nitric oxide (NO); the former can then lead to the release of pro-inflammatory tissue factor (TF). Resveratrol seems to disrupt this pathway, although there is some disagreement about how these effects are accomplished. Tsai *et al* (33) described inhibition of NO generation accompanied by down-regulation of NF-KB in a macrophage cell line stimulated by lipopolysaccharide (LPS) at a resveratrol concentration of 30 μM. Wadsworth and Koop (34) reported that, in concentrations in the range of 50-100 μM, resveratrol did not inhibit LPS-induced activation of NF-KB in the same cell line. It did reduce LPS-induced NO release but enhanced LPS-induced production of TNFα. Oxidized lipoproteins activate NF-KB binding to the promoter region of target genes in PC12 cells, a rat pheochromocytoma cell line, but resveratrol protects the cells against this activation and apoptotic cell death that follows (35). All three groups measured NF-KB activation by the same technique (electrophoretic mobility shift assay).

A further set of investigators found that resveratrol displayed a dose-dependent inhibition of TF expression in endothelial cells stimulated by a variety of agonists, including TNFα and LPS (36). They also showed that resveratrol inhibited LPS-induced expression of TNFα and IL-1β in endothelial cells and monocytes. However, these phenomena could not be attributed to activation of transcription factors (including NF-KB) necessary for induction of the TF promoter in these cells. Resveratrol has also been reported to block the dioxin-induced increase of IL-1β in an endometrial adenocarcinoma cell line (37). Further, production of phorbolester-induced TGF-β1 in mouse skin was inhibited by resveratrol (9,10), although these authors were unable to detect an increased TNFα content in these cells. To summarize, it does appear that resveratrol can attenuate the production of cytokines by vascular cells and peripheral blood cells, but the mechanisms involved remain to be elucidated, especially the issue of whether these effects are indirectly due to radical scavenging activity or whether they are associated with direct alteration of gene expression.

The possibility that resveratrol may modulate lipid metabolism was first proposed by Arichi *et al* (38) who provided resveratrol both orally and intraperitoneally to rats and mice fed a high cholesterol diet, and noted reduced deposition of cholesterol and triglyceride in the livers of these animals, as well as a diminished rate of hepatic triglyceride synthesis. Our group utilized the human hepatoma cell line Hep G2 to study the effects of resveratrol upon lipid and lipoprotein metabolism (19,39). The intracellular content of cholesteryl esters and the rate of secretion of both cholesteryl esters and triglycerides were reduced in a dose-dependent manner over concentrations of 1-50 μM. Under these conditions the intracellular content and rates of secretion of apolipoprotein B (the main protein of VLDL and LDL) and of apolipoprotein AI (the main protein of HDL) were also reduced; since the former change would tend to prevent and the latter to augment atherosclerosis, these effects would seem to cancel each other out. When wines of high and low resveratrol content were administered to healthy humans for a period of 4 weeks, there was no major difference in the plasma lipid and apolipoprotein responses between the two experimental groups (40). An absence of change in serum lipoprotein patterns in the rat following the intraperitoneal injection of large doses of resveratrol has also been reported (41). On balance, it appears that resveratrol does not have a beneficial effect on circulating lipid or lipoprotein concentrations and that its anti-atherosclerotic properties *in vivo*, if any, are not attributable to such effects. Indeed a disturbing report published a few years ago described an *increase* in the area of aortic atherosclerosis visualized in resveratrol-fed hypercholesterolemic rabbits compared with controls (42). The resveratrol was given in a dose of 0.6 mg/kg during the first 5 days and 1 mg/kg from days 6-60, but this amount (up to 3 mg) was stated to be dissolved in 0.05 ml of ethanol, vastly in excess of its solubility.

CELL GROWTH, PROLIFERATION, AND CANCER

When added to cultured Hep G2 cells in concentrations ranging from 1-50 μM, resveratrol did not alter the following functions over time periods up to 7 days: number of cells per plate; cell viability as gauged by trypan blue exclusion and lactate dehydrogenase efflux; incorporation of [^{14}C]-leucine into cell proteins. However, [^{14}C]-thymidine incorporation into DNA was stable for 3 days and showed a sharp increase at day 7, but only at 50 μM concentration (39). Two years later Jang *et al* (7) reported that resveratrol (1-25 μM) inhibited the initiation and promotion of hydrocarbon-induced skin cancer in the mouse as well as the progression of breast cancer in the same animal. A potent antimutagenic activity of resveratrol was also demonstrated (43). Subsequently, resveratrol has been shown to behave as an antiproliferative agent in estrogen-dependent as well as estrogen-independent human breast epithelial cells (44), in a human oral cancer cell line (45), in androgen-responsive and androgen-nonresponsive human prostate cancer cell lines (46), and in the Yoshida AH-130 ascites hepatoma inoculated into rats (47).

One mechanism responsible for this behaviour seems to be induction by resveratrol of apoptosis. This was first described in resveratrol-treated HL-60 cells, a human leukemia cell line, and to be mediated by a dose-dependent increase in intracellular caspases as well as CD-95L expression (48). Apoptosis of Yoshida AH-130 ascites tumour cells in response to resveratrol was demonstrated by flow cytometric analysis (47). By contrast, normal human lymphocytes were unaffected. In cells expressing wild-type p53, but not in p53-deficient cells, resveratrol suppression of tumor promoter-induced cell transformation is accompanied by apoptosis together with transactivation of p53 activity and expression of p53 protein (49). The dose responses for these apparently related phenomena manifest a similar pattern. Androgen-responsive human prostate cancer cells also undergo apoptosis in response to resveratrol (46). Paradoxically, resveratrol was reported to block apoptosis induced by oxidized lipoproteins in PC-12 cells, an outcome that is preceded by NF-KB activation and binding to DNA (35).

Arrest of cell division is an alternative mechanism for resveratrol-induced inhibition of cell growth, and may be accompanied by enhanced differentiation or similar phenotypic changes in growth-arrested cells. This was first demonstrated for HL-60 cells that, at a concentration of 30 μM, became arrested at S-phase concomitant with significant increase of cyclins A and E and of cdc 2 in the inactive phosphorylated forms (44). However, rat hepatic stellate cells did not show any increase in these cyclins in response to resveratrol, although cyclin D1 content was reduced (16). Differentiation of the HL-60 cells towards a myelo-monocytic phenotype simultaneously occurred (50). These findings are consistent with an earlier report that resveratrol inhibits ribonucleotide reductase (IC_{50} around 4 μM), the enzyme that provides proliferating cells with deoxyribonucleotides required for DNA synthesis during early S-phase (51). Indeed, its potency on a molar basis was orders of magnitude greater than that of hydroxyurea, another inhibitor of the same enzyme that has been used therapeutically as an anticancer and anti-HIV agent. Resveratrol also leads to an increase in the proportion of androgen-nonresponsive human prostate cancer cell lines in S-phase, but this does not occur with androgen-responsive cells (46). It will be recalled that the latter undergo apoptosis in response to resveratrol whereas the former do not. Resveratrol inhibits another important enzyme involved in DNA synthesis, DNA polymerase (52), and causes cleavage of DNA in the presence of Cu^{2+} ions (53). At variance with the above findings is a report that resveratrol in low concentrations (10^{-9}- 10^{-7} M) dose-dependently increased DNA synthesis, proliferation, and differentiation of osteoblastic MC 3T3-E1 cells (11). This action was blocked by the antiestrogenic compound tamoxifen.

In addition to its putative antimutagenic, pro-apoptotic, and DNA antisynthetic properties, resveratrol may target another biological system involved in carcinogenesis. Aryl hydrocarbons such as dioxin and dimethylbenzanthracene are taken up by a specific cytosolic receptor (AHR) in susceptible cells. The complex translocates to the nucleus where it dimerizes with another protein and initiates the transcription of a number of genes involved in carcinogenesis. The best characterized of these is the *CYP1A1* gene that encodes a cytochrome P_{450}-dependent microsomal enzyme; the *CYP1A1* gene product hydroxylates aryl hydrocarbons to genotoxic metabolites that bind DNA with consequent mutational events. Ciolino and colleagues reported that resveratrol in concentrations between 0.5 and 20 μM inhibited the induction of CYP1A1 protein, mRNA and enzyme activity by the halogenated dioxin derivative TCDD in Hep G2 cells in a dose-dependent manner (54). It also prevented the TCDD-induced transformation of cytosolic AHR to its nuclear DNA-binding form and blocked its binding to promoter sequences that regulate CYP1A1 transcription. It did not modulate the binding of TCDD to cytosolic AHR.

These results were partially confirmed by Casper *et al* in a human breast cancer cell line, but with some differences (37). They found that resveratrol displaced labelled dioxin from AHR with an IC_{50} of 6 μM. Neither nuclear translocation or DNA binding of AHR were altered by resveratrol, but its transcriptional activity for CYP1A1 was blocked. The most novel and exciting aspect of this report was the finding that resveratrol, when given in doses of 1 and 5 mg/kg to rats, inhibited the expression of CYP1A1 in lung and kidney induced by benzpyrene and dimethylbenzanthracene. The likely tissue concentrations of resveratrol were three orders of magnitude less than those required for CYP1A1 inhibition in the *in vitro* experiments, suggesting that resveratrol may be converted *in vivo* to a metabolite one thousand-fold more active than the parent compound. It should be added that resveratrol in concentrations <1 µM inhibited a range of cytochrome P_{450}-linked enzymes in hamster liver microsomes *in vitro* (55), but it also induced the mRNA for CYP1A1 in cultured Hela cells derived from a human cervical carcinoma (56). Finally, modulation of c-fos gene expression has been postulated to be an important target for the anticancer activity of resveratrol, at least in the mouse skin carcinogenesis model (9,10).

An important and practical conundrum surrounding the interaction of resveratrol with cancer cells is whether the former is able to suppress the production by the latter of tumor-specific cancer marker proteins. Hsieh and Wu (45) reported a decrease in the intracellular and secreted prostate-specific antigen (PSA) content of an androgen-sensitive prostate cancer cell line. Utilizing human breast cancer cell lines, we have been unable to demonstrate an effect of resveratrol upon the secretion of either PSA or carcinoembryonic antigen (CEA) in four different breast carcinoma cell lines. Nor could we demonstrate any changes in cancer-associated p53 gene expression even though the presence of genetic mutations in these cell lines was structurally determined by DNA analysis.

ANTIOXIDANT ACTIVITY

The ability of *trans*-resveratrol to function as an antioxidant was first demonstrated by Frankel *et al* (57). On a molar basis it was less effective than a number of flavonoids in preventing the copper-mediated oxidation of human LDL, but it was much more potent than α-tocopherol. Frankel *et al* (58) examined the relative contribution of individual wine phenolics to the inhibition of LDL oxidation, based upon their concentrations in the wines utilized, and concluded that resveratrol did not correlate with this activity. Later, Soleas *et al* (59) reported that resveratrol contributed significantly to the total antioxidant activity of wine as evaluated using the Randox *in vitro* assay.

Belguendouz *et al* carried out an extensive examination of the inhibition by resveratrol of porcine LDL oxidation in the presence of the free radical generator AAPH or copper ions (60). The slope of the propagation phase and the prolongation of the lag phase were much greater with the latter than with the former. Formation of thiobarbitiuric acid-reactive substances (TBARS) was completely inhibited up to 200 min in the copper-mediated system by 1 µM resveratrol, more effective than trolox or the flavonoids tested. The relevant mechanisms appeared to be a combination of copper chelation and free radical scavenging; surprisingly, resveratrol was unable to chelate iron. In subsequent experiments it proved to be more effective than flavonoids as a chelator of copper and less effective as a free-radical scavenger (61). Resveratrol added to plasma was distributed between the lipoprotein classes according to their lipid content in the order VLDL > LDL > HDL (62). The authors' suggestion that resveratrol may be effective in a lipid as well as in an aqueous environment was supported by experiments showing that resveratrol blocked the formation of TBARS by AAPH in phospholipid liposomes. Using a different system (inhibition of cytochrome C oxidation by hydroxyl radicals generated by photolysis of H_2O_2), Turrens *et al* (41) reported that *trans*-resveratrol manifested antioxidant activity, the EC_{50} concentration being 33 µM. These findings were extended by Fauconneau *et al* (63) who reported that *trans*-resveratrol protected rat liver microsomes against Fe^{2+}-mediated lipid peroxidation and human LDL against Cu^{2+}-mediated lipid peroxidation. The EC_{50} concentrations were 3.0 and 2.6 µM, respectively: in the same range as anthocyanins but around 2-fold higher than catechins and the stilbene astringinin. The activity of resveratrol in scavenging the stable free radical DPPH (EC_{50} 74 µM) was much higher than that of the other previously mentioned compounds.

Resveratrol appears to be a potent antioxidant in a number of other biological systems. It was more effective than vitamins C or E in preventing oxidative damage and death in a rat pheochromocytoma cell line (64). It protects the same cells against damage induced by oxidized lipoproteins (65), and also proved to be a powerful inhibitor of reactive oxygen species production in murine macrophages (Figure 3), human monocytes and human

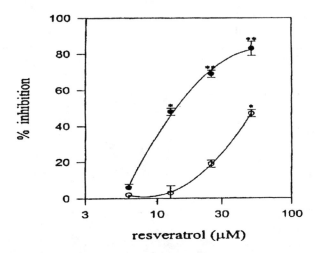

Figure 3. Inhibition by resveratrol of O_2 consumption (Solid Circles) and ROS production (Open Circles) in stimulated murine macrophages. (From Ref. 66, with permission).

neutrophils, although the IC_{50} values for these effects ranged from 17 to 23 µM (66). Jang and Pezzuto (9,10) have attributed its anticancer activity in the mouse skin carcinogenesis model, at least in part, to its antioxidant properties, since phorbol ester-mediated increases in myeloperoxidase, superoxide dismutase and H_2O_2 production were restored to control levels by treatment with resveratrol. Related stilbenes also have antioxidant properties. *Cis*-resveratrol and resveratrol glucosides demonstrated protection against lipid peroxidation in mouse liver microsomes and human LDL, although the IC_{50} values were an order of magnitude greater than that of *trans*-resveratrol (63,67). Oxyresveratrol is a potent inhibitor of dopa oxidase activity (68).

VASCULAR RELAXATION AND NITRIC OXIDE PRODUCTION

Nitric oxide (NO) is produced in a wide range of cells. At least two different enzymes, nitric oxide synthase (NOS), are involved in its synthesis. One, iNOS, is inducible in response to inflammatory stimulants such as LPS in macrophages and other cells involved in inflammatory reactions. In this scenario, NO is pro-oxidant and potentially noxious. Its production by iNOS is inhibited by resveratrol in rat hepatic stellate cells (15), and macrophages (10,33,34).

The second, cNOS, is a constitutive enzyme in vascular endothelial cells. NO produced in this location prevents adherence of platelets to the endothelial surface and diffuses distally to promote relaxation of the smooth muscle layer, in part attributable to its antagonism of the vasoconstricting agent endothelin. Using rat aortic rings, Fitzpatrick *et al* (69) showed that red wine extracts were able to abolish vasoconstrictive events; a number of wine constituents (including quercetin) could reproduce this phenomenon but resveratrol was inactive in this regard. Subsequently, Chen and Pace-Asciak

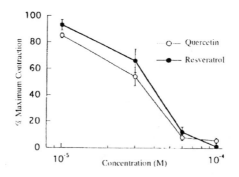

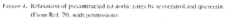

Figure 4. Relaxation of precontracted rat aortic rings by resveratrol and quercetin. (From Ref. 70, with permission).

(70) were able to demonstrate quite effective vasorelaxation by resveratrol in a similar system (Figure 4), but could not offer any explanation for the discordance between these and the previous results. A recent report (71) lends strong support to the findings of Chen and Pace-Asciak (70) by demonstrating dose-dependent inhibition by resveratrol of histamine and fluoride-induced contractions in isolated porcine coronary arteries at very low EC_{50} concentrations of <1 nmol/l.

ESTROGENIC ACTIVITY

Following the knowledge that pinosylvin, a stilbene containing one less OH group than resveratrol, is estrogenic in human breast cancer cell lines (72), Gehm et al (73) were the first to report the interaction of resveratrol with estrogen and its receptor. At 3-10 µM concentrations, resveratrol inhibited the binding of labeled estradiol to the estrogen receptor in human breast cancer cells, and activated transcription of estrogen-responsive reporter genes transfected into these cells. This transcriptional activation was estrogen receptor-dependent, required an estrogen response element in the reporter gene, and was inhibited by specific estrogen antagonists. Depending on the cell type, it produced activation greater than, equal to or less than that of estradiol. It also increased the expression of native estrogen-regulated genes and stimulated the proliferation of an estrogen-dependent human breast carcinoma cell line.

A subsequent report described resveratrol as lacking the ability to bind to estrogen receptor in a pituitary cell line (74). Unlike other phytoestrogens tested in the same system, resveratrol did not stimulate the growth of these cells, but like them it was able to stimulate prolactin secretion by these cells in a dose and time-dependent manner. When tested in concentrations ranging from approximately 2.5-200 µM, resveratrol inhibited the growth and proliferation of human breast cancer cell lines irrespective of their estrogen responsiveness (44). These results were extended by Lu and Serrero (75) who also grew estrogen receptor-positive breast cancer cells (MCF-7) in the presence of resveratrol. At concentrations of 1µM and above, the latter antagonized the growth-promoting effect of 17-beta-estradiol (1nM) upon these cells (Figure 5), as well as its stimulation of progesterone receptor gene expression. At higher concentrations (100 µM), resveratrol blocked the expression of mRNA for TGFα and ILGF-I receptor but increased mRNA for $TGF_{\beta 2}$ in MCF-7 cells. The increase in DNA synthesis and stimulation by resveratrol of an osteoblastic cell line was inhibited by the antiestrogen tamoxifen (11).

Although its role as a phytoestrogen has been invoked to account, at least in part, for its protection against atherosclerosis (76), recent *in vivo* experiments cast doubt about the extrapolation of these *in vitro* antiestrogenic effects to whole animals. When given to rats by oral gavage or subcutaneous injection, resveratrol in doses ranging up to the equivalent in a 70 kg human of 2800 l of wine daily did not show any activity in an assay using uterine estrogen receptors (77). In fact, *in vitro* studies carried out by this group and reported in the same paper described the affinity of resveratrol for rat uterine estrogen receptors as 5 orders of magnitude lower than that of estradiol or diethyl-stilbestrol. Similar conclusions were reached with experiments utilizing estrogen receptor-transfected yeast cells and cos-1 cells. Finally,

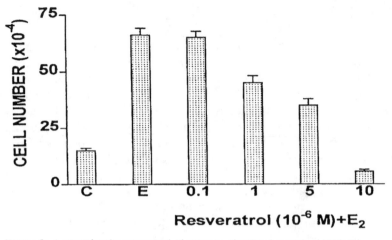

Figure 5: Antagonism by resveratrol of estrogen stimulated growth of MCF-7 human breast cells after 6 days. C, control; E, estrogen; remaining bars are various concentrations of resveratrol in presence of estrogen.
(From Ref. 75, with permission).

Turner et al (78) carried out an extensive investigation on the effect of orally-administered resveratrol (graded doses equivalent to 0.5-500 ml of red wine per day for 6 days to weanling rats) upon estrogen target tissues assessed by growth rate, body weight, serum cholesterol and radial bone growth, all of which were enhanced by equivaient doses of estradiol. Resveratrol did not alter any of these parameters.

Before accepting these negative conclusions, two caveats are worthy of consideration. Firstly, it is conceivable that the affinity of resveratrol for estrogen receptors is subject to some tissue specificity, being more potent for breast than for uterus; moreover, since Ashby et al (77) had found that the affinity of resveratrol for uterine estrogen receptors was 5 orders of magnitude less than that of estradiol, it is surprising that they employed similar doses of both agonists in their whole animal experiments. Secondly, the parameters selected by Turner et al (78) may have been appropriate for estradiol, but conceivably not for resveratrol, whose widespread biological actions, including those on cell growth and DNA synthesis, may have masked its possible role as a phytoestrogen, as judged by these criteria.

ABSORPTION AND BIOAVAILABILITY

The disappointing results of human and whole animal experiments designed to reproduce the *in vitro* actions of resveratrol give urgency to the question whether it is efficiently absorbed and if so, whether its metabolic and excretory patterns are consistent with tissue concentrations adequate to achieve desirable effects. The prerequisite to such investigations was the development of assays sensitive enough to allow the measurement of resveratrol in blood, as well as its distribution between plasma or serum and formed elements of the blood. Our group was the first to describe investigations relevant to these issues (79,80). Using a HPLC method, we found that *trans*-resveratrol added to whole human blood was >90% recoverable and partitioned as follows: serum 54.8%; erythrocytes 36.0%; leukocytes and platelets 6.1%. However, taking protein content into account, the latter fraction was the most highly enriched in resveratrol.

A subsequent report, incorrectly claiming to be the first method developed to measure resveratrol in animal and human samples, presented results that were not quite consistent with these findings (81). Washed human and rat erythrocytes, rat platelets and human LDL incorporated approximately 50%, 10% and 17.5% respectively of *trans*-resveratrol when incubated at room temperature for 15-30 min. Two HPLC methods for the measurement of plasma resveratrol have been described with detection limits of 20 µg/l (82) and 5 µg/l (83), respectively. Only the former has actually been applied in whole animals; 15 min after unspecified administration of 2 mg/kg to rats, the plasma resveratrol concentration was stated to be 175 µg/l, almost 10% of the dose given, a result completely at variance with all other literature reports on this topic (82).

Bertelli and colleagues developed a HPLC method to determine resveratrol concentrations in rat serum, and claimed a detection limit of 1ng/ml. They found that after 4 ml of red wine containing 26 µg of resveratrol given to the animals by gavage, the blood resveratrol concentration peaked around 60 min at about 15 ng/ml, or 5.8×10^{-2} percent of the dose administered, and returned to baseline by 4 hours (84). In a further experiment, they gave 13 µg of total *trans* and *cis*-resveratrol per day to a second group of rats for 15 days, at which time the concentrations of resveratrol in plasma (7.6 ng/ml), urine (66 ng/ml), heart (3 ng/ml), liver (54 ng/ml) and kidneys (44 ng/ml) were well below those required for pharmacologic activity based upon *in vitro* studies (85). A kinetic analysis revealed that relative tissue bioavailability, calculated as *Area Under the Curve* (AUC) for tissues expressed as a percentage of AUC for plasma, accorded with the following ratios: heart, 24; liver, 218; kidneys, 295. However, they subsequently claimed that by the administration of red wine, they were able to achieve resveratrol concentrations compatible with the inhibition of platelet aggregation (86).

Table 2. Recovery of Labelled Resveratrol 24 Hours After Gastric Administration in Rats [a]

Matrix	Total (%)	Stool (%)	Urine (%)
Grape Juice	61.1 ± 4.9	10.8 ± 0.9	50.3 ± 5.7
V-8 Juice	73.6 ± 3.5	14.1 ± 1.0	59.5 ± 4.5
Alcohol	62.2 ± 2.3	13.2 ± 1.4	49.0 ± 3.1

[a]Mean of 8 experiments ±SEM

Our group has recently completed an investigation in which we gave 298 nCi of $[H^3]$-resveratrol added to 10% ethanol, white grape juice or vegetable homogenate (V-8) by stomach tube to male Wistar rats (avg. weight 300g), following which the animals were held in metabolic cages for collection of urine and feces independently. After 24 hours, they were sacrificed with collection of blood, various organs, and the contents of colon and bladder that were added to stool and urine, respectively. Only traces of radioactivity were detected in the blood after 24 hours, or in groups of rats sacrificed at 30 min intervals over the first 2 hours. Urine and bladder accounted for 50-60%, and stool and colon for 11-14% of the radioactivity after 24 hours (Table 2). There were no significant differences between the three beverages. Only traces of radioactivity were detected in spleen, liver, kidney, or the cellular elements of the blood. Using ethanol as the vehicle, competition experiments were performed with cold resveratrol as well as unlabelled catechin and quercetin (two flavonoid poyphenols present in red wine that share some similar structural features with resveratrol). None of these compounds altered the amount of radioactivity in stool or urine after 24 hours. We conclude, based upon urine measurements, that around 50-60% of the *trans*-resveratrol entering the rat intestine is absorbed, probably by bulk fluid transfer rather than by receptor-mediated mechanisms, and that its clearance from the blood stream is very rapid. This percentage may be closer to 90 if we assume that all of the radioactivity not recovered in the stool was actually absorbed. 25-40% of tracer could not be accounted for and may have been deposited in adipose tissue and brain in view of its lipophilic nature. Finally, the presence of alcohol does not seem to be necessary for effective absorption to take place.

MISCELLANEOUS

Three papers have appeared that testify to efforts underway for the large-scale production of resveratrol and its glucosides, presumably for pharmaceutical purposes. Orsini *et al* have reported the synthesis of a range of resveratrol derivatives, including polydatin (piceid) by means of Wittig reactions followed by glucosylation under phase-transfer catalysis (87). Polydatin has also been generated on a preparative scale through the microbial transformation of resveratrol by a strain of *Bacillus cereus* (88). Resveratrol is much more stable than other polyphenols in grape skins and pomace after fermentation when stored at room temperature for relatively lengthy periods (89), raising the expectation that these materials will be excellent sources for its extraction and purification on a commercial scale.

An interesting set of observations was made by Busam *et al* (90) on the phenomenon of systemic acquired resistance in grapes. Treatment of cell-suspension cultures of *Vitis vinifera* with fungi or a number of chemicals caused the accumulation of resveratrol. Simultaneously, the expression of S-adenosyl-L-methionine: trans-caffeoyl-coenzyme A 3-0-methyl transferase, as well as of stilbene synthase, was increased. Phenolic esterification, in addition to the synthesis of stilbenes, may play an important role in disease resistance of grapevines.

Given the interest in the possibility that antioxidant flavonoids may prevent dementia and improve cerebral function, it is worth drawing attention to a recent paper describing an induction by resveratrol of phosphorylation of several protein kinases (mitogen-activated and extracellular signal-regulated) in differentiated and undifferentiated human neuroblastoma cells (91).

CONCLUSION

Since our first review on resveratrol (2), many more biological effects of the compound have been demonstrated *in vitro*. Further, the molecular and biochemical basis for several of these effects has been elucidated. One of the paradoxes, as true to-day as it was several years ago, is the difficulty of reproducing these biological activities in whole animals or humans. A concern at that time was the issue of whether resveratrol can actually undergo intestinal absorption. This now seems to have been affirmatively resolved. However, its excretion appears to be fairly rapid; even when quite large amounts are given, its concentrations in blood and tissues fall well below the levels required for most biological activities, and suggestions that long term administration may lead to cumulatively higher concentrations are not convincing. Given the levels in naturally-produced red wines, it seems unlikely that biologically useful concentrations will be achieved from this source alone, although one report does provide evidence that resveratrol may be converted *in vivo* to metabolites with much greater activity (36).

Our finding that resveratrol appears to be absorbed as effectively in matrices that do not contain alcohol as in those that do lends credibility to the notion that it could feasibly be provided as a capsule or elixir, joining the rank of natural health preparations that are increasingly invading our retail outlets. Alternatively, wine makers may wake up to the realization that enriching their products with resveratrol may give them a market advantage, provided that there are no adverse organoleptic characteristics as a result. The future of resveratrol as a non-patentable natural product will depend upon the delicate interplay of scientific and commercial forces. At any time in the future the balance could change dramatically if synthetic analogues with greater potency are developed.

ACKNOWLEDGMENTS

We thank Mrs. Sheila Acorn and Mrs. Patricia Machado for their help in preparing this manuscript. The personal work cited in this paper has been generously supported by the National Research Council of Canada (IRAP) and the Wine Institute, San Francisco.

REFERENCES

1.   Siemann EH, Creasy LL. Concentration of the phytoalexin resveratrol in wine. Am J Enol Vitic 1992; 43:49-52.
2.   Soleas GJ, Diamandis EP, Goldberg DM. Resveratrol: A molecule whose time has come? And gone? Clin Biochem 1997; 30:91-113.
3.   Daniel O, Meier MS, Schlatter J, Frischknecht P. Selected phenolic compounds in cultivated plants: Ecologic functions, health implications, and modulation of pesticides. Environ Health Perspect 1999; 107 Suppl 1:109-114.
4.   Constant J. Alcohol, ischemic heart disease, and the French paradox. Coron Artery Dis 1997; 8:645-649.
5.   Ross R. Atherosclerosis – An inflammatory disease. N Engl J Med 1999; 340:115-126.
6.   Nicholson AC, Hajjar DP. Herpesviruses in atherosclerosis and thrombosis: etiologic agents or ubiquitous bystanders? Arterioscler Thromb Vasc Biol 1998; 18:339-348.
7.   Jang M, Cai L, Udeani GO, *et al.* Cancer chemopreventive activity of resveratrol, a natural product derived from grapes. Science 1997; 275:218-220.
8.   Subbaramaiah K, Chung WJ, Michaluart P, *et al.* Resveratrol inhibits cyclooxygenase-2 transcription and activity in phorbol ester-treated human mammary epithelial cells. J Biol Chem 1998; 273:21875-21882.
9.   Jang M, Pezzuto JM. Effects of resveratrol on 12-O-tetradecanoylphorbol-13-acetate-induced oxidative events and gene expression in mouse skin. Cancer Lett 1998; 134:81-89.

10. Jang M, Pezzuto JM. Cancer chemopreventive activity of resveratrol. Drugs Exp Clin Res 1999; 25:65-77.

11. Mizutani K, Ikeda K, Kawai Y, Yamori Y. Resveratrol stimulates the proliferation and differentiation of osteoblastic MC3T3-E1 cells. Biochem Biophys Res Commun 1998; 253:859-863.

12. Johnson JL, Maddipati KR. Paradoxical effects of resveratrol on the two prostaglandin H synthases. Prostaglandins Other Lipid Mediat 1998;56:131-143.

13. Lee SH, Shin NH, Kang SH et al. Alpha-viniferin: a prostaglandin H2 synthase inhibitor from root of Carex humilis. Planta Med 1998; 64:204-207.

14. Shin NH, Ryu SY, Lee H, Min KR, Kim Y. Inhibitory effects of hydroxystilbenes on cyclooxygenase from sheep seminal vesicles. Planta Med 1998; 64:283-284.

15. Knight J, Taylor GW, Wright P, Clare AS, Rowley AF. Eicosanoid biosynthesis in an advanced deuterostomate invertebrate, the sea squirt (Ciona intestinalis). Biochim Biophys Acta 1999; 1436:467-478.

16. Kawada N, Seki S, Inoue M, Kuroki T. Effect of antioxidants, resveratrol, quercetin, and N-acetylcysteine, on the functions of cultured rat hepatic stellate cells and Kupffer cells. Hepatology 1998; 27:1265-1274.

17. Chen T, Li J, Cao J, Xu Q, Komatsu K, Namba T. A new flavanone isolated from rhizoma smilacis glabrae and the structural requirements of its derivatives for preventing immunological hepatocyte damage. Planta Med 1999; 65:56-59.

18. Kimura Y, Okuda H, Arichi S. Effects of stilbenes on arachidonate metabolism in leukocytes. Biochim Biophys Acta 1985; 834:275-278.

19. Goldberg DM, Soleas GJ, Hahn SE, Diamandis EP, Karumanchiri A. Identification and assay of trihydroxystilbenes in wine and their biological properties. In: Watkins T, ed. *Wine composition and health benefits.* American Chemical Society, Washington DC, 1997; pp. 24-43.

20. Kimura Y, Okuda H, Kubo M. Effects of stilbenes isolated from medicinal plants on arachidonate metabolism and degranulation in human polymorphonuclear leukocytes. J Ethnopharmacol 1995; 45:131-139.

21. Shan CW. Effects of polydatin on platelet aggregation of rabbits. Acta Pharmacol Sin 1988; 23:394-396.

22. Shan CW, Yang SQ, He HD, Shao SL, Zhang PW. Influences of 3,4,5-trihydroxy stilbene-3-β-mono-D-glucoside on rabbits' platelet aggregation and thromboxane B_2 production *in vitro*. Acta Pharmacol Sin 1990; 11:527-530.

23. Chung M-I, Teng C-M, Cheng K-L, Ko F-N, Lin C-N. An antiplatelet principle of *Veratrum formosanum*. Planta Med 1992; 58:274-276.

24. Pace-Asciak CR, Hahn S, Diamandis EP, Soleas G, Goldberg DM. The red wine phenolics *trans*-resveratrol and quercetin block human platelet aggregation and eicosanoid synthesis: Implications for protection against coronary heart disease. Clin Chim Acta 1995; 235:207-219.

25. Bertelli AAE, Giovannini L, Giannessi D. et al. Antiplatelet activity of synthetic and natural resveratrol in red wine. Int J Tiss React 1995; 17:1-3.

26. Bertelli AAE, Giovannini L, De Caterina R. et al. Antiplatelet activity of *cis*-resveratrol. Drugs Exp Clin Res 1996; 22:61-63.

27. Orsini F, Pelizzoni F, Verotta L, Aburjai T, Rogers CB. Isolation, synthesis, and antiplatelet aggregation activity of resveratrol 3-O-beta-D-glucopyranoside and related compounds. J Nat Prod 1997; 60:1082-1087.

28. Cavenagh JD, Cahill MR, Kelsey SM. Adhesion molecules in clinical medicine. Crit Rev Clin Lab Sci 1998; 34:415-459.

29. Chia MC. The role of adhesion molecules in atherosclerosis. Crit Rev Clin Lab Sci 1998; 35:573-602.

30. Ferrero ME, Bertelli AE, Fulgenzi A. et al. Activity *in vitro* of resveratrol on granulocyte and monocyte adhesion to endothelium. Am J Clin Nutr 1998; 68:1208-1214.

31. Rotondo S, Rajtar G, Manarini S, *et al.* Effect of *trans*-resveratrol, a natural polyphenolic compound, on human polymorphonuclear leukocyte function. Br J Pharmacol 1998; 123:1691-1699.
32. Cheong H, Ryu SY, Kim KM. Anti-allergic action of resveratrol and related hydroxystilbenes. Planta Med 1999; 65:266-268.
33. Tsai SH, Lin-Shiau SY, Lin JK. Suppression of nitric oxide synthase and the down-regulation of the activation of NfkappaB in macrophages by resveratrol. Br J Pharmacol 1999; 126:673-680.
34. Wadsworth TL, Koop DR. Effects of the wine polyphenolics quercetin and resveratrol on pro-inflammatory cytokine expression in RAW 264.7 macrophages. Biochem Pharmacol 1999; 57:941-949.
35. Draczynska-Lusiak B, Chen YM, Sun AY. Oxidized lipoproteins activate NF-kappaB binding activity and apoptosis in PC12 cells. Neuroreport 1998; 9:527-532.
36. Pendurthi UR, Williams JT, Rao LV. Resveratrol, a polyphenolic compound found in wine, inhibits tissue factor expression in vascular cells: A possible mechanism for the cardiovascular benefits associated with moderte consumption of wine. Arterioscler Thromb Vasc Biol 1999; 19:419-426.
37. Casper RF, Quesne M, Rogers IM, *et al.* Resveratrol has antagonist activity on the aryl hydrocarbon receptor: Implications for prevention of dioxin toxicity. Mol Pharmacol 1999; In Press.
38. Arichi H, Kimura Y, Okuda H, Baba K, Kozawa M, Arichi S. Effects of stilbene components of the roots of *Polygonum cuspidatum* Sieb. et Zucc. on lipid metabolism. Chem Pharm Bull 1982; 30:1766-1770.
39. Goldberg DM, Hahn SE, Parkes, JG. Beyond alcohol: Beverage consumption and cardiovascular mortality. Clin Chim Acta 1995; 237:155-187.
40. Goldberg DM, Garovic-Kocic V, Diamandis EP, Pace-Asciak, CR. Wine: does the colour count? Clin Chim Acta 1996; 246:183-193.
41. Turrens JF, Lariccia J, Nair MG. Resveratrol has no effect on lipoprotein profile and does not prevent peroxidation of serum lipids in normal rats. Free Radic Res 1997; 27:557-62.
42. Wilson T, Knight TJ, Beitz DC, Lewis DS, Engen RL. Resveratrol promotes atherosclerosis in hypercholesterolemic rabbits. Life Sci 1996; 59:15-21.
43. Uenobe F, Nakamura S-I, Miyazawa M. Antimutagenic effect of resveratrol against Trp-P-1. Mutat Res 1997; 373:197-200.
44. Mgbonyebi OP, Russo J, Russo IH. Antiproliferative effect of synthetic resveratrol on human breast epithelial cells. Int J Oncol 1998; 12:865-869.
45. ElAttar TM, Virji AS. Modulating effect of resveratrol and quercetin on oral cancer cell growth and proliferation. Anticancer Drugs 1999; 10:187-193.
46. Hsieh TC, Wu JM. Differential effects on growth, cell cycle arrest, and induction of apoptosis by resveratrol in human prostate cancer cell lines. Exp Cell Res 1999; 249:109-115.
47. Carbo N, Costelli P, Baccino FM, Lopez-Soriano FJ, Argiles JM. Resveratrol, a natural product present in wine, decreases tumour growth in a rat tumour model. Biochem Biophys Res Commun 1999; 254:739-743.
48. Clement MV, Hirpara JL, Chawdhury SH, Pervaiz S. Chemopreventive agent resveratrol, a natural product derived from grapes, triggers CD95 signaling-dependent apoptosis in human tumor cells. Blood 1998; 92:996-1002.
49. Huang C, Ma MY, Goranson A, Dong Z. Resveratrol suppresses cell transformation and induces apoptosis through a p53-dependent pathway. Carcinogenesis 1999; 20:237-242.
50. Ragione FD, Cucciolla V, Borriello A, *et al.* Resveratrol arrests the cell division cycle at S/G2 phase transition. Biochem Biophys Res Commun 1998; 250:53-58.
51. Fontecave M, Lepoivre M, Elleingand E, Gerez C, Guittet O. Resveratrol, a remarkable inhibitor of ribonucleotide reductase. FEBS Lett 1998; 421:277-279.

52. Sun NJ, Woo SH, Cassady JM, Snapka RM. DNA polymerase and topoisomerase II inhibitors from Psoralea corylifolia. J Nat Prod 1998; 61:362-366.

53. Fukuhara K, Miyata N. Resveratrol as a new type of DNA-cleaving agent. Bioorg Med Chem Lett 1998; 8:3187-3192.

54. Ciolino HP, Daschner PJ, Yeh GC. Resveratrol inhibits transcription of CYP1A1 in vitro by preventing activation of the aryl hydrocarbon receptor. Cancer Res 1998; 58:5707-5712.

55. Teel RW, Huynh H. Modulation by phytochemicals of cytochrome P450-linked enzyme activity. Cancer Lett 1998; 133:135-141.

56. Frotschl R, Chichmanov L, Kleeberg U, Hildebrandt AG, Roots I, Brockmoller J. Prediction of aryl hydrocarbon receptor-mediated enzyme induction of drugs and chemicals by mRNA quantification. Chem Res Toxicol 1998; 11:1447-1452.

57. Frankel EN, Waterhouse AL, Kinsella JE. Inhibition of human LDL oxidation by resveratrol. Lancet 1993; 341:1103-1104.

58. Frankel EN, Waterhouse AL, Teissedre PL. Principal phenolic phytochemicals in selected California wines and their antioxidant activity in inhibiting oxidation of human low-density lipoproteins. J Agric Food Chem 1995; 43:890-894.

59. Soleas GJ, Tomlinson G, Diamandis EP, Goldberg, DM. Relative contributions of polyphenolic constituents to the antioxidant status of wines: Development of a predictive model. J Agric Food Chem 1997; 45:3995-4003.

60. Belguendouz L, Fremont L, Linard A. Resveratrol inhibits metal ion-dependent and independent peroxidation of porcine low-density lipoproteins. Biochem Pharmacol 1997; 53:1347-1355.

61. Frémont L, Belguendouz L, Delpal S. Antioxidant activity of resveratrol and alcohol-free wine polyphenols related to LDL oxidation and polyunsaturated fatty acids. Life Sci 1999; 64:2511-2521.

62. Belguendouz L, Fremont L, Gozzelino MT. Interaction of trans-resveratrol with plasma lipoproteins. Biochem Pharmacol 1998; 55:811-816.

63. Fauconneau B, Waffo-Teguo P, Huguet F, Barrier L, Decendit A, Merillon JM. Comparative study of radical scavenger and antioxidant properties of phenolic compounds from Vitis vinifera cell cultures using in vitro tests. Life Sci 1997; 61:2103-2110.

64. Chanvitayapongs S, Draczynska-Lusiak B, Sun AY. Amelioration of oxidative stress by antioxidants and resveratrol in PC12 cells. Neuroreport 1997; 8:1499-1502.

65. Draczynska-Lusiak B, Doung A, Sun AY. Oxidized lipoproteins may play a role in neuronal cell death in Alzheimer disease. Mol Chem Neuropathol 1998; 33:139-148.

66. Jang DS, Kang BS, Ryu SY, Chang IM, Min KR, Kim Y. Inhibitory effects of resveratrol analogs on unopsonized zymosan-induced oxygen radical production. Biochem Pharmacol 1999; 57:705-712.

67. Waffo-Teguo P, Fauconneau B, Deffieux G, Huguet F, Vercauteren J, Merillon JM. Isolation, identification, and antioxidant activity of three stilbene glucosides newly extracted from vitis vinifera cell cultures. J Nat Prod 1998; 61:655-657.

68. Shin NH, Ryu SY, Choi EJ, et al. Oxyresveratrol as the potent inhibitor on dopa oxidase activity of mushroom tyrosinase. Biochem Biophys Res Commun 1998; 243:801-803.

69. Fitzpatrick DF, Hirschfield SL, Coffey RG. Endothelium-dependent vasorelaxing activity of wine and other grape products. Am J Physiol 1993; 265:H774-H778.

70. Chen CK, Pace-Asciak CR. Vasorelaxing activity of resveratrol and quercetin in isolated rat aorta. Gen Pharmacol 1996; 27:363-366.

71. Jager U, Nguyen-Duong H. Relaxant effect of trans-resveratrol on isolated porcine coronary arteries. Arzneimittelforschung 1999; 49:207-211.

72. Mellanen P, Petanen T, Lehtimaki J, et al. Wood-derived estrogens: studies in vitro with breast cancer cell lines and in vivo in trout. Toxicol Appl Pharmacol 1996; 136:381-388.

73. Gehm BD, McAndrews JM, Chien PY, Jameson JL. Resveratrol, a polyphenolic compound found in grapes and wine, is an agonist for the estrogen receptor. Proc Natl Acad Sci USA 1997; 94:14138-14143.

74. Stahl S, Chun TY, Gray WG. Phytoestrogens act as estrogen agonists in an estrogen-responsive pituitary cell line. Toxicol Appl Pharmacol 1998; 152:41-48.

75. Lu R, Serrero G. Resveratrol, a natural product derived from grape, exhibits antiestrogenic activity and inhibits the growth of human breast cancer cells. J Cell Physiol 1999; 179:297-304.

76. Kopp P. Resveratrol, a phytoestrogen found in red wine. A possible explanation for the conundrum of the 'French paradox'? Eur J Endocrinol 1998; 138:619-620.

77. Ashby J, Tinwell H, Pennie W, *et al.* Partial and weak oestrogenicity of the red wine constituent resveratrol: consideration of its superagonist aactivity in MCF-7 cells and its suggested cardiovascular protective effects. J Appl Toxicol 1999; 19:39-45.

78. Turner RT, Evans GL, Zhang M, Maran A, Sibonga JD. Is resveratrol an estrogen agonist in growing rats? Endocrinology 1999; 140:50-54.

79. Tham L, Goldberg DM, Diamandis P, Karumanchiri A, Soleas GJ. Extraction of resveratrol from human blood. Clin Biochem 1995; 28:339 (Abst).

80. Goldberg DM, Tham L, Diamandis EP, Karumanchiri A, Soleas GJ. The assay of resveratrol and its distribution in human blood. Clin Chem 1995; 41:S115 (Abst).

81. Blache D, Rustan I, Durand P, Lesgards G, Loreau N. Gas chromatographic analysis of resveratrol in plasma, lipoproteins and cells after in vitro incubations. J Chromatogr B Biomed Sci Appl 1997; 702:103-110.

82. Juan ME, Lamuela-Raventos RM, de la Torre-Boronat MC, Planas JM. Determination of *trans*-resveratrol in plasma by HPLC. Anal Chem 1999; 71:747-750.

83. Zhu Z, Klironomos G, Vachereau A, Neirinck L, Goodman DW. Determination of *trans*-resveratrol in human plasma by high-performance liquid chromatography. J Chromatogr B Biomed Sci Appl 1999; 724:389-392.

84. Bertelli AA, Giovannini L, Stradi R, Bertelli A, Tillement JP. Plasma, urine and tissue levels of *trans*- and *cis*-resveratrol (3,4',5-trihydroxystilbene) after short-term or prolonged administration of red wine to rats. Int J Tissue React 1996; 18:67-71.

85. Bertelli AA, Giovannini L, Stradi R, Urien S, Tillement JP, Bertelli A. Kinetics of *trans*- and *cis*-resveratrol (3,4',5-trihydroxystilbene) after red wine oral administration in rats. Int J Clin Pharmacol Res 1996; 16:77-81.

86. Bertelli A, Bertelli AA, Gozzini A, Giovannini L. Plasma and tissue resveratrol concentrations and pharmacological activity. Drugs Exp Clin Res 1998; 24:133-138.

87. Orsini F, Pelizzoni F, Bellini B, Miglierini G. Synthesis of biologically active polyphenolic glycosides (combretastatin and resveratrol series). Carbohydr Res 1997; 301:95-109.

88. Cichewicz RH, Kouzi SA. Biotransformation of resveratrol to piceid by Bacillus cereus. J Nat Prod 1998; 61:1313-1314.

89. Bertelli AA, Gozzini A, Stradi R, Stella S, Bertelli A. Stability of resveratrol over time and in the various stages of grape transformation. Drugs Exp Clin Res 1998; 24:207-211.

90. Busam G, Junghanns KT, Kneusel RE, Kassemeyer HH, Matern U. Characterization and expression of caffeoyl-coenzyme A 3-O-methyltransferase proposed for the induced resistance response of Vitis vinifera L. Plant Physiol 1997; 115:1039-1048.

91. Miloso M, Bertelli AA, Nicolini G, Tredici G. Resveratrol-induced activation of the mitogen-activated protein kinases, ERK1 and ERK2, in human neuroblastoma SH-SY5Y cells. Neurosci Lett 1999; 264:141-144.

14

THE EFFECTS OF RESVERATROL ON *CYP1A1* EXPRESSION AND ARYL HYDROCARBON RECEPTOR FUNCTION *IN VITRO*

Henry P. Ciolino and Grace Chao Yeh

Cellular Defense and Carcinogenesis Section, Basic Research Laboratory, National Cancer Institute-Frederick Cancer Research and Development Center Frederick, MD

INTRODUCTION

The aryl hydrocarbon receptor (AHR) is a ligand-activated transcription factor of the basic helix-loop-helix family.[1] It binds and is activated by a number of compounds, including polycyclic aromatic hydrocarbons (PAH) such as benzo[a]pyrene (B[a]P), which are generated during the combustion of fossil fuels and are present in tobacco smoke and smoked meats. The AHR also binds halogenated aromatic hydrocarbons such as 2,3,7,8-tetrachlorodibenzodioxin (TCDD), which is a contaminant formed during the manufacture of chlorophenols (for chemical structures see Fig. 1). Both these classes of AHR ligands are persistent environmental pollutants and cause a variety of toxic and carcinogenic effects that are mediated by the AHR.

The ubiquitously expressed AHR exists as a cytosolic receptor in a complex with the 90-kDa heat shock protein and several other proteins of unknown function. Upon ligand binding, the AHR disassociates from the complex and translocates to the nucleus. In the nucleus it complexes with the

Nutrition and Cancer Prevention, edited under the auspices of AICR
Kluwer Academic / Plenum Publishers, New York, 2000.

aryl hydrocarbon receptor nuclear translocator (ARNT). This heterodimer binds to specific enhancer sequences termed the xenobiotic-response element (XRE) present within the promoter region of a number of genes. The best characterized molecular response to ligands of the AHR is the induction of transcription of the gene *CYP1A1*.[2] It encodes cytochrome P450 1A1 (CYP1A1), an important carcinogen activating (Phase 1) enzyme. This enzyme catalyzes the 1-electron reduction of PAHs such as B[a]P or dimethylbenzanthracene (DMBA), generating highly reactive epoxide metabolites which bind DNA and cause mutations which lead to cellular transformation.[3] The carcinogen activating pathway mediated by the AHR is, therefore, a central biochemical component in the initiation stage of carcinogenesis induced by PAHs. Inhibition of the AHR pathway, either by preventing the induction of *CYP1A1* transcription by the AHR, or by inhibiting CYP1A1 enzyme activity, is an important mechanism of chemoprevention.

Epidemiological studies have clearly established that diets rich in fruits and vegetables are associated with a reduced risk for several types of cancer.[4,5] Modulation of AHR function and the pathway it regulates by dietary components may be an important mechanism in preventing carcinogenesis caused by environmental carcinogens, and may be part of the established chemopreventive effect of plant-based diets. Recently we have investigated the effect of a number of phytochemicals on AHR activity and *CYP1A1* expression.[6-9] Resveratrol, a phytoalexin present in grapes and grape products such as wine, was recently shown to inhibit tumorigenesis caused by PAHs in rodents[10]. We therefore examined the effect of resveratrol on the AHR and *CYP1A1* activity expression *in vitro*,[11,12] using the HepG2 human liver carcinoma cell line, an established model for AHR studies.

Resveratrol

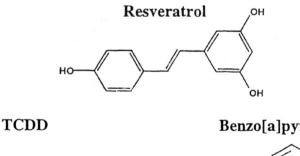

TCDD

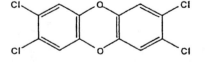

Benzo[a]pyrene

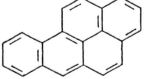

Figure 1. Structures of Resveratrol, TCDD, and benzo[a]pyrene.

1. RESVERATROL AND CYP1A1 ACTIVITY

We examined the effect of resveratrol on CYP1A1 enzyme activity, as measured by the ethoxyresorufin-*O*-deethylase (EROD) assay. HepG2 cells have no detectable activity in the absence of any treatment, but exposure of the cells to B[a]P or TCDD causes a profound increase in EROD activity (Figure 2). In cells co-incubated with resveratrol, there is a dose-dependent decrease in enzyme activity (Fig 2). The resveratrol concentration at which activity was inhibited by 50% (IC_{50}) was approximately 1 µM.

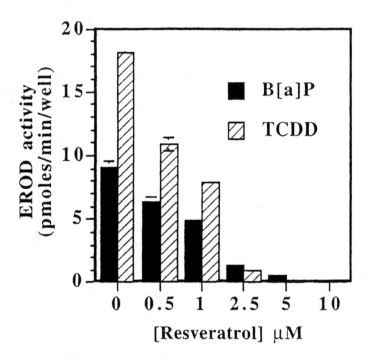

Figure 2. Effect of resveratrol on B[a]P- or TCDD-induced CYP1A1 activity. HepG2 cells were incubated with B[a]P (100 nM) or TCDD (1 nM) for 24 h in the presence of DMSO (control) or the indicated concentrations of resveratrol and CYP1A1 enzyme activity in the intact cells was determined by EROD assay. N = 4 ± standard error (SE). There was a significant difference in activity in cells co-incubated with all concentrations of resveratrol compared to control ($p < 0.05$).

Several phytochemicals have been found to inhibit CYP1A1 enzyme activity by directly interacting with the enzyme in a competitive or noncompetitive manner.[6-9,13] To determine whether the effect of resveratrol on enzyme activity is the result of a direct effect on CYP1A1, we isolated microsomes from B[a]P-treated cells and measured EROD activity of the microsomal CYP1A1 in the presence of resveratrol. Figure 3 demonstrates that resveratrol directly inhibits CYP1A1 activity. Kinetic analysis by double-reciprocal plot (Fig 3B) shows that this inhibition is predominately of the competitive nature, indicating that resveratrol binds to the substrate binding site of the enzyme and prevents substrate binding.

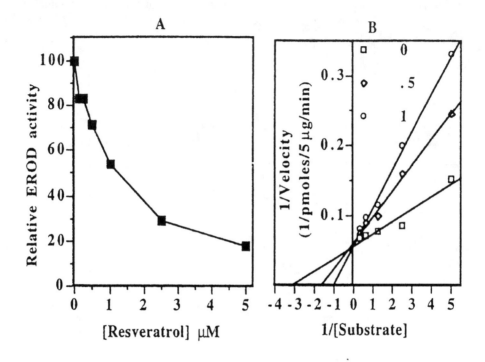

Figure 3. Effect of resveratrol on microsomal CYP1A1 activity. CYP1A1 EROD activity was measured in microsomes isolated from B[a]P-treated HepG2 cells in the presence of different resveratrol concentrations (A) or in the presence of different substrate and resveratrol concentrations (B). For B, data was graphed as a double-reciprocal (Lineweaver-Burk) plot. For both, n = 4.

Inhibition of CYP1A1 by resveratrol should prevent the activation of B[a]P, since CYP1A1 is the major PAH-activating enzyme in HepG2 cells. The effect of resveratrol on B[a]P metabolism by HepG2 microsomes was measured by incubating microsomes with [³H]B[a]P in the presence of NADPH. As shown in Figure 4, approximately 16 fmoles/10 min of [³H]-B[a]P were converted to water-soluble metabolites in DMSO-treated microsomes. The presence of resveratrol in the reaction mixture caused a dose-dependent decrease in B[a]P metabolism (Fig. 4).

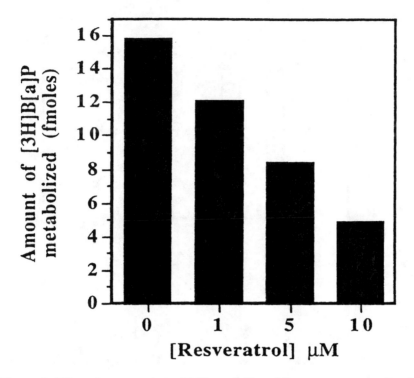

Figure 4. Effect of resveratrol on B[a]P metabolism. Microsomes were incubated with [^{3}H]B[a]P in the presence of NADPH and the indicated concentrations of resveratrol for 10 min and the amount of B[a]P metabolized to water-soluble compounds was determined. n = 4 $\pm$ SE.

Figures 2-4 demonstrate that resveratrol can directly inhibit CYP1A1 enzyme activity, resulting in a decrease in the activation of B[a]P.

2. RESVERATROL AND *CYP1A1* EXPRESSION

Although the decrease in B[a]P-induced CYP1A1 enzymatic activity in intact cells (Fig. 2) may be due to the direct inhibitory effect of resveratrol towards CYP1A enzymatic activity, it may also result from inhibition of the transcriptional activation of the *CYP1A1* gene in response to B[a]P or TCDD. We therefore examined the effect of resveratrol on *CYP1A1* expression in HepG2 cells. As shown in Fig. 5, treatment of cells transfected with a CAT reporter vector controlled by the *CYP1A1*-promoter with B[a]P or TCDD causes an increase in transcription. In cells co-incubated with resveratrol, there was a dose-dependent decrease in the amount of transcription.

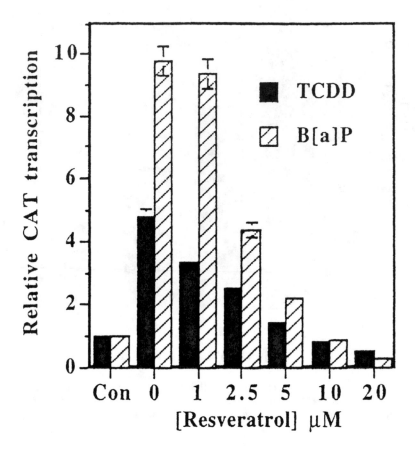

Figure 5. Effect of resveratrol on *CYP1A1*-promoter controlled transcription. HepG2 cells were transfected with a chloramphenicol reporter vector containing the *CYP1A1* promoter and a vector containing β-galactosidase. Transfected cells were treated for 6 h with DMSO (Con), B[a]P (100 nM), or TCDD (1 nM) in the presence of the indicated concentrations of resveratrol. CAT transcription was normalized to β-galactosidase transcription. N = 4 ± SE.

If *CYP1A1* transcription is inhibited by resveratrol, one would expect a decrease in the amount of CYP1A1 mRNA present in cells treated with resveratrol. CYP1A1 mRNA was measured using reverse-transcription polymerase chain reaction (RT-PCR). As shown in Fig. 6, there was a 6-fold increase in the amount of CYP1A1 mRNA in HepG2 cells treated with B[a]P compared to DMSO controls. In cells co-treated with resveratrol, there was a dose-dependent decrease in the amount of CYP1A1 mRNA. Since the HepG2 cells line also expresses another important carcinogen activating enzyme, CYP1A2, we also examined the effect of resveratrol on its expression, with similar results (Fig. 6).

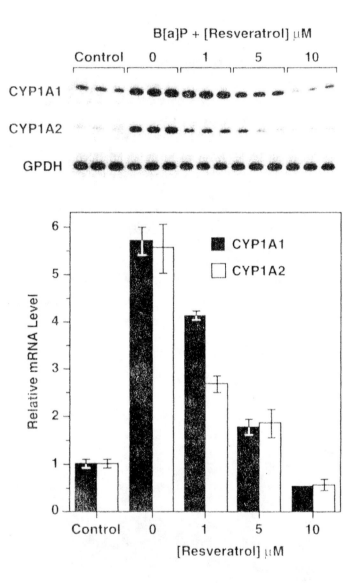

Figure 6. Effect of resveratrol on B[a]P-induced CYP1A1 and CYP1A2 mRNA. HepG2 cells were treated with DMSO (Control) or B[a]P (100 nM) for 6 h in the presence of the indicated concentrations of resveratrol. The amount of mRNA was determined by RT-PCR. The PCR product was subjected to electrophoresis and phosphoimaging. For graph, the amount of CYP1A mRNA was normalized to the level of the housekeeping gene glyceraldehyde-3-phosphate dehydrogenase (GPDH). N = 3 ± SE.

Resveratrol also inhibited the amount of CYP1A1 and CYP1A2 mRNA in cells treated with TCDD (data not shown).

3. RESVERATROL AND AHR FUNCTION

As mentioned in the introduction, the ligand-activated AHR binds to an enhancer sequence of the *CYP1A1* promoter termed the XRE, up-regulating transcription. We determined the effect of resveratrol on the binding of the activated AHR with the XRE using electro-mobility shift assay (EMSA). Nuclear extracts from HepG2 cells were prepared and incubated with radiolabeled XRE oligonucleotide and subjected to electrophoresis (Fig. 7). In the absence of treatment, there was little binding of AHR to the XRE. In extracts from cells treated with B[a]P, on the other hand, there was a distinct band shift that was significantly inhibited by excess unlabeled XRE or by an antibody to the AHR, demonstrating the specificity of this band shift. In cells co-treated with resveratrol, there was a dose-dependent decrease in AHR-XRE binding.

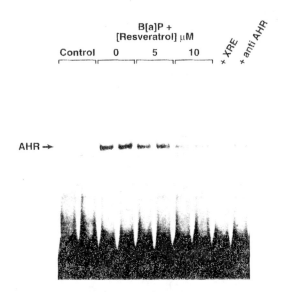

Figure 7. Effect of resveratrol on B[a]P-induced binding of the AHR to the XRE of *CYP1A1*. HepG2 cells were treated for 2 h with DMSO (control) or 1 μM B[a]P in the presence of DMSO or the indicated concentrations of resveratrol. Nuclear protein was isolated, and the amount of activated AHR in 5 μg of protein was measured by EMSA. For competition studies, nuclear protein from B[a]P-treated cells was preincubated with a 200-fold excess of unlabeled XRE or with 0.9 μg of a polyclonal antibody to the AHR. This experiment was repeated two times with similar result.

Resveratrol also inhibited TCDD-induced binding of AHR to the XRE (data not shown). These results indicate that resveratrol disrupts the binding of AHR to the *CYP1A1* promoter, thereby preventing the upregulating of gene transcription that normally results from the activation of the AHR by its ligand.

Several inhibitors of *CYP1A1* transcription are known to function by binding to the ligand binding site of the AHR, blocking the binding of other ligands and thereby preventing AHR activation.[7,13] To determine whether the inhibition of AHR-XRE binding by resveratrol shown in Fig. 7 results from blocking binding of B[a]P to the AHR, HepG2 cytosol was incubated with [³H]B[a]P in the presence of excess resveratrol and the specific binding was measured using sucrose density gradient centrifugation. As shown in Fig. 8, excess resveratrol, even at 1000-fold higher concentration than [³H]B[a]P, did not significantly reduce binding to the AHR. Furthermore, [³H]resveratrol did not bind to the receptor. This result indicates that resveratrol does not directly interact with the receptor and does not prevent receptor activation by ligand.

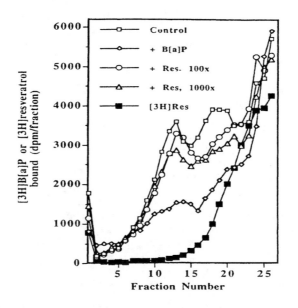

Figure 8. Effect of resveratrol on the binding of [³H]B[a]P to HepG2 cytosol. HepG2 cytosol was incubated with 5 nM [³H]B[a]P in the presence of DMSO (control), 5 μM unlabeled B[a]P, 0.5 μM (100x) resveratrol, or 5 μM (1000x) resveratrol, or with 5 nM [³H]resveratrol. The specific binding of [³H]B[a]P or [³H]resveratrol was analyzed by sucrose density gradient centrifugation. This experiment was repeated three times with different cytosolic preparations with similar results. Res, resveratrol. The gradients were calibrated with catalase (11S; fraction 10) and bovine serum albumin (4S; fraction 20).

SUMMARY AND FUTURE DIRECTIONS

The data presented in this chapter demonstrate that resveratrol affects the carcinogen activation pathway *in vitro* at two levels: it directly inhibits the activity of carcinogen activation enzymes, and it inhibits the increase in *CYP1A1* and *CYP1A2* expression caused by PAHs by inhibiting the activity of the AHR. In concert, these two activities may be responsible for the chemopreventive effect of resveratrol towards PAH-induced carcinogenesis. Several questions remain to be answered. One, how does resveratrol inhibit AHR function? It does not inhibit binding of the ligand to the receptor, nor does it directly bind to the receptor. Its effects must therefore be indirect, i.e., it may prevent translocation of the activated receptor to the nucleus, or prevent dimerization of the AHR with its partner ARNT. Two, does resveratrol have chemopreventive activity towards carcinogenesis in different *in vivo* cancer models? The chemopreventive effect of resveratrol towards PAH-induced carcinogenesis was first demonstrated by Jang et al.[10] To date there have been few subsequent *in vivo* studies. Based on the *in vitro* data presented in this chapter, one might predict that resveratrol would be effective in model systems in which the carcinogen studied requires metabolic activation by CYP1A1 to induce cancer.

REFERENCES

1. Rowlands, J.C., and Gustafsson, J.A. Aryl hydrocarbon receptor-mediated signal transduction. Crit. Rev. Toxicol., 27: 109-134, 1997.
2. Whitlock, J. P. Jr, Chichester, C. H., Bedgood, R. M., Okino, S. T., Ko, H. P., Ma, Q., Dong, L., Li, H., and Clarke-Katzenberg, R. Induction of drug-metabolizing enzymes by dioxin. Drug Metab. Rev., 29: 1107-1127, 1997.
3. Peltonen, K., and Dipple, A. Polycyclic aromatic hydrocarbons: chemistry of DNA adduct formation. J. Occup. Environ. Med., 37: 52-58, 1995.
4. Block, G., Patterson, B., and Subar, A. Fruit, vegetables, and cancer prevention: a review of the epidemiological evidence. Nutr. Cancer, 18: 1-29, 1992.
5. Steinmetz, K. A., and Potter, J. D. Vegetables, fruit, and cancer prevention: a review. J. Am. Diet Assoc., 96: 1027-1039, 1996.
6. Ciolino H.P., Wang T.T., and Yeh G.C. Diosmin and diosmetin are agonists of the aryl hydrocarbon receptor that differentially affect cytochrome P450 1A1 activity. Cancer Res., 58: 2754-2760, 1998.
7. Ciolino H.P., Daschner P.J., Wang T.T., and Yeh G.C. Effect of curcumin on the aryl hydrocarbon receptor and cytochrome P450 1A1 in MCF-7 human breast carcinoma cells. Biochem. Pharmacol., 56: 197-206, 1998.
8. Ciolino H.P., and Yeh G.C. The flavonoid galangin is an inhibitor of CYP1A1 activity and an agonist/antagonist of the aryl hydrocarbon receptor. Br. J. Cancer, 79: 1340-1346, 1999.
9. Ciolino H.P., Daschner P.J., and Yeh G.C. Dietary flavonols quercetin and kaempferol are ligands of the aryl hydrocarbon receptor that affect CYP1A1 transcription differentially. Biochem. J., 40: 715-722, 1999.
10. Jang, M., Cai, L., Udeani, G.O., Slowing, K.V., Thomas, C.F., Beecher, C.W., Fong, H.H., Farnsworth, N.R., Kinghorn, A.D., Mehta, R.G., Moon, R.C., and Pezzuto,

J.M. Cancer chemopreventive activity of resveratrol, a natural product derived from grapes. Science, 275: 218-220, 1997.

11. Ciolino H.P., Daschner P.J., and Yeh G.C. Resveratrol inhibits transcription of CYP1A1 in vitro by preventing activation of the aryl hydrocarbon receptor. Cancer Res., 58: 5707-5712, 1998.

12. Ciolino H.P and Yeh G.C Inhibition of aryl hydrocarbon-induced cytochrome P-450 1A1 enzyme activity and *CYP1A1* expression by resveratrol. Mol. Pharmacol., 56: 760-767, 1999

13. Santostefano, M., Merchant, M., Arellano, L., Morrison, V., Denison, M.S., and Safe, S. (α)-Naphthoflavone-induced CYP1A1 gene expression and cytosolic aryl hydrocarbon receptor transformation. Mol. Pharmacol., 43: 200-206, 1993.

15

HERBALS AND CANCER

Michael J. Wargovich

Department of Pathology
University of South Carolina School of Medicine and
South Carolina Cancer Center Columbia, SC 29203

INTRODUCTION

By some recent estimates up to 30% of Americans routinely use some form of dietary supplement. In attempts to comply with government and public health messages about the health benefits of including fruits and vegetables in the diet many interpret this to include the use of vitamins, herbals, and other dietary supplements in addition to, or, as a substitute for fruits and vegetables. The use of herbal and botanical supplements has been meteoric, with sales approaching $4 billion in 1999. Gingko, St. John's Wort, ginseng, garlic, echinacea, and saw palmetto are among the most popular herbs used in this country (1). While they may be consumed with the hopes of improving memory, combating depression, stimulating the immune system, and a plethora of other health benefits, it is increasingly likely that some herbal and botanical products may also have cancer preventive activities, as well. It is also estimated that as many as 1 in 2 cancer patients use complementary and alternative medicines (CAM) in addition to, or following the failure of standard therapy (2).

DEFINITIONS OF HERBALS AND BOTANICALS

Nutrition and Cancer Prevention, edited under the auspices of AICR
Kluwer Academic / Plenum Publishers, New York, 2000.

"Phytomedicine" is a new term connoting a medical benefit from the use of plant-derived substances. Phytomedicines are the final step in the preparation of botanicals that begin with the fresh or dried herb that is subsequently extracted with water or alcohol to develop herbal extract and tinctures. Standardized extracts, now found in many health food stores and pharmacies are extracts that have been prepared to consistent criteria, often indicated by the presence or absence of a marker phytochemical. Phytomedicines, however, imply a benefit beyond nutritional value, and these may be associated with the cure or prevention of disease, or, alleviation of the disease's symptoms. Seeking medicine from plant-derived sources is not a new idea. As many as 60% of modern medicinals have plant origins. Given that the ingestion of some plant foods is associated with reduced risk for cancer, researchers have delved into the identification of phytochemicals responsible for cancer preventive activity in cell culture, animal models, and in human populations (3). Generally, phytochemicals can be minimally grouped into four mechanisms of chemopreventive action as shown in Table 1.

Table 1. Mechanism of Action of Phytochemicals in Cancer Prevention

Agent	Food Source	Anti-oxidant and/or Anti-inflammatory	Modifiers of Carcinogen Metabolism	Modifiers of Tumor Biology	Inducers Of Differentiation
Carnosol	Rosemary	✓			
Carotenoids	Carrots				✓
Curcumin	Tumeric	✓	✓		
Diallyl sulfide	Garlic		✓		
Ginkolides	Gingko	✓			
Isothiocyanates	Crucifers		✓		
Limonene	Citrus				
Menthol	Mint			✓	
Perillyl alcohol	Cherries			✓	
Quercetin	Onion	✓			
Resveratrol	Grape seed	✓			
Rosmarinic acid	Rosemary	✓			
Silymarin	Milk thistle	✓			
Soy isoflavones	Soybean			✓	
Sulphoraphane	Crucifers		✓		
Tea Catechins	Tea	✓			
Ursolic acid	Rosemary	✓			

From the agents listed above several are found in sources of botanicals commonly used as supplements. In the search for sources of chemopreventive agents it is rare to find actual experiments conducted with fresh or dried botanicals except when the agent has been derived from a plant food. Such has been the case with early studies that showed that feeding of Brassica and

Allium vegetables produced reductions in the incidence of experimentally induced tumors in rodents (4,5). Most experimental protocols use extracted, isolated and purified phytochemicals in the determination of chemopreventive efficacy. The reasons are two-fold: first, to discover a chemical entity or entities that mechanistically explains the anti-tumor effect, and second, to produce an active agent in concentrated and purified form that might be secondarily tested in clinical trials. Preclinical studies often focus on the chemical identity of possible cancer preventive agents, short-term pharmacology studies and an assessment of toxicity. Agents that are within tolerable safety limits are then advanced to clinical trial testing.

Mechanisms of Chemopreventive Action in Botanicals

From Table 1 one can surmise that there are herbal and botanicals with the ability to inhibit tumorigenesis at any point along the linear timeframe of a tumor's development. Antioxidant botanicals, for instance, may directly protect the genome from oxidative damage and mutation, or aid in disrupting the endogenous formation of chemical carcinogens, early steps in the carcinogenic process. Many antioxidants are also anti-inflammatory, a mechanism that might, as discussed below, have utility in the prevention of colon cancer. Thus, even the earliest stages of cancer causation may be prevented by antioxidant botanicals. Botanicals that have been identified as strong antioxidants include several of the polyphenolic compounds found in green and black tea, the compound curcumin in the spice tumeric, ursolic and carnosol in the spice rosemary, resveratrol in red grapes and other red fruits, and quercetin and rutin in onions. Tea polyphenols (also called tea catechins) have shown promising chemopreventive activity in a number of animal tumor models, with skin cancer most strongly curbed by tea (6,7). Equally potent is the compound curcumin, which accounts for the intense color of the culinary spice tumeric. Curcumin inhibits cancers of the skin, colon, and oral cavity in animals (8-10). Resveratrol, a phytoalexin, in red grape juice and wine is a potent antioxidant in vitro, and was found to inhibit mammary cancer in rats (11). Ursolic acid from rosemary shows strong preventive activity in mouse skin cancer models, and quercetin, demonstrated to be a powerful antioxidant inhibits several animal carcinogenesis models (12,13).

Vegetables, fruits, herbs, and other botanicals, also seem to have a strong influence on how carcinogens are metabolized, activated to DNA damaging species, or detoxified. In this category the organosulfur compounds in allium vegetables and isothiocyanates in crucifers have been shown to be moderate to strong inducers of glutathione-S-transferases (14). For some time our laboratory and others have investigated the effects of allium vegetables on Phase 1 and Phase 2 drug metabolism. One of the most interesting effects of organosulfur compounds from garlic and onion is their predilection for inhibition of the carcinogens metabolized by cytochrome P420 2E1 (Cyp

2E1). Studies in our laboratory and others have identified the allylic structure in sulfur volatiles and non-volatiles as a determinant of chemopreventive modulation of Cyp 2E1 (15,16). Carcinogens known to be metabolized by Cyp2E1- mediated reactions include many potent nitrosamines such as the liver carcinogen, dimethylnitrosamine, the oral-pharyngeal carcinogen, NNK, and the esophageal carcinogen, NMBA, and the colon specific carcinogens dimethylhydrazine and azoxymethane. Garlic volatiles are all strongly chemopreventive in these animal models (17-20).

Some natural compounds have the ability to interrupt key molecular events by which a tumor cell has escaped normal regulation on its growth and proliferation. Probably the most notable compounds .in this class are the monoterpenes found in citrus and other fruits. Monoterpenes may operate at several levels in cancer prevention. One mechanism ascribes an ability to interfere with the farnesylation of the ras oncoprotein, while another has shown the monoterpenes limonene and perillyl alcohol to be effective inducers of apoptosis (21-23).

The last mechanism by which botanical agents can subvert the tumorigenesis is by re-induction of the normal process of differentiation. For many years carotenoids, the natural pigments in red-colored vegetables, and the synthetic retinoids, derivatives of retinoic acid, have been investigated as cancer chemopreventives in animals and in human clinical trials (24). These agents show very promising activity in regressing certain premalignant lesions, but the effects are limited to the duration of treatment and side effects such as chaffing, itching, and desquamation of the skin are common, limiting use only in the highest risk patients for recurrent cancer.

ANTIOXIDANT/ANTI-INFLAMMATORY HERBALS AND BOTANICALS IN THE PREVENTION OF CANCER OF THE COLON

Probably one of the most exciting areas of cancer chemoprevention is the effect of anti-inflammatory compounds in colon cancer. Almost a dozen case-control and cohort studies from around the world have concluded that the daily or alternate day consumption of aspirin over extended periods results in a halving one's risk for colon cancer (25). Several prospective studies are underway to assess specifically if daily consumption of aspirin affects the recurrence rates of colonic adenomas in high-risk subjects for colon cancer. These studies strongly suggest that eicosanoids, especially prostaglandins, figure prominently in colorectal carcinogenesis (26). Two genes encode the two major forms of cyclooxygenase, the enzyme responsible for the metabolic conversion of dietary arachidonate to prostaglandins, thromboxanes, and leukotrienes. COX-1, the constitutive form is present in many cell types. COX-2, the isoform inducible by growth factors and tumor promoters, is rarely found in the normal gastrointestinal epithelium, but is over-expressed in colon tumors (27). Since COX-1 is a housekeeping gene, drugs directed to interfering with this isoform result in side effects. Most strongly affected by overuse of aspirin and other NSAIDs (non-steroidal anti-inflammatory drugs) are kidney function, platelet aggregation, and the integrity of the stomach lining (28). These limit the widescale application of NSAIDs in the general public for the chemoprevention of colon cancer. But the paradox is that NSAIDs are excellent chemopreventives in animal models for colon cancer.

Our laboratory has evaluated the effects of oral-dosing of many of the most commonly used NSAIDs in preventing aberrant crypt foci (ACFs), preneoplastic lesions leading to colon cancer in rats. Aspirin, ibuprofen, indomethacin, sulindac, naproxen, and ketoprofen are potent inhibitors of ACFs and have proven to be just as effective in the long-term, full length carcinogenesis assays (29). Despite the strong evidence that NSAIDs are chemopreventives the benefit is out-weighed by the potential adverse effects, notably, gastric and small bowel ulceration. The advent of COX-2 selective drugs such as Celebrex® and Vioxx®, may prove to be highly effective NSAIDs for long-term human use since the constitutive functions of COX-1 are unaffected. At the present time, such COX-2 selective drugs are not 100% specific, still in the process of research evaluation, and expensive.

Herbal NSAIDs?

The plant world is apparently rich in sources of cyclooxygenase inhibitors. Many botanicals are routinely tested for anti-inflammatory properties in the hopes of finding new sources of medicinals for the treatment of chronic inflammatory conditions. Several of these have been found to inhibit cancer in animal models. Some of the more promising botanicals are shown in Table 2. Curcumin has been shown to inhibit COX activity in the

Table 2. Plant-based Sources of Anti-inflammatory Compounds

Plant source	Compound	Chemopreventive Effects in Animal Models	Reference
Tumeric	Curcumin	Inhibitory-skin, colon	(10, 30)
Tea	EGCG	Inhibitory-skin	(31)
Rosemary	Carnosol	Inhibitory-skin, mammary	(12, 13)
Milk thistle	Silymarin	Weakly inhibitory-skin	(32)
Ginger	Ginger extracts	Inhibitory-skin	(33)
Grape seed	Resveratrol	Inhibitory-skin, mammary	(11)

skin, and strongly suppresses skin cancer in the SENCAR mouse model. Tea, given to human volunteers in a clinical trial, reduced PGE2 activity in the rectal mucosa. Resveratrol is a potent inhibitor of cyclooxygenases and is an inhibitor in the mouse skin and rat mammary cancer models. Silymarin was also found to inhibit skin cancer, while cancer prevention activity on carnosol and ginger compounds, both COX inhibitors, has yet to be fully gathered. As indicated in Table 2 a number of compounds remain to be tested in animal models for the most common cancers such as colon, mammary, prostate, and lung.

CONCLUSIONS

In the last five years the use of herbal medicines has risen dramatically in the United States and Europe. In fact the meteoric growth in the use of botanicals in the US has lagged behind use in Europe where phytomedicines are commonly prescribed. Some of the more popular botanicals used for purported health benefits ranging from modulation of cholesterol levels to restoration of urinary tract function are also among those with cancer suppressive properties. For example, polyphenolics in tea are potent inhibitors of experimentally-induced skin cancer, organosulfur compounds in garlic have been shown to suppress the gastrointestinal cancers, and phytoalexins in grapes and cherries have been found to inhibit mammary cancer in rats. As of now much more research is needed to truly establish that certain botanicals will be of use in preventing human cancer. Currently the epidemiologic evidence is suggestive of green tea polyphenols reducing risk for some forms of cancer, while data for other commonly used herbs such as garlic is less convincing. Part of the problem lies in precise quantitation of food-borne phytochemicals where multiple dietary sources of a particular phytochemical is involved, as in recent studies relating dietary quercetin to prevention of heart disease.

Future investigations may focus on specific botanicals with a propensity to intervene in critical pathways in carcinogenesis as demonstrated by the possible use of "natural" NSAIDs in the prevention of colon cancer and the soy-based phytoestrogens in the prevention of breast cancer. Clearly much is to be learned by collaboration between ethnopharmacologists and cancer researchers probing dietary prevention of cancer.

REFERENCES

1.   Brevoort P. The booming US botanical market: a new overview. Herbalgram 1998; 44, 33-46.
2.   Eisenberg DM, Davis RB, Ettner SL, Appel S, Wilkey S, Van Rompay M et al. Trends in alternative medicine use in the United States, 1990-1997: results of a follow-up national survey. JAMA 1998; 280(18):1569-1575.
3.   Craig WJ. Phytochemicals: guardians of our health. J Am Diet Assoc 1997; 97(10 Suppl 2):S199-S204.
4.   Wattenberg LW. Inhibitors of chemical carcinogenesis. Adv Cancer Res 1978; 26:197-226.

5. Fahey JW, Zhang Y, Talalay P. Broccoli sprouts: an exceptionally rich source of inducers of enzymes that protect against chemical carcinogens. Proc Natl Acad Sci U S A 1997; 94(19):10367-10372.
6. Katiyar SK, Mukhtar H. Tea consumption and cancer. World Rev Nutr Diet 1996; 79:154-184.
7. Dreosti IE, Wargovich MJ, Yang CS. Inhibition of carcinogenesis by tea: the evidence from experimental studies. Crit Rev Food Sci Nutr 1997; 37(8):761-770.
8. Rao CV, Reddy BS. Inhibition by dietary curcumin of azoxymethane-induced ornithine decarboxylase, tyrosine protein kinase, arachidonic acid metabolism and aberrant crypt foci formation in the rat colon. Carcinogenesis 1993; 14:2219-2225.
9. Nagabhushan M, Bhide SV. Curcumin as an inhibitor of cancer. J Am Coll Nutr 1992; 11:192-198.
10. Conney AH, Lou YR, Xie JG, Osawa T, Newmark HL, Liu Y et al. Some perspectives on dietary inhibition of carcinogenesis: studies with curcumin and tea. Proc Soc Exp Biol Med 1997; 216(2):234-245.
11. Jang M, Cai L, Udeani GO, Slowing KV, Thomas CF, Beecher CW et al. Cancer chemopreventive activity of resveratrol, a natural product derived from grapes. Science 1997; 275(5297):218-220.
12. Huang MT, Ho CT, Wang ZY, Ferraro T, Lou YR, Stauber K et al. Inhibition of skin tumorigenesis by rosemary and its constituents carnosol and ursolic acid. Cancer Res 1994; 54(3):701-708.
13. Singletary KW, Nelshoppen JM. Inhibition of 7,12-dimethylbenz[a]anthracene (DMBA)-induced mammary tumorigenesis and of in vivo formation of mammary DMBA-DNA adducts by rosemary extract. Cancer Lett 1991; 60(2):169-175.
14. Dalvi RR. Alterations in hepatic phase I and phase II biotransformation enzymes by garlic oil in rats. Toxicol Lett 1992; 60:299-305.
15. Yang CS, Brady JF, Hong JY. Dietary effects on cytochromes P450, xenobiotic metabolism, and toxicity. FASEB J 1992; 6:737-744.
16. Brady JF, Wang MH, Hong JY, Xiao F, Li Y, Yoo JS et al. Modulation of rat hepatic microsomal monooxygenase enzymes and cytotoxicity by diallyl sulfide. Toxicol Appl Pharmacol 1991; 108:342-354.
17. Wargovich MJ. "Inhibition of gastrointestinal cancer by organo-sulfur compounds in garlic". In: *Cancer chemoprevention.* L.W.Wattenberg M .Lipkin M, CW Boone , GJ Kelloff, editors. CRC Press: Boca Raton, FL, 1992.
18. Wargovich MJ, Imada O, Stephens LC. Initiation and postinitiation chemopreventive effects of diallyl sulfide in esophageal carcinogenesis. Cancer Lett 1992; 64:39-42.
19. Hong JY, Wang ZY, Smith TJ, Zhou S, Shi S, Pan J et al. Inhibitory effects of diallyl sulfide on the metabolism and tumorigenicity of the tobacco-specific carcinogen 4-(methylnitrosamino)-1-(3-pyridyl)-1-butanone (NNK) in A/J mouse lung. Carcinogenesis 1992; 13:901-904.
20. Sparnins VL, Barany G, Wattenberg LW. Effects of organosulfur compounds from garlic and onions on benzo[a]pyrene-induced neoplasia and glutathione S-transferase activity in the mouse. Carcinogenesis 1988; 9:131-134.
21. Haag JD, Lindstrom MJ, Gould MN. Limonene-induced regression of mammary carcinomas. Cancer Res 1992; 52:4021-4026.
22. Elegbede JA, Elson CE, Qureshi A, Tanner MA, Gould MN. Inhibition of DMBA-induced mammary cancer by the monoterpene d-limonene. Carcinogenesis 1984; 5:661-664.
23. Lantry LE, Zhang Z, Gao F, Crist KA, Wang Y, Kelloff GJ et al. Chemopreventive effect of perillyl alcohol on 4-(methylnitrosamino)-1-(3-pyridyl)-1-butanone induced tumorigenesis in (C3H/HeJ X A/J)F1 mouse lung. J Cell Biochem Suppl 1997; 27:20-25.
24. Lippman SM, Davies PJ. Retinoids, neoplasia and differentiation therapy. Cancer Chemother Biol Response Modif 1997; 17:349-362.

25. Gupta RA, DuBois RN. Aspirin, NSAIDS, and colon cancer prevention: mechanisms? Gastroenterology 1998; 114(5):1095-1098.
26. Smalley WE, DuBois RN. Colorectal cancer and nonsteroidal anti-inflammatory drugs. Adv Pharmacol 1997; 39:1-20.
27. Sheehan KM, Sheahan K, O'Donoghue DP, MacSweeney F, Conroy RM, Fitzgerald DJ et al. The relationship between cyclooxygenase-2 expression and colorectal cancer. JAMA 1999; 282(13):1254-1257.
28. Graham DY, Smith JL. Aspirin and the stomach. Ann Int Med 1986; 104(3):390-398.
29. Wargovich MJ, Chen CD, Harris C, Yang E, Velasco M. Inhibition of aberrant crypt growth by non-steroidal anti-inflammatory agents and differentiation agents in the rat colon. Int J Cancer 1995; 60:515-519.
30. Rao CV, Rivenson A, Simi B, Reddy BS. Chemoprevention of colon carcinogenesis by dietary curcumin, a naturally occurring plant phenolic compound. Cancer Res 1995; 55(2):259-266.
31. Steele VE, Bagheri D, Balentine DA, Boone CW, Mehta R, Morse MA et al. Preclinical efficacy studies of green and black tea extracts. Proc Soc Exp Biol Med 1999; 220(4):210-212.
32. Lahiri-Chatterjee M, Katiyar SK, Mohan RR, Agarwal R. A flavonoid antioxidant, silymarin, affords exceptionally high protection against tumor promotion in the SENCAR mouse skin tumorigenesis model. Cancer Res 1999; 59(3):622-632.
33. Lee E, Park KK, Lee JM, Chun KS, Kang JY, Lee SS et al. Suppression of mouse skin tumor promotion and induction of apoptosis in HL-60 cells by Alpinia oxyphylla Miquel (Zingiberaceae). Carcinogenesis 1998; 19(8):1377-1381.

16

THE ROLE OF DIETARY SUPPLEMENTS IN HEALTH
An Overview in the United States

Bernadette M. Marriott

Northern Arizona University
4375 East Burning Tree Loop
Flagstaff, AZ 86004

INTRODUCTION

Dietary supplements are in widespread use in the United States (Eisenberg et al., 1998). This use continues to grow as more and more people become concerned about their health care and turn to supplemental self-medication. Information on the supplement use comes from many sources but there are limited data that incorporate the reason for supplement selection and employ sampling techniques that are representative of the breadth and diversity of the United States' population. Yet the widespread use of supplements cannot be ignored or disregarded by health care providers because choice and dose of supplements can directly impact other treatment regimes and nutrient bioavailability from food (Drew and Meyers, 1997; Ernst, 1998). This chapter will provide an overview of the history and current situation with dietary supplements in the United States including the role of the National Institutes of Health Office of Dietary Supplements. Research data on selected botanical supplements commonly used by cancer patients will be reviewed. Finally, sources of information on botanical supplements will be provided.

Nutrition and Cancer Prevention, edited under the auspices of AICR
Kluwer Academic / Plenum Publishers, New York, 2000.

A BRIEF OVERVIEW OF DIETARY SUPPLEMENT REGULATION IN THE UNITED STATES

In 1994 the United States Congress passed the Dietary Supplement Health and Education Act (DSHEA, Public law 103-417, October 25, 1994, 103rd Congress). This law modified the Food, Drug and Cosmetic Act and expanded the definition of dietary supplements to include botanical ingredients, hormones, and a diverse array of related products in addition to vitamins and minerals. The DSHEA also specified the role of the United States Food and Drug Administration (FDA) in regulating dietary supplements, mandated the creation of a Presidential Commission on Dietary Supplement Labeling, and authorized the establishment of the Office of Dietary Supplements at the National Institutes of Health (NIH). The main elements of the definition of dietary supplements from the DSHEA are listed in Table 1.

For products that are regulated by the FDA, the "intended use" is the turnkey that determines whether an item is broadly classified as a food or a drug. Dietary supplements, no matter how they are presented, if intended to be used to supplement the diet, are reviewed by the Office of Special Nutritionals and related offices in the Center for Food Safety and Applied Nutrition (CFSAN) at FDA. The DSHEA included a number of provisions that apply to dietary supplements alone. As a result of the DSHEA the premarket safety evaluations that are required for new food ingredients or new uses of approved food ingredients do not apply to dietary supplements. The DSHEA authorized the FDA to establish good manufacturing practice (GMP) guidelines for dietary supplements and dietary supplement ingredients and the DSHEA provided guidelines for the display of literature used to market dietary supplement products.

Table 1. Key elements of the Definition of a Dietary Supplement from the DSHEA

A Dietary Supplement can be:
•   a product (other than tobacco) intended to supplement the diet that bears or contains one or more of the following dietary ingredients:
- a vitamin, mineral, amino acid, herb or other botanical; OR
- a dietary substance for use to supplement the diet by increasing the total dietary intake; OR
- a concentrate, metabolite, constituent, extract, or combination of any ingredient described above;
Use:
•   intended for ingestion in the form of a capsule, powder, softgel, or gelcap; and
•   not represented as a conventional food or as a sole item of a meal or the diet.

When a manufacturer wishes to market a dietary supplement or dietary supplement ingredient, they must submit information attesting to the safety of the new ingredient to the FDA 75 days prior to the product availability. This petition must indicate that the ingredient does not present a significant risk of illness or injury based on the conditions of use specified on the product label. This DSHEA-based process for dietary supplements differs from the requirements for food additives and new food products, ingredients or uses for food ingredients. These products must be reviewed through FDA's premarket approval process, which includes the submission to FDA of the results from a specified array of safety studies. Once a dietary supplement is on the shelf, the FDA must demonstrate that the product or its ingredients are unsafe for the agency to take action. Since the passage of the DSHEA, the FDA has taken two major stands regarding dietary supplements. In 1997 the FDA requested manufacturers to limit the amount of ephedrine alkaloids in dietary supplements as a result of reports of adverse events including in the extreme cases heart attacks, strokes, seizures, and death. Also in 1997, the presence of a harmful herb, *Digitalis lanata*, as a contaminant in selected batches of an herbal product containing plantain, resulted in the industry and FDA joining forces to identify and remove the contaminated products from stores nationwide (Slifman et al., 1998).

Both manufacturers and the FDA have been moving forward to assure the safety of dietary supplements. While the FDA has made progress to fulfill the mandates of the DSHEA regarding guidance, labeling and GMPs, many companies have begun to self regulate their products and adopt the same manufacturing practices used for foods. Of particular concern to the consumer, is the fact that botanical supplements and supplement ingredients are derived from plant materials that may be grown throughout the world and shipped to the United States for capsulation and packaging. Collection and processing of natural plant materials introduces many additional concerns that need to be addressed for good consumer information on the quality of the products. There are plant variables such as identification of the plant species, the plant part (young leaf versus mature leaf, stem, etc.), the presence of potentially toxic pesticide residues, and purity concerns such as the potential for contamination with bacteria, fungal growths, etc. There are manufacturing variables including the processing of the plant material, extraction procedures, product formulation, and product packaging (exposure to light). Also to be considered are post-manufacturing variables including appropriate shipping and product stability during storage or on the shelf. A shelf life designation is not required for dietary supplements.

The Presidential Commission on Dietary Supplement Labeling issued its report in 1997 and the resulting labeling requirements for dietary supplements went into effect on March 23, 1999. The label is modeled after the label on food products and includes a "Supplement Facts" box of specified size that must include information about the serving size, amount of primary ingredient, other ingredients in descending order and the name and contact information of the supplier. The identity of the product, net quantity and any structure-function claims for the product are elsewhere on the label. If the manufacturer chooses to include a structure-function claim, there must also then be the disclaimer: "This statement has not been evaluated by the Food and Drug Administration. This product is not intended to diagnose, treat, cure, or prevent any disease." An example of the dietary supplement label is included in Figure 1 a, b.

A structure-function claim on a dietary supplement is a statement about how the product may affect the structure or function of the body. An example of a structure-function claim that is used as an example by the FDA is "Calcium builds strong bones". Another that might be used related to the functioning of the body is "Amino acids are essential for normal brain functioning." Structure-function claims do not have to be approved by the FDA.

In contrast, health claims on products must be authorized by the FDA. The FDA has authorized eleven health claims for foods, three of which can be used for supplements if the product meets the minimum content requirements.

How To Read A Dietary Supplement Label
(Information Panel)

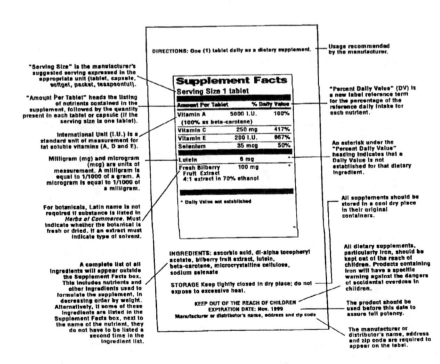

Figure 1a. How to read a dietary supplement label (Information Panel).

How to Read A Dietary Supplement Label
(Principal Display Panel)

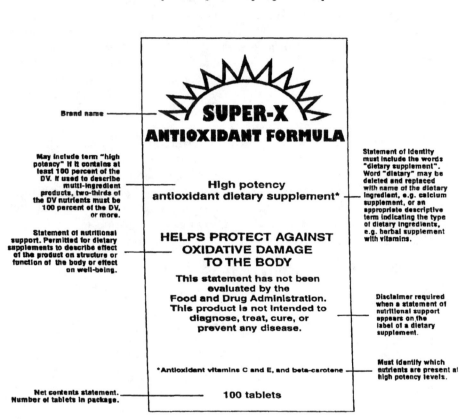

Brand name

May include term "high potency" if it contains at least 100 percent of the DV. If used to describe multi-ingredient products, two-thirds of the DV nutrients must be 100 percent of the DV, or more.

Statement of nutritional support. Permitted for dietary supplements to describe effect of the product on structure or function of the body or effect on well-being.

Net contents statement. Number of tablets in package.

SUPER-X

ANTIOXIDANT FORMULA

High potency
antioxidant dietary supplement*

HELPS PROTECT AGAINST
OXIDATIVE DAMAGE
TO THE BODY

This statement has not been
evaluated by the
Food and Drug Administration.
This product is not intended to
diagnose, treat, cure, or
prevent any disease.

*Antioxidant vitamins C and E, and beta-carotene

100 tablets

Statement of identity must include the words "dietary supplement". Word "dietary" may be deleted and replaced with name of the dietary ingredient, e.g. calcium supplement, or an appropriate descriptive term indicating the type of dietary ingredients, e.g. herbal supplement with vitamins.

Disclaimer required when a statement of nutritional support appears on the label of a dietary supplement.

Must identify which nutrients are present at high potency levels.

Figure1b. How to read a dietary supplement label, principal display panel (prepared by the Council on Responsible Nutrition).

Health claims link the product or ingredients in the product, whether food or supplements, to a disease or health condition. Health claims can be found on calcium with the reduction in risk of osteoporosis, and folic acid, and psyllium husk fiber with reduction in risk of neural tube defects, and heart disease, respectively.

While the steps for handling the regulatory process for supplements are evolving, there are new products classes on the market that further confuse the picture. Standard snack foods such as potato chips can be found that include botanical ingredients such as ginseng, kava kava, etc. Beverages, performance enhancement food bars, and teas also boast the addition of botanical ingredients with structure-function claims on the products. True to the DSHEA definition of dietary supplement most of these products are indeed foods with non-regulated food additives incorporated into them. However, most are being marketed as dietary supplements.

On October 26, 1999 the FDA authorized the use of health claims about the role of soy protein in reducing the risk of coronary heart disease (CHD) through cholesterol lowering. To qualify for the health claim the food item must include 6.25 grams of soy protein per serving. This amount is based on the assumption of four servings per day and because 25 grams per day has been shown to significantly lower cholesterol. This new health claim is an example of one in which the amount of soy protein in the product may result in health claims for dietary supplement food products such as snack bars, beverages, etc. How the FDA will regulate these types of products as well as the growing market of functional foods remains to be seen. It appears, however, that the approach of "intended use" may no longer be a clear turn key for distinguishing among the ever evolving array of products that are blurring the distinction among food, drug and dietary supplement.

USE OF DIETARY SUPPLEMENTS IN THE UNITED STATES

The use of dietary supplements in the United States has grown dramatically since the passage of the DSHEA. Well-stratified statistical samples of the use of dietary supplements by the United States population have yet to be conducted. The most recent National Health and Nutrition Examination Survey (NHANES), which began in 1999, includes a comprehensive set of questions on dietary supplement use. The previous NHANES were designed and conducted prior to the passage of the DSHEA and included questions about vitamin and mineral supplement use by Americans, but did not collect information on the use of botanical supplements and other ingredients newly reclassified as dietary supplements by the DSHEA. Current information on supplement use in the United States stems primarily from market information and studies that have focused on specific populations.

Supplement Sales in the United States

It is estimated that from 30-53% of Americans use dietary supplements on a regular basis (several times each week) or 100 million people. In 1996 sales of dietary supplements totaled $9.8 billion and represented 51% of the total sales in the nutrition industry in the United States. Sales of dietary supplements in natural food stores comprised 44% of the total, and mass-market retail accounted for 26% of the total with the remainder in direct marketing through the mail or Internet. Overall sales for dietary supplements grew 9% in 1996 (Aarts, 1997). Sales continued to grow in 1997 and 1998 to a new record level for total sales of dietary supplements of $13.9 billion in 1998, which was a 10% increase over sales in 1997. Of this market, specialty supplements, in particular, glucosamine, grew 23%, botanical supplements sales increased 13%, and sports-oriented supplements, as exemplified by energy bars, grew 12%. In contrast, vitamin and mineral sales grew less dramatically at the rate of 6% and 8% respectively (NBJ, 1999a). Online internet sales for dietary supplements represented the "fastest growing distribution channel" which totaled $40 million in 1998 and was a significant increase over the $12 million online sales total for 1997 (NBJ, 1999b).

In 1997 botanical supplements sales from all distribution channels totaled $3.6 billion with multi-herbal products comprising 27% of the total. The top five single botanical products sold in 1997 were Echinacea (9%, $324 million), Ginseng (8%, $288 million), Ginkgo (7%, $252 million), Garlic (6%, $216 million), and St. John's wort (6%, $216 million) (NBJ, 1998).

Use of Nutrient Supplements Based on Representative Samples of Specific Groups

The National Health Interview Surveys conducted in 1987 and 1992 surveyed Americans' use of vitamin and mineral supplements over the previous 12-month period. Data from this survey indicated that the prevalence of use remained unchanged between the two surveys. Forty-six percent of adults stated that they used vitamin and mineral supplements in the last year and 24 percent reported regular use (Slesinski et al., 1995). Those who used nutrient supplements, as recorded by the 1992 survey, had overall diets that were lower in fat, higher in fiber and higher in specific vitamins and minerals than non-users of supplement (Slesinski et al., 1996). Data from the NHANES similarly indicated that nutrient supplement users had a higher mean intake of nutrients from their diets, higher incomes and higher education levels than non-users (Koplan, 1986; Looker, 1988). In a survey that assessed the health habits of a representative sample of older residents in the state of Georgia, which included persons in their 60's, 80's and 76 individuals over the age of 100, those who used nutrient supplements were more physically active and more consistently followed the United States Dietary Guidelines for Americans (Houston et al., 1997).

In contrast to nutrient supplement users, those who use botanical supplements present a different profile. In a random sample of 1,035 Americans, those who used botanical supplements were more highly educated but in generally poorer health, specifically they reported a higher prevalence of back pain, chronic pain and anxiety than those who did not use supplements (Astin, 1998).

Overall, representatives of health professional groups tend to use nutrient supplements in similar patterns to the general population. Of 1732 nurses surveyed in the Nurses Health Study, 38% reported regularly taking multivitamins. Use of single nutrient supplements was less prevalent: vitamin C (23%), vitamin E (15%) and vitamin A (4%) (Willett, 1981). Forty-seven per cent of 692 pharmacy students queried in a study by Ranelli et al. (1993) reported using nutrient supplements within the previous two weeks. Among 181 cardiologists, 44% reported routinely taking antioxidants, 42% were routinely taking aspirin and 28% reported regular use of both products (Mehta, 1997). Dietitians appear to use supplements to a greater degree than other health professionals do. Of 665 dietitians polled in Washington State, 60% reported using some form of dietary supplement (Worthington-Roberts, 1984).

Two nationally representative random household telephone surveys in the 1990's that measured the use of alternative medicinal practices by Americans included questions on dietary supplements. Between 1990 and 1997 there was a dramatic increase in the use of high dose vitamins (130% increase) and botanical supplements (380 % increase) by adults (Eisenberg et al., 1998). Most other data on botanical supplement use in the United States are industry-sponsored, consumer-based surveys. In a 500 household survey conducted by the Celestial Seasons Company in partnership with the Harris Organization, 33% of households regularly used botanical supplements (cited by Brevoort, 1998). A larger survey of 43,000 households reported the use of specific botanical supplements as garlic (19%), Ginseng (10%), Ginkgo (9%), and Echinacea (7%) (as cited in Brevoort, 1998). A Gallup interview of 704 individuals about attitudes toward and usage of botanical supplements cited fatigue, stress and menopause/PMS as the three most frequently cited reason for use of botanical supplements (Gallup, 1997, as cited in Brevoort, 1998). A survey by Prevention magazine of their readership indicated that 32% of those who responded used botanical supplements and spent an average of $54 per year on botanical supplement purchases. Sixty-five of the respondents indicated that they used botanical supplements because they believed these products were safer than drugs (Prevention Magazine, 1997, as cited in Brevoort, 1998).

In general, comprehensive information on the use of dietary supplements, as defined in the DSHEA, is limited to select population-based studies. The current NHANES includes questions on the type and amount of supplement used and will therefore provide a stratified sample of these factors within the sampling model of the overall project. However, the necessary breadth of the NHANES results in a limited set of questions related to dietary supplements. For more detailed information on determinants of supplement selection, rationale for supplement use, relation of price to choice patterns, specifics of use, etc. more targeted research is needed.

COMMONLY USED BOTANICAL SUPPLEMENTS BY CANCER PATIENTS

Not unexpectedly, a large percentage of cancer patients incorporate alternative medical therapies as adjuvant to conventional treatments. In a cohort of 480 patients who were newly diagnosed with early-stage breast cancer, 10.6 % of the women had used alternative medicine prior to their diagnosis and 28.1% initiated the use of alternative medicine after surgery. Alternative medicine was defined in this study to include botanical supplements. There was no difference among alternative medicine users and nonusers on quality of life measures at the time of surgery, however, at three months post surgery, use of alternative practices was associated with depression, fear measures, lowered mental health ratings, and lowered sexual satisfaction (Burstein et al., 1999). A secondary breast cancer prevention trial of 435 women who had completed medical treatment used four 24-hour dietary recalls over a two-week period to identify dietary patterns. In this study, 80.9% of the women reported dietary supplement use on a regular basis, which is approximately double that of the general population. Women who used supplements, whether nutrient, botanical or biological, consumed diets with more dietary fiber and less dietary fat than non-users (Rock et al., 1997). In a localized breast cancer follow up trial in postmenopausal women, 71% of the first 724 patients randomized on the study were regularly taking dietary supplements. In a subset of 116 consecutive women on the same study, 82% were taking at least one dietary supplement but the variety of the supplements taken each day varied from 1 to 10 and the number of pills consumed per day ranged from 1 to 26. Of those women who reported regular intake of dietary supplements, 22% were taking botanical supplements and biologicals (Winters et al., 1997). Ongoing work by these two groups is the main source of growing understanding of the parameters of use of dietary supplements by cancer patients.

The role of components derived from native plants and foods from around the world in the potential treatment and prevention of cancer has been a major focus of the National Cancer Institute for many years. Botanical supplements that are currently used most commonly as adjuvant therapy for cancer include *Astralgalus membranaceus* (Astralagus, huang-qi), *Serenoa repens* (saw palmetto), *Uncaria tomentosa* (cat's claw), *Viscum album* (mistletoe), *Silybum marianum gaertn* (milk thistle), and shitake mushrooms.

Astralgalus membranaceus Bunge (*Astralagus*, huang-qi) is a Chinese herb that is cultivated for its roots as an immunostimulant (Foster, 1996). In a small in vitro study, the function of T lymphocytes in cells from 13 cancer patients improved by 260% when compared with untreated cells and there was an improvement of 160% in comparison with cells of healthy donors (Chu et al., 1988). Using a mouse model, Lau et al, (1994) have shown that a combination of extracts from *Astralagus* and *Ligustrum lucidum* led to a 57% cure rate with a tumor load of 2x105 and a 100% cure rate when the initial tumor load was 1x105. The authors attribute the antitumor activity to augmentation of phagocyte and LAK cell activities. More studies are in progress but preliminary indications are that the reputed immunostimulant activity of *Astralagus* continues to be supported in model systems and in human case studies. Current research emphases include exploration of other biological responses (Khoo and Ang, 1995), identification of the active constituents (Yu and Liu, 1993), and growth conditions that affect the amounts of these constituents (Shibata et al., 1996). Clinical studies in humans in the United States are needed. Reported adverse effects to *Astralagus* include lowered blood pressure, and with high doses, immunosuppression.

The botanical supplement, *Serenoa repens* (saw palmetto) is derived from the fruit of a small shrub in the palm family that is native to the United States. This supplement is at the center of a controversy over its efficacy for the treatment of benign prostatic hyperplasia (BPH). Wilt et al (1998) reported the results of a systematic review and meta-analysis of the existing randomized trials. Eighteen randomized controlled trials that included 2939 men met the criteria for inclusion in the quantitative meta-analysis. The authors found that the average study duration in the trials was short – only nine weeks and there was significant variability in the study designs, preparations and manner which outcomes were measured. Nonetheless, the data indicated that *Serenoa repens* provided improvement in urinary tract symptom scores and urine flow. It is clear that a longer-term trial with clear outcome measures is needed to assess the efficacy of *S. repens* for long term treatment of BPH. NIH currently supports 129 active clinical trials for BPH research and is contemplating a clinical trial with saw palmetto. There are no known serious adverse effects with saw palmetto.

Uncaria tomentosa (U. guianensis) (cat's claw) is derived from the root and stem of two woody vines found in the Amazon. Traditional uses for *U. tomentosa* in South America include intestinal ailments, gastric ulcers and cancer, among others (Foster, 1996). *U.tomentosa* root contains six active alkaloids that have been explored for their potential to treat cancer. Also identified are other compounds with potential antioxidant activity (Spaulding-Albright, 1997). Studies in cell culture have indicated that one alkaloid, uncarine F, has potential for treatment of acute leukemia through inhibition of tumor cell growth (Stuppner et al., 1993). Trials in humans are ongoing. Cat's claw that is found on the United States market as a dietary supplement can be composed of stems and roots from the two *Uncaria* species and several other species that have the same common name from the Caribbean and South America. European physicians use *U. tomentosa* as an immunostimulant in treatment of cancer. However, in Germany and Austria where this treatment is used, *U. tomentosa* is a standardized product that is available only by prescription. Concern exists about the varying degrees of potency and adulteration of products in the United States market, and the potential for adverse effects if used by patients with diseases of the immune system in including HIV infection (Foster, 1996; Spaulding-Albright, 1997). Therefore, physician consultation is recommended when using cat's claw.

Leaf extracts from *Viscum album* (European mistletoe) have shown promise for treatment of cancer in human trials. A review of the efficacy of 11 controlled studies reported that patient survival was extended in ten of the eleven studies (Kleijnen and Knipchild, 1994). One factor contributing to the success of *Viscum album* as a treatment may be DNA repair. Kovacs et al., 1991(as cited in Spaulding-Albright, 1997) indicated that 12 of 14 breast cancer patients treated parentally with a standardized extract product called Iscador, demonstrated a 2.7 times higher DNA repair rate. Most research with *V. album* has been conducted in Europe. Mistletoe berries are toxic. Since contaminated product is a possibility as a result of the parasitic growth habit of *V.* album, self-dosing with this species is not recommended (Spaulding-Albright, 1997).

Seeds from *Silybum marianum gaertn* (milk thistle) have been used for over 2,000 years to treat liver disorders. Numerous studies in the last 30 years have identified silymarin as the active compound that acts primarily on the cells of the liver membrane to inhibit chemical transport (Foster, 1996). Topical application of silymarin prevented skin tumor growth in mice (Agarwalet al., 1994). More studies of the potential use of this agent in skin cancer prevention and treatment are needed. The anti-hepatotoxic activity of silymarin shows potential as an adjunct for persons receiving chemotherapy (Spaulding-Albright, 1997) particularly as adverse effects are few. A recent study indicated that treatment with silymarin did not reduce the effectiveness of anti-tumor drug therapy in rodent models (Bokemayer et al., 1996).

Shiitake mushrooms contain the polysaccharide, lentinan, that has been shown to stimulate the production of T lymphocytes and natural killer cells (Chihara, 1987). In mice receiving chemotherapy, lentinan was effective in reducing ethrythroid toxicity (Takasuki et al., 1996). Shiitake mushrooms have no known side effects and a long history of ingestion in Asia. Human studies to measure specific outcomes are needed.

A number of the botanical supplements that have been discussed above and demonstrate significant promise in the treatment and prevention of recurrence of cancer are in use for these purposes in Europe. The major difference is that in those countries these compounds are available by prescription as registered pharmaceuticals. The concern in the United States is that cancer patients may self-medicate with these botanical supplements without discussing their use with their physician. It is important to urge all health care providers, especially those who work with cancer patients, to ask patients, as a routine part of each health care visit, whether or not they are using dietary supplements. Patients who are using supplements should be asked to bring the supplement labels to their health care provider to insure that none of the products may interact adversely with treatment (Marriott, 1997).

INTERNET SOURCES OF INFORMATION ON SUPPLEMENTS

The Office of Dietary Supplements (ODS) was authorized at the NIH as part of the DSHEA legislation. This office was formally started in late 1995 with the mandate to serve as a source of research support, inter-government advice, and science-based information on dietary supplements. The ODS has worked extensively with the other NIH institutes, centers, and offices to partner in identifying the most fruitful areas for research in dietary supplements and to serve as a source of information for scientists, industry and the public. The ODS website (http://dietary-supplements.info.nih.gov) includes a readily searchable database of scientific articles on dietary supplements and will contain peer reviewed information pages on nutrient and botanical supplements that can be printed or downloaded. The ODS site also includes links to other reputable sites with dietary supplement information on the Internet. The ODS has recently funded two Dietary Supplement Research Centers that will be focused on research on botanical supplements and health outcomes.

Also through NIH, the National Center for Complementary and Alternative Medicine's website (http://nccam.nih.gov) includes information about their current clinical trials in botanical supplements. Of course, the National Cancer Institute (NCI), the American Institute for Cancer Research, and the American Cancer Society all provide information on cancer prevention and treatment through their websites. Of particular interest for cancer patients is the NCI listing of ongoing clinical cancer trials that are open for participants to join (http://www.nih.gov/health/trials/index.htm). This database allows the patient or health care provider to search the trials database by details of cancer type, geographic location and specific therapy. NIH has a combined health information database (http://chid.nih.gov) that is a good initial source of general information.

The FDA provides current information on the regulatory status of dietary supplements, summary reports of adverse effects and general information about supplements in a question and answer format on their WebPages at (http://vm.cfsan.fda.gov/~dms/supplmnt.html). Adverse effects of supplement use should be reported directly to the FDA through their MedWatch phone line: 800-332-1088. The Federal Trade Commission (FTC) is responsible for accurate advertising of supplement products. The activities of the FTC related to supplement product advertising can be found on their website at http://ftc.gov. The American Dietetic Association (http://eatright.irg) and the National Council Against Health Fraud (http://www.primenet.com~nchf/) are additional resources.

Basic information on plant species can be found on websites of the American Botanical Council http://www.herbalgram.org/abcmisson.html), the Council for Responsible Nutrition (http://www.crn.org). the Herb Research

Foundation (http://www.herbs.org/index.html), and the American Herbal Products Association (htte://www.apha.com). The latter has produced two books of particular interest. One includes a listing of the plant species from which ingredients are marketed in the United States (*Herbs of Commerce*) and the other takes the species from that listing and identifies the known safety concerns. Both books are available through their website. Figures related to dietary supplement industry sales can be found on the Nutrition Business website (http://www.nutritionbusiness.com). These last five groups have direct ties to the supplement industry so any specific advice to consumers found on their websites must take their organizational function into consideration.

CONCLUSION

Dietary supplements in the United States include a wide array of ingredients and products that are broadly available in the marketplace. While these products are presented in formats that give the appearance of standard over-the-counter (OTC) medications such as aspirin, their manufacturers are not required to provide the same level of pre-market safety data or adhere to the same level of good manufacturing practices as are manufacturers of OTC products. Botanical supplements in particular are directly derived from wild, or in some cases, commercially grown plants and therefore are more subject to product variability due to plant contamination, and manufacturing and post-manufacturing variables that are currently not regulated. Patients who chose to use these supplements should not do so as replacement for prescribed therapy. If they choose to augment their therapy with dietary supplements they should do so after discussing it with their physician, and pharmacist. It is also advised that name brand products that are widely available should be selected and that ingestion closely follows the doses and instructions on the labels.

REFERENCES

1. Astin JA. Why patients use alternative medicine: results of a national study. JAMA 1998; 279:1548-53.
2. Bokemayer C, Fels LM, Dunn T, Voight W, Gaedeke I, Schmoll HJ, Stolte H, LentzenH. Silibimin protects against cisplatin-induced nephrotoxicity without compromising cisplatin or ifosfmide anti-tumour activity. Br J Cancer 1996; 74:2036-41.
3. Brevoort P. The booming U.S. botanical market: a new overview. Herbalgram 1998; 44:33-47.
4. Burstein HJ, Gelber S, Guadagnoli E, Weeks JC. Use of alternative medicine by women with early-stage breast cancer. N Engl J Med 1999; 340:1733-39.
5. Chihara G. Anti-tumor and metastasis-inhibitory activities of lentinan as an immunomodulator. Cancer Detect Prev Suppl 1987:423-43.

6. Chu DT, Wong WL, Mavlight GM. Immunotherapy with Chinese medicinal herbs: immune restoration of local zenogeneic graft-versus-host reaction in cancer patients by fractionated Astragalus membranacueus in vitro. J Clin Lab Immunol. 1988; 25(3):1, 19-23.

7. Drew AK, Myers SP. Safety issues in herbal medicine: implications for the health professions. MJA 1997; 166:538-41.

8. Eisenberg DM, Davis RB, Ettner SL, Appel S, Wilkey S, Rompay MV, Kessler RC. Trends in alternative medicine use in the United States, 1990-1997. JAMA 1998; 280:1569-75.

9. Ernst E, MD. Harmless herbs? A review of the recent literature. Am J Med. 1998; 104:170-8.

10. Foster S. *Herbs for Your Health*. Loveland, Colorado: Interweave Press, 1996.

11. Gallup Study of attitudes toward and usage of herbal supplements. 1995, 1996, 1997., as cited in Brevoort P. The booming U.S. botanical market: a new overview. Herbalgram 1998; 44:33-47.

12. Houston DK, Johnson MA, Daniel TD, Poon LW. Health and dietary characteristics of supplement users in an elderly population. International J Vit and Nutr Res 1997; 67:183-91.

13. Khoo KS, Ang PT. Extract of *Astragalus membranaceus* and *Ligustrum lucidum* does not prevent Cyclophosphamide-induced myelosuppression. Singapore Medical Journal 36(4); 1995:387-90.

14. Kleijnen J, Knipchild P. Mistletoe treatment for cancer: review of controlled trials in humans. Phytomedicine 1994; 13: 255-60.

15. Koplan JP, Annest JL, Layde PM, Rubin GL. Nutrient intake and supplementation in the United States (NHANES II). Am J Public Health 1986; 76:287-89.

16. Kovacs RE, Hajto T, Kostanska K. Improvement of DNA repair in lymphocytes of breast cancer patients treated with Viscum album extract (Iscador). Europ J Cancer 1991; 27: 1672-6.

17. Lau BHD, Ruckle HC, Botolazzo T, Lui PD. Chinese medicinal herbs inhibit growth of murine renal cell carcinoma. Cancer biotherapy 9(2) 1994:153-61.

18. Looker A, Sempos CT, Johnson C, Yetley EA. Vitamin-mineral supplement use: association with dietary intake and iron status of adults. J Am Dietetic Assn 1998; 88:808-14.

19. Marriott BM. Vitamin D Supplementation: A Word of Caution. Annals Int Med 1997; 127(3): 231-3.

20. Mehta J. Intake of antioxidants among American cardiologists. Am J Cardiol 1997; 79:1558-60.

21. Nutrition Business Journal. Consumer sales 1997. 1998: Web site http://www.nutritionbusiness.com.

22. Nutrition Business Journal. 1998 Internet sales of supplements hits $40 million. 1999a:Web site http://www.nutritionbusiness.com.

23. Nutrition Business Journal. Nutrition industry generates $25.8Bn in sales. 1999b:Web site http://www.nutritionbusiness.com.

24. Ranelli PL, Dickerson RN, White KG. Use of vitamin and mineral supplements by pharmacy students. Am J Hosp Pharm 1993; 50:674-78.

25. Rock CL, Newman V, Flatt SW, Faerber S, Wright FA, Pierce JP. Nutrient intakes from foods and dietary supplements in women at risk for breast cancer recurrence. Nutrition and Cancer 1997; 29: 133-9.

26. Shibata TSE, Asetai NKM. Growth and glycoside contents of *Astragalus membranaceus* (Leguminosae) cultivated in different soil groups. Natural Medicines 1996; 50(4): 296-99.

27. Slesinski MJ, Subar AF, Kahle LL. Dietary intake of fat, fiber and other nutrients is related to the use of vitamin and mineral supplements in the United States: The 1992 National Health Interview Survey. J Nutrition 1996; 126:3001-8.

28. Sleinski MJ, Subar AF, Kahle LL. Trends in use of vitamin and mineral supplements in the United States: The 1987 and 1992 National Health Interview Surveys. J Am Diet Assoc 1995; 95:921-3.

29. Slifman NR, Obermeyer WR, Aloi BK, Musser SM, Correll WA, Cichowicz SM, Betz JM, Love LA. Contamination of botanical dietary supplements by *Digitalis lanata*. N Engl J Med 1998; 339: 806-10.

30. Spaulding-Albright N. A review of some herbal and related products commonly used in cancer patients. J Am Diet Assoc 1997; 97(suppl2): S208-15.

31. Stuppner H, Sturm S, Geisen G, Zillian U, Konwalinka G. A differential sensitivity of oxindole alkaloids to normal and leukemic cell lines. Planta Med 1993; Supplement A: 583.

32. Tslsysuki F, Miyasaka Y, Kikuchi T, Suzuki M, Hamuro J. Improvement of erythroid toxicity by lentinan and erythorpoietin in mice treated with chemotherapeutic agents. Exp Hematol 1996; 24:416-22.

33. Willett W, Samson L, Bain C. Vitamin supplement use among registered nurses. Am J Clin Nutr 1981; 34:1121.

34. Wilt TJ, Ishani A, Stark G, MacDonald R, Lau J, Mulrow C. Saw palmetto extracts for treatment of benign prostatic hyperplasia. JAMA 1998; 280:1604-9.

35. Winters B, Grosevenor M, Chon Y, Blackburn G, Copeland T, Chlebowski R, Marsoobian V, Shapiro A, Wynder E. Dietary supplement use by breast cancer participants in the women's intervention nutrition study (WINS). FASEBJ 1997; 11(3): A160.

36. Worthington-Roberts B, Breskin M. Supplementation patterns of Washington state dietitians. J Am Diet Assoc 1984; 84:795-800.

37. Yu ZK, Liu KJ. Studies of active constituents of *Astragalus membranaceus* (Fisch) Bunge. Journal of Plant Resources and Environment 1993; 2(4): 40-3.

17

THE BETA-CAROTENE STORY

Peter Greenwald[1] and Sharon S. McDonald[2]

[1]Division of Cancer Prevention
National Cancer Institute, National Institutes of Health
[2]The Scientific Consulting Group, Inc.

INTRODUCTION

Considered to be an effective antioxidant, beta-carotene, a carotenoid that occurs naturally in many vegetables and fruits and that converts to vitamin A in the body, has been the subject of intensive cancer prevention research for decades,[1] and is a commonly found supplement on the shelves of most supermarkets. This compound recently attracted significant national and international attention when results from two large-scale trials using beta-carotene—the Alpha-Tocopherol, Beta-Carotene Cancer Prevention (ATBC) Study[2] and the Beta-Carotene and Retinol Efficacy Trial (CARET),[3] discussed later in this chapter—showed adverse treatment effects in terms of increased lung cancer incidence. These findings called into question the safety of supplementation with beta-carotene in high-risk individuals such as smokers and underscored the need for further research on beta-carotene, particularly to investigate possible mechanism(s)-of-action. The story of beta-carotene serves as an excellent example of the carefully designed, step-wise research strategy that must be carried out to provide clear direction for planning and implementing effective cancer-preventive public health applications. This strategy comprises a systematic review of existing epidemiologic and laboratory evidence to form cancer prevention hypotheses followed by methods development and efficacy studies to test intervention hypotheses in well-

Nutrition and Cancer Prevention, edited under the auspices of AICR   **219**
Kluwer Academinc / Plenum Publishers, New York, 2000.

characterized populations before application to a general population and, ultimately, widespread implementation in national prevention programs.[4]

THE EPIDEMIOLOGIC EVIDENCE

Although the value of epidemiologic evidence has been questioned by some,[5] epidemiologic studies remain essential to the hypothesis-building process by providing initial clues that can spark scientific interest and suggest directions for future research; such studies often are the only pragmatic or ethically acceptable way to link exposures to human disease.[6] Critical evaluation and meaningful distillation of epidemiologic study results have played and will continue to play a key role in the identification of dietary factors related to cancer risk. Weighing the evidence from the many epidemiologic studies in the 1970s that linked high intake of vegetables and fruits—an index of beta-carotene intake—with reduced cancer risk, Peto and colleagues, in 1981, published a comprehensive review of the collective epidemiologic evidence that correlated either blood levels or dietary intake of carotenoids (mostly beta-carotene) with cancer risk.[7] The review concluded that sufficient epidemiologic evidence existed to suggest that investigating the potential anticancer effects of beta-carotene, and possibly other carotenoids, was warranted. The encouraging epidemiologic evidence, as well as corroborating laboratory investigations, provided a strong rationale for the conduct of randomized, controlled clinical intervention trials with beta-carotene. Such trials, described more fully later in this chapter, were initiated in the early 1980s, and were carried out concurrently with continuing epidemiologic and laboratory studies.

More recent published reviews of epidemiologic studies that also focused primarily on indices of beta-carotene consistently have continued to find strong support for a significant protective effect of dietary beta-carotene on lung cancer.[1,8-11] One review[10] noted that associations of either high intakes of vegetables and fruits rich in beta-carotene or high blood concentrations of beta-carotene with reduced cancer risk were most consistent for lung and stomach cancer. Data for esophageal cancer showed limited but promising risk reduction.[10] Reported results for the effects of beta-carotene were equivocal for prostate cancer[12] and indicated a possible protective effect of beta-carotene for breast cancer.[13] For colon cancer, some case-control studies reported significantly reduced risk at high intakes,[14] but, overall, data suggested only a modest risk reduction.[10] The comprehensive review of studies on nutrition, food, and cancer commissioned by the World Cancer Research Fund and the American Institute for Cancer Research concluded that carotenoid intake—measured as beta-carotene in the majority of studies—probably decreases lung cancer risk and possibly decreases the risk of esophageal, stomach, colorectal, breast, and cervical cancers; data on prostate cancer risk was judged to be equivocal.[1]

It is important to remember that data from these epidemiologic studies do not prove a direct benefit from beta-carotene in vegetables and fruits. Many other potentially beneficial compounds (including other carotenoids, as discussed in a later section), acting either alone or more likely in combination, could contribute to the cancer-protective properties of plant-based foods. For lung cancer, however, the body of evidence provided by epidemiologic investigations of disease risk in relation to consumption of vegetables and fruits rich in beta-carotene and serum beta-carotene concentrations is highly persuasive, with respect to both the magnitude and the consistency of the observed protective association.[15]

EARLY CLINICAL EFFICACY TRIALS

Early clinical efficacy trials on oral cancer showed evidence of benefit from beta-carotene. In Filipino betel nut chewers, who are at very high risk for oral cancer, the percentage of buccal mucosa cells with micronuclei—evidence of genotoxic damage—was significantly lower in people given beta-carotene for 9 weeks than in those given canthaxanthin, a carotenoid with no vitamin A activity.[16] One study that examined the effect of beta-carotene on leukoplakia, a precancerous oral lesion, reported that 17 of 24 patients showed significant reversal of lesions after 6 months of treatment.[17] In another study, however, low-dose 13-*cis*-retinoic acid was significantly more effective than beta-carotene in maintaining the stability of leukoplakia reversed by high-dose 13-*cis*-retinoic acid.[18] Also, a trial of beta-carotene to prevent nonmelanoma skin cancer in persons previously treated for skin cancer demonstrated no beneficial effect.[19]

Trials to prevent colorectal polyps showed no evidence of benefit—and no evidence of harm—from beta-carotene. In a study in which 864 people, who previously had polyps removed, received either beta-carotene, vitamins C and E, all three antioxidants, or placebo for 4 years, no reduction in polyp incidence was demonstrated for any of the interventions.[20] Similarly, an Australian polyp prevention trial, in which approximately 400 patients with previous polyps received either beta-carotene or placebo along with usual diet, low-fat diet, high-wheat bran diet, or low-fat/high-wheat bran diet, found no significant polyp reduction.[21] Data suggested, however, that the low-fat/high-wheat bran diet may inhibit the transition from smaller to larger polyps, which have greater malignant potential.

LARGE-SCALE, RANDOMIZED CLINICAL INTERVENTION TRIALS

The large-scale, randomized, controlled clinical trial, with a cancer endpoint, is considered the best means available to determine the efficacy of preventive interventions. This section presents results for several large-scale, randomized beta-carotene trials that have either been completed (Linxian Trials, Physicians' Health Study [PHS]) or for which accrual has been closed; long-term followup is continuing for these trials. The epidemiologic and laboratory data that linked high intakes of foods containing beta-carotene and high blood levels of beta-carotene to reduced risk of lung cancer provided strong hypotheses for the interventions used in the trials described here. Although the results were not as expected for the ATBC Study and CARET, these trials demonstrated the difficulty of isolating a single component of a healthful diet as the one beneficial element and exemplified the need for large-scale clinical trials to determine safety as well as efficacy, before recommendations for dietary intake of single components are formulated for the public.[22]

The Linxian Trials, conducted by the NCI in collaboration with the Chinese Institute of the Chinese Academy of Medical Sciences, were two randomized, double-blind chemoprevention trials designed to determine whether daily ingestion of vitamin/mineral supplements would reduce incidence and mortality rates for esophageal cancer in a high-risk population in Linxian, China, where approximately 20% of all deaths result from esophageal cancer. The General Population Trial, which began in 1986, randomized more than 30,000 individuals to eight treatment groups to provide a one-half replicate of a 2^4 factorial design that tested the effects of four combinations of nutrients. Combinations included retinol and zinc (A); riboflavin and niacin (B); vitamin C and molybdenum (C); and beta-carotene, vitamin E, and selenium (D). The eight treatment groups received either placebo, AB, AC, AD, BC, BD, CD, or ABCD each day for 5.25 years, at doses equivalent to one to two times the U.S. Recommended Daily Allowances (RDAs).[23] The second study, the Dysplasia Trial, enrolled 3,318 individuals with evidence of severe esophageal dysplasia; subjects were randomized to receive either a placebo or a daily supplement of 14 vitamins and 12 minerals, including beta-carotene, at two to three times the U.S. RDAs, for 6 years.

Results of the General Population Trial indicated a significant benefit for those receiving the beta-carotene/vitamin E/selenium combination—a 13% reduction in cancer mortality, resulting largely from a 21% drop in stomach cancer mortality.[24] Also, this group experienced a 9% reduction in deaths from all causes, a 10% decrease in deaths from strokes, and a 4% decrease in deaths from esophageal cancer. The effects of the beta-carotene/vitamin E/selenium combination began to appear within 1 to 2 years after the intervention began and continued throughout the study; the three other combinations did not affect cancer risk. It should be noted that the benefits of individual components of supplement D—beta-carotene, vitamin E, and selenium—cannot be evaluated independently in this design; it is possible that components may have had either an additive or a multiplicative effect on cancer risk. An end-of-intervention endoscopy survey, carried out in a small sample of subjects as part of the General Population Trial, showed no significant reductions in prevalence of either esophageal or gastric dysplasias. However, prevalence of esophageal cancer was 42% lower in those receiving supplement D, and prevalence of stomach cancer was 62% lower in those receiving supplement A.[23] A nonsignificant, 16% reduction in mortality from esophageal cancer was reported for the Dysplasia Trial.[25] The results of these trials are encouraging but may not be directly applicable to Western cultures, which tend to be well nourished and not deficient in multiple micronutrients, in contrast to the Linxian community.

The Physicians' Health Study (PHS), a general population trial in 22,000 U.S. physicians that evaluated the effect of aspirin and beta-carotene supplementation on the primary prevention of cardiovascular disease and cancer, began in 1982. The aspirin component of PHS ended in 1987, because a benefit of aspirin on risk of first heart attack (44% reduction) was found. The treatment period for beta-carotene continued until December 1995; data showed no significant evidence of benefit or harm from beta-carotene for either cardiovascular disease or cancer.[26]

Both the ATBC Study and CARET were carried out in populations at high risk for lung cancer. The ATBC Study investigated the efficacy of vitamin E (alpha-tocopherol) alone, beta-carotene alone, or a combination of the two compounds in preventing lung cancer among more than 29,000 male cigarette smokers ages 50 to 69, with an average treatment/followup of 6 years. Unexpectedly, this study showed a 16 percent higher incidence of lung cancer in the beta-carotene group. However, 34 percent fewer cases of prostate cancer and 16 percent fewer cases of colorectal cancer were diagnosed among men who received vitamin E.[2,27] In the ATBC Study, the adverse effects of beta-carotene were observed at the highest two quartiles of ethanol intake, initially indicating that alcohol consumption may enhance the actions of beta-carotene.[27] However, further analysis of 7.7 years of followup data for drinkers found no association between lung cancer and either total ethanol or specific beverage (beer, wine, spirits) intake, after adjustment for potential confounders.[28] Also, there was no evidence of modification of an alcohol effect by either beta-carotene or alpha-tocopherol supplementation. CARET tested the efficacy of a combination of beta-carotene and retinol (as retinyl palmitate) in former and current heavy smokers and in men with extensive occupational asbestos exposure. This trial was terminated in January 1996 after 4 years of treatment, when data showed an overall 28 percent higher incidence of lung cancer in participants receiving the beta-carotene/retinyl palmitate combination.[3] Male current smokers in CARET, excluding those exposed to asbestos, showed a 39 percent higher incidence,[22] compared with the 16 percent higher incidence in the ATBC study,[27] suggesting a possible adverse effect for supplemental retinol. Further, the trend for increased lung cancer incidence was similar to that in ATBC—this was a major factor in the decision to stop CARET.

Results of these trials may seem discouraging with regard to the future use of beta-carotene in cancer preventive interventions. However, before making the decision that beta-carotene is of no value in reducing cancer risk, a better understanding of the reasons for the unanticipated findings from ATBC and CARET is needed, especially considering that no increase in lung cancer incidence was observed in the 11 percent of men in the PHS who were current smokers.[26] Several possible explanations for the unanticipated outcomes of these beta-carotene trials have been considered, including inappropriate timing of the intervention,[3,29,30] a too-short followup time,[3,30] differing effects of beta-carotene on initiation versus promotion,[29,30] competitive inhibition by beta-carotene of the activities of other dietary carotenoids[31] and prooxidant effects of beta-carotene in combination with cigarette smoke and/or asbestos exposure.[29,30,32]

A recent literature review indicates that supplementation with high doses of beta-carotene might disturb the carotenoid balance, that is, affect absorption and plasma concentrations of other carotenoids.[31] Evidence suggests interactions between beta-carotene and several carotenoids, including lycopene, lutein, and canthaxanthin. However, findings among studies are contradictory—with regard to both magnitude of interactions and whether the interactions facilitate or inhibit the absorption and activities of other carotenoids—and do not provide a ready explanation for the adverse effects of beta-carotene observed in the ATBC Study and CARET.

Although beta-carotene and other carotenoids have been characterized as effective antioxidants and free radical scavengers *in vitro*, there is little evidence on which to base extrapolation of these findings to *in vivo* circumstances.[33] In fact, available data currently demonstrate that the antioxidant activity of carotenoids can shift into prooxidant activity, depending on the redox potential of the compound and the biological environment, including carotenoid concentration, oxygen tension, and interactions with other antioxidants.[34] Prooxidant effects have been reported *in vitro* when beta-carotene was used at high concentrations. Also, available evidence shows that beta-carotene acts as an antioxidant at low oxygen tension but, with increasing oxygen tension, it is readily autooxidized and exhibits prooxidant behavior, which can result in reactive oxygen metabolites that induce cell damage in normal cells. In tumor cells, however, prooxidant behavior of beta-carotene could be beneficial, producing tumor cytotoxic effects.[34] Further studies are needed to clarify the importance of prooxidant effects of beta-carotene *in vivo* and their relevance to cancer. One recent *in vivo* study found a highly significant increase in carcinogen-metabolizing enzymes in the lungs of rats supplemented with high doses of beta-carotene; the authors suggested that this increase was associated with the generation of oxidative stress.[35] In humans, high levels of these enzymes would predispose individuals to cancer risk from bioactivated tobacco-smoke carcinogens, particularly individuals with genetic polymorphisms such as the exon 7 CYP1A1 variant, which is associated with higher polyaromatic hydrocarbon (PAH)-DNA levels.[36]

It is noteworthy that participants with higher serum beta-carotene concentrations at entry into the ATBC study[27] and CARET[22] developed fewer lung cancers during the course of the trial, even among those who received beta-carotene supplements. Baseline serum concentrations of beta-carotene reflect total intake of vegetables and fruits, which contain numerous other antioxidants, as well as many naturally occurring potential anticarcinogens that may exert their effects through diverse mechanisms; the beta-carotene serum levels may simply be a marker for the actual protective agents. Thus, this finding is in agreement with epidemiologic evidence that links diets high in vegetables and fruits that contain beta-carotene with reduced lung cancer risk and reaffirms the importance of including an abundance of plant foods in our diets.[15,27,32]

DIETARY CAROTENOIDS: PART OF THE STORY

It is important to remember that beta-carotene is only one of the many carotenoids found in vegetables and fruits, and that findings from research on beta-carotene, *per se*, should be interpreted in that context. Common green, yellow/red, and yellow/orange vegetables and fruits contain more than 40 carotenoids in addition to beta-carotene that are commonly consumed and that can be absorbed and metabolized by humans, including lutein, zeaxanthin, cryptoxanthin, lycopene, alpha-carotene, phytofluene, phytoene, astaxanthin, canthaxanthin, and crocetin.[37] About 20 of these are present in quantifiable amounts in human serum and tissues.[11] A recently published, comprehensive monograph by the International Agency for Research on Cancer (IARC)[38] has summarized the current state-of -knowledge regarding carotenoids—including data from the ATBC Study and CARET—with an emphasis on evaluation of the cancer-preventive effects of these compounds. Mechanisms-of-action of carotenoids that may contribute to their potential cancer-preventive effects include antioxidant activity, modulation of carcinogen metabolism, effects on cell transformation and differentiation, effects in cell-to-cell communication, inhibition of cell proliferation and oncogene expression, effects on immune function, and inhibition of endogenous formation of carcinogens.[38] The ability of carotenoids to upregulate the expression of connexin 43, a gene that codes for one of the structural proteins of the gap junction and thus facilitates direct intercellular gap junctional communication (GJC), has been recently reviewed by Bertram.[39] Improved or restored GJC , which is deficient in many human tumors, is associated with decreased proliferation.

The epidemiologic evidence linking carotenoids and various cancers is well documented in the IARC monograph.[38] Findings from several relatively recent studies are included here. Using a carotenoid database compiled for more than 2,400 vegetables, fruits, and multicomponent foods containing vegetables and fruits,[40] Ziegler and colleagues[41] reanalysed data from a population-based study conducted in New Jersey during 1980 and 1981 to evaluate the hypothesis that beta-carotene may be protective against lung cancer. The reanalysis estimated smoking-adjusted risk of lung cancer in white male current and recent cigarette smokers by intakes of alpha-carotene, beta-carotene, beta-cryptoxanthin, lutein/zeaxanthin, lycopene, alpha-carotene + beta-carotene + lutein/zeaxanthin, and total carotenoids. Men in the lowest quartile of alpha-carotene intake had more than twice the risk of men in the highest quartile. The corresponding risks associated with intakes of beta-carotene and lutein/zeaxanthin were increased only about 60 percent, suggesting that beta-carotene may be not the dominant protective factor in vegetables and fruits for lung cancer.[41] Ecological data suggested that an inverse association with lutein (but not with alpha- or beta-carotene) accounted for 14 percent of the variation in lung cancer incidence in Fiji, where rates are markedly lower than for other South Pacific islands.[42] Data from a nested case-control study of serum micronutrient levels (highest vs. lowest tertiles) in a cohort of Japanese-American men indicated that alpha-carotene (RR=0.19), beta-carotene (RR=0.10), beta-cryptoxanthin (RR=0.25), and total carotenoids (RR=0.22) all significantly reduce the risk of aerodigestive tract cancers.[43]

Findings from a large prospective epidemiologic cohort study suggested that significant reduction in prostate cancer may be associated with increased dietary intake levels of lycopene (RR=0.79, highest vs. lowest quintile) and tomato-based foods (RR=0.65), which are high in lycopene.[44] Analysis of prostate tissue has determined that lycopene is present in biologically active concentrations, supporting the hypothesis that lycopene could have direct cancer-protective effects within the prostate.[45] Results from a study of serum carotenoids in a cohort of American men of Japanese descent did not support a reduced prostate cancer risk for any carotenoid, including lycopene.[46] In a nested case-control study of men enrolled in the PHS, however, the risk for all prostate cancer decreased with increasing quintile of plasma lycopene (OR = 0.75) and there was a stronger inverse association for aggressive cancers (OR = 0.56).[47] A recent review of 72 studies of tomatoes, tomato-based products, lycopene and cancer found that evidence of a benefit was strongest for cancers of the prostate, lung, and stomach and that data suggested a benefit for cancers of the pancreas, colon and rectum, esophagus, oral cavity, breast, and cervix.[48]

The IARC Monograph concluded that, at present, clear evidence of cancer-protective effects is not available for any of the carotenoids, including beta-carotene, and that supplemental carotenoids should not be recommended for use in cancer prevention for the general population. Further, it should not be assumed that the protective benefits of diets rich in carotenoid-containing vegetables and fruits are linked to any individual carotenoid.[38]

FUTURE DIRECTIONS

There is general agreement in the scientific community that diets rich in carotenoid-containing vegetables and fruits do protect against cancer. Epidemiologic evidence strongly and consistently supports such an effect. But, where do we go from here? Is it possible to determine which constituents of carotenoid-containing vegetables and fruits are the effective agents? It is likely that many constituents have important, but different, roles with respect to carcinogenesis, depending on cancer site, cancer stage, and prevailing risk factors.[49] Also, effects will be determined in part by genetic metabolic profiles that vary across populations and within individuals. Considering the variety of phytochemicals in commonly consumed plant foods, their interactive effects could be significant, as well as complex and difficult to separate. Although sorting out the cancer-related effects and mechanisms-of-action of vegetable and fruit constituents may appear to pose a formidable challenge, the potential benefits of such research endeavors for human health are enormous.

Large gaps exist in our basic knowledge of even the most widely studied phytochemicals. Beta-carotene and the other dietary carotenoids illustrate this point well. Basic information is lacking about digestion and absorption of carotenoids from foods, carotenoid bioavailability and metabolic fate, carotenoid interactions, the role of *cis*-carotene isomers as provitamin A, effects of carotenoids on cellular metabolism and immunity, gene/carotenoid interactions, *in vivo* antioxidant value of carotenoids, composition of carotenoids in foods, and effects of simple food preparation techniques on carotenoid chemistry. Also, inadequate clinical research data are available about which types of cancer might be responsive to carotenoids, optimal carotenoid mixtures and dose levels, timing of dose in relationship to carcinogenic stages, characteristics of individuals who might be responsive, and appropriate pharmacokinetic and safety data.[29,31,33,34,38,39]

Comprehensive, yet well-targeted, clinical trials that aim to answer such questions are essential so that appropriate cancer preventive interventions can be designed and implemented. The value of the statistical power afforded by large-scale, randomized clinical trials should not be underestimated. In the ATBC Study, lung cancer incidence in the group supplemented with beta-carotene was approximately 6 cases per 1,000 person-years compared with 5 cases per 1,000 person-years in the placebo group[2]—a difference too small to be apparent in an epidemiologic study. If the beta-carotene supplementation trials had not been carried out, it is possible that, based on the strong epidemiologic evidence, specific dietary guidelines for beta-carotene might have been considered.[15] Clearly, definitive clinical evidence is needed about individual vegetable and fruit constituents, including the carotenoids, before dietary guidelines more specific than those promoting greater consumption of vegetables and fruits can be formulated.

Meanwhile, as research proceeds, interest in nutraceutical products and biotechnology approaches that incorporate new findings deemed to be beneficial to human health continues to grow among consumers and those in the food industry. For example, plant molecular biologists have genetically engineered a golden-colored rice that contains beta-carotene and iron.[50] The rice carries four foreign genes that encode enzymes that give rice grains the ability to make beta-carotene and three genes that allow the grains to accumulate extra iron in a form that the human body can absorb. Three hundred grams of the cooked rice per day would provide almost the entire daily vitamin A requirement. Although this rice was developed to nutritionally enhance the diets of people in underdeveloped countries, it is an excellent example of where technology is headed. As another example, beta-carotene—because of its antioxidant properties—currently is being promoted by some in the industry for use in food fortification at levels of 1.5 mg per serving (assuming 4 servings per day),[51] a level lower than the 20 mg and the 30 mg daily supplements used in the ATBC Study[2] and CARET,[3] respectively. This proposed application of beta-carotene serves to remind us that development of new products by industry and their adoption by the general population do not always wait for an evidence-based rationale regarding their efficacy and safety.

REFERENCES

1.   World Cancer Research Fund. Food, Nutrition and the Prevention of Cancer: A Global Perspective. World Cancer Research Fund. 1997. Washington, DC, American Institute for Cancer Research.
2.   Alpha-Tocopherol Beta-Carotene Cancer Prevention Study Group, Heinonen OP, Huttunen JK, Albanes D. The effect of vitamin E and beta carotene on the incidence of lung cancer and other cancers in male smokers. N Eng J Med 1994;330(15):1029-1035.

3. Omenn GS, Goodman GE, Thornquist MD, Balmes J, Cullen MR, Glass A, Keogh JP, Meyskens FL, Jr., Valanis B, Williams JH, Jr., Barnhart S, Hammar S. Effects of a combination of beta carotene and vitamin A on lung cancer and cardiovascular disease. N Eng J Med 1996;334:1150-1155.
4. Greenwald P. Introduction: history of cancer prevention and control. Greenwald P, Kramer BS,Weed DL. Cancer Prevention and Control. 1995(1):1-7. New York, Marcel Dekker.
5. Taubes G. Epidemiology faces its limits: the search for subtle links between diet, lifestyle, or environmental factors and disease is an unending source of fear - but often yields little certainty. Science 1995;269:164-169.
6. Weed DL, Kramer BS. Induced abortion, bias, and breast cancer: why epidemiology hasn't reached its limit. J Natl Cancer Inst 1996;88(23):1698-1700.
7. Peto R, Doll R, Buckley JD, Sporn MB. Can dietary beta-carotene materially reduce human cancer rates? Nature 1981;290:201-208.
8. Ziegler RG. Vegetables, fruits, and carotenoids, and the risk of cancer. Am J Clin Nutr 1991;53:251s-259s.
9. Ziegler RG, Mayne ST, Swanson CA. Nutrition and lung cancer. Cancer Causes Control 1996;7:157-177.
10. Van Poppel G, Goldbohm RA. Epidemiologic evidence for β-carotene and cancer prevention. Am J Clin Nutr 1995;62:1393S-1402S.
11. Cooper DA, Eldridge AL, Peters JC. Dietary carotenoids and lung cancer: a review of recent research. Nutrition Rev 1999;57(5):133-145.
12. Kolonel LN. Nutrition and prostate cancer. Cancer Causes Control 1996;7:83-94.
13. Hunter DJ, Willett WC. Nutrition and breast cancer. Cancer Causes Control 1996;7:56-68.
14. Enger SM, Longnecker MP, Chen M-J, Harper JM, Lee ER, Frankl HD, Haile RW. Dietary intake of specific carotenoids and vitamins A, C, and E, and prevalence of colorectal adenomas. Cancer Epidemiol Biomarkers Prev 1996;5:147-153.
15. Albanes D. β-Carotene and lung cancer: a case study. Am J Clin Nutr 1999;69 (suppl):1345S-1350S.
16. Stich HF, Rosin MP, Vallejera MO. Reduction with vitamin A and beta-carotene administration of the proportion of micronucleated buccal mucosal cells in Asian betel nut and tobacco chewers. Lancet 1984;2:1204-1206.
17. Garewal HS, Meyskens FL, Jr., Killen D, Reeves D, Kiersch TA, Elletson H, Strosberg A, King D, Steinbronn K. Response of oral leukoplakia to beta-carotene. J Clin Oncol 1990;8(10):1715-1720.
18. Lippman SM, Batsakis JG, Toth BB, Weber RS, Lee JJ, Martin JW, Hays GL, Goepfert H, Hong WK. Comparison of low-dose isotretinoin with beta carotene to prevent oral carcinogenesis. N Eng J Med 1993;328:15-20.
19. Greenberg ER, Baron JA, Stukel TA, Stevens MM, Mandel JS, Spencer SK, Elias PM, Lowe N, Nierenberg DW, Bayrd G, Vance JC, Freeman DH, Jr., Clendenning WE, Kwan T, The Skin Cancer Prevention Study Group. A clinical trial of beta carotene to prevent basal-cell and squamous cell cancers of the skin. N Eng J Med 1990;323:789-795.
20. Greenberg ER, Baron JA, Tosteson TD, Freeman DH, Jr., Beck GJ, Bond JH, Colacchio TA, Coller JA, Frankl HD, Haile RW, Mandel JS, Nierenberg DW, Rothstein R, Snover DC, Stevens MM, Summers RW, van Stolk RU. A clinical trial of antioxidant vitamins to prevent colorectal adenoma. N Eng J Med 1994;331:141-147.
21. MacLennan R, Macrae F, Bain C, Battistutta D, Chapuis P, Gratten H, Lambert J, Newland RC, Ngu M, Russell A, Ward M, Wahlqvist ML. Randomized trial of intake

of fat, fiber, and beta carotene to prevent colorectal adenomas. J Natl Cancer Inst 1995;87(23):1760-1766.

22. Omenn GS, Goodman GE, Thornquist MD, Balmes J, Cullen MR, Glass A, Keogh JP, Meyskens FL, Jr., Valanis B, Williams JH, Jr., Barnhart S, Cherniack MG, Brodkin CA, Hammar S. Risk factors for lung cancer and for intervention effects in CARET, the Beta-Carotene and Retinol Efficacy Trial. J Natl Cancer Inst 1996;88(21):1550-1559.

23. Taylor PR, Li B, Dawsey SM, Li J-Y, Yang CS, Guo W, Blot WJ, Linxian Nutrition Intervention Trials Study Group. Prevention of esophageal cancer: the nutrition intervention trials in Linxian, China. Cancer Res (supplement) 1994;54:2029s-2031s.

24. Blot WJ, Li J-Y, Taylor PR, Guo W, Dawsey SM, Wang G-Q, Yang CS, Zheng S-F, Gail MH, Li G-Y, Yu Y, Liu B-Q, Tangrea JA, Sun Y-H, Liu F, Fraumeni JF, Jr., Zhang Y-H, Li B. Nutrition intervention trials in Linxian, China: supplementation with specific vitamin/mineral combinations, cancer incidence, and disease-specific mortality in the general population. J Natl Cancer Inst 1993;85:1483-1492.

25. Li J-Y, Taylor PR, Li B, Dawsey SM, Wang G-Q, Ershow AG, Guo W, Liu S-F, Yang CS, Shen Q, Wang W, Mark SD, Zou X-N, Greenwald P, Wu Y-P, Blot WJ. Nutrition intervention trials in Linxian, China: multiple vitamin/mineral supplementation, cancer incidence, and disease-specific mortality among adults with esophageal dysplasia. J Natl Cancer Inst 1993;85:1492-1498.

26. Hennekens CH, Buring JE, Manson JE, Stampfer M, Rosner B, Cook NR, Belanger C, LaMotte F, Gaziano JM, Ridker PM, Willett W, Peto R. Lack of effect of long-term supplementation with beta carotene on the incidence of malignant neoplasms and cardiovascular disease. N Eng J Med 1996;334:1145-1149.

27. Albanes D, Heinonen OP, Taylor PR, Virtamo J, Edwards BK, Rautalahti M, Hartman AM, Palmgren J, Freedman LS, Haapakoski J, Barrett MJ, Pietinen P, Malila N, Tala E, Liippo K, Salomaa E-R, Tangrea JA, Teppo L, Askin FB, Taskinen E, Erozan Y, Greenwald P, Huttunen JK. α-tocopherol and β-carotene supplements and lung cancer incidence in the Alpha-Tocopherol, Beta-Carotene Cancer Prevention Study: effects of base-line characteristics and study compliance. J Natl Cancer Inst 1996;88(21):1560-1570.

28. Woodson K, Albanes D, Tangrea J, Rautalahti M, Virtamo J, Taylor PR. Association between alcohol and lung cancer in the alpha-tocopherol, beta-carotene cancer prevention study in Finland. Cancer CausesControl 1999;10:219-226.

29. Erdman JW, Jr., Russell RM, Mayer J, Rock CL, Barua AB, Bowen PE, Burri BJ, Curran-Celentano J, Furr H, Mayne ST, Stacewicz-Sapuntzakis M. Beta-carotene and the carotenoids: beyond the intervention trials. Nutrition Rev 1996;54(6):185-188.

30. Rautalahti M, Albanes D, Virtamo J, Taylor PR, Huttunen JK, Heinonen OP. Beta-carotene did not work: aftermath of the ATBC study. Cancer Lett 1997;114:235-236.

31. van den Berg H. Carotenoid interactions. Nutrition Rev 1999;57(1):1-10.

32. Mayne ST, Handelman GJ, Beecher G. β-carotene and lung cancer promotion in heavy smokers - a plausible relationship? J Natl Cancer Inst 1996;88(21):1513-1515.

33. Rice-Evans CA. Why do we expect carotenoids to be antioxidants *in vivo*? Free Rad Res 1997;26:381-398.

34. Palozza P. Prooxidant actions of carotenoids in biologic systems. Nutrition Rev 1998;56(9):257-265.

35. Paolini M, Cantelli-Forti G, Perocco P, Pedulli GF, Abdel-Rahman SZ, Legator MS. Co-carcinogenic effect of β-carotene. Nature Apr 29, 1999;398:760-761.

36. Mooney LA, Bell DA, Santella RM, Van Bennekum AM, Ottman R, Paik M, Blaner WS, Lucier GW, Covey L, Young T-L, Cooper TB, Glassman AH, Perera FP. Contribution of genetic and nutritional factors to DNA damage in heavy smokers.

Carcinogenesis 1997;18(3):503-509.

37. Khachik F, Nir Z, Ausich RL, Steck A, Pfander H. Distribution of carotenoids in fruits and vegetables as a criterion for the selection of appropriate chemopreventive agents. Ohigashi H, Osawa T, Terao J, Watanabe S,Yoshikawa T. Food Factors for Cancer Prevention. 1997:204-208. New York, Springer Verlag.

38. IARC Working Group on the Evaluation of Cancer Preventive Agents. IARC Handbooks of Cancer Prevention - Carotenoids. 1998(2):1-326.

39. Bertram JS. Carotenoids and Gene Regulation. Nutrition Rev 1999;57(6):182-191.

40. Chug-Ahuja JK, Holden JM, Forman MR, Mangels AR, Beecher GR, Lanza E. The development and application of a carotenoid database for fruits, vegetables, and selected multicomponent foods. J Am Diet Assoc 1993;93(3):318-323.

41. Ziegler RG, Colavito EA, Hartge P, McAdams MJ, Schoenberg JB, Mason TJ, Fraumeni JF, Jr. Importance of α-carotene, β-carotene, and other phytochemicals in the etiology of lung cancer. J Natl Cancer Inst 1996;88(9):612-615.

42. Le Marchand L, Hankin JH, Bach F, Kolonel LN, Wilkens LR, Stacewicz-Sapuntzakis M, Bowen PE, Beecher GR, Laudon F, Baque P, Daniel R, Seruvatu L, Henderson BE. An ecological study of diet and lung cancer in the South Pacific. Int J Cancer 1995;63:18-23.

43. Nomura AMY, Ziegler RG, Stemmermann GN, Chyou P-H, Craft NE. Serum micronutrients and upper aerodigestive tract cancer. Cancer Epidemiol Biomarkers Prev 1997;6:407-412.

44. Giovannucci E, Ascherio A, Rimm EB, Stampfer MJ, Colditz GA, Willett WC. Intake of carotenoids and retinol in relation to risk of prostate cancer. J Natl Cancer Inst 1995;87(23):1767-1776.

45. Clinton SK, Emenhiser C, Schwartz SJ, Bostwick DG, Williams AW, Moore BJ, Erdman JW, Jr. *cis-trans* lycopene isomers, carotenoids, and retinol in the human prostate. Cancer Epidemiol Biomarkers Prev 1996;5:823-833.

46. Nomura AMY, Stemmermann GN, Lee J, Craft NE. Serum micronutrients and prostate cancer in Japanese Americans in Hawaii. Cancer Epidemiol Biomarkers Prev 1997;6:487-491.

47. Gann PH, Ma J, Giovannucci E, Willett W, Sacks FM, Hennekens CH, Stampfer MJ. Lower prostate cancer risk in men with elevated plasma lycopene levels: results of a prospective analysis. Cancer Res 1999;59:1225-1230.

48. Giovannucci E. Tomatoes, tomato-based products, lycopene, and cancer: review of the epidemiologic literature.J Natl Cancer Inst 1999;91(4):317-331.

49. Block G. Micronutrients and cancer: time for action? [editorial]. J Natl Cancer Inst 1993;85(11):846-848.

50. Gura T. New genes boost rice nutrients. Science 1999;285:994-995.

51. Elliott JG. Application of antioxidant vitamins in foods and beverages. Food Tech 1999;53(2):46-48.

18

DIETARY INTERVENTION STRATEGIES: VALIDITY, EXECUTION AND INTERPRETATION OF OUTCOMES

Phyllis E. Bowen

University of Illinois at Chicago
1919 West Taylor Street
Chicago, IL 60612

1. INTRODUCTION

Experimental research designs that use single chemical entities have been the cornerstone of careful scientific research. Therefore the use of total diet patterns, or whole foods, which contain hundreds of chemical components, would appear to lack sufficient control to yield productive information. However, cancer prevention and control may be an area where well-designed diet intervention strategies may be an efficient research approach. This chapter will present arguments for the necessity of diet and whole food supplementation research studies and descriptions of strategies for their implementation. Additionally, the components of effective diet intervention studies will be discussed. Whether the research involves cell media, animal diets or human diets, the whole diet should be considered an important factor in any research design where the ultimate aim is cancer prevention and control.

Nutrition and Cancer Prevention, edited under the auspices of AICR
Kluwer Academic / Plenum Publishers, New York, 2000.

2. WHY ARE DIETARY INTERVENTION STUDIES A NECESSARY APPROACH TO EFFECTIVE CANCER PREVENTION AND CONTROL?

There are three major reasons for including diet intervention studies in any organized research program aimed at effective cancer prevention and control in human populations.

2.1. The Major Diet/Cancer Hypotheses Have Been Derived from Food Consumption Patterns

Our interest in diet, as an important source of cancer risk and prevention, stems from the remarkable variance in cancer incidence from one country to another, varying 2 to 100 fold for a single cancer type from the highest to the lowest cancer incidence region.[1] Although this variance is well known, it is under-appreciated as a front-line tactical arena to save people's health and lives. A recent example of this variance is the remarkably low lung cancer incidence in Indian and Native Fiji Islanders compared to other South Pacific Islanders despite a high rate of smoking in each of these subgroups (Table 1)[2].   What is special about the Fijian lifestyle? Although the authors note that smoking habit was associated with 61% of the individual variance in the South Pacific men as a whole, it certainly does not explain the low Fijian incidence as a group. Lutein intake (a carotenoid prevalent in dark green leafy vegetables) accounted for 14% of the variance for all South Pacific men but

Table 1. Variations in Lung Cancer Incidence in South Pacific Males

Region	Number of Men	Incidence Rate per 100,000[1]	Current Smoker Percent
Fijian	83	2.7	59.0
Fijian-Indian	88	0.7	50.0
Cook Islander	98	27.6	43.6
Hawaiian-Japanese	114	37.5	29.0
Hawaiian-Caucasian	64	66.1	25.0
Tahitian	102	76.9	49.0
New Caledonian	84	87.0	51.8
Hawaiian	37	84.9	35.1

[1] Average annual age-adjusted incidence rate/100,000 for 1983-86 (Hawaii), 1988-91 (New Caledonia), 1989-90 (Tahiti), 1984-90 (Cook Island), 1985-91 (Fiji). *Adapted from Le Marchand et al. Int J Cancer 1995;63:18-23.*

cannot explain the 39-fold difference in cancer incidence between Fijian Indian men and Cook Islander, which had the next lowest cancer rate. The Fijian gap in cancer incidence is so dramatic that it is likely due to multiple factors and their interactions, which are difficult to segment in population studies. Diet patterns, food preparation and storage practices are only interactive components in a complex array of genetic propensities, infections, carcinogen exposure, and individual practices that range from the level of physical activity to the use of tobacco and alcohol.

The temptation to ascribe greatest importance to gene/environment interactions is mitigated by the widespread evidence for changes in cancer rates in migrant populations within the lifetime of the immigrant. The study by McMichael et al.[3] (Table 2) is an example of this type showing shifts in colon cancer mortality rates toward those of Australia, the host country, from high rate countries (Scotland) and low rate countries (Yugoslavia, Greece,

Table 2. Age-Sex-Standardized Relative Risk of Death from Cancers of the Colon in Migrants to Australia, Aged 30-plus by Duration of Residence (Number of migrant deaths in brackets)

Country of Origin	Duration ≤ 16 years	Duration > 16 years
Australia *	1.0	1.0
England	0.99 (497)	1.04 (2337)
Scotland	1.47 (126)	1.24[1] (675)
Ireland	0.62 (26)	1.06 (218)
Poland	1.02 (33)	1.14 (106)
Yugoslavia	0.47 (21)	0.66 (37)
Greece	0.36 (24)	0.69[1] (58)
Italy	0.37 (65)	0.70[1] (183)

, *Adapted from McMichael et al. Int J Cancer 1980; 25:431-37.*
* Australia-born population rate set at 1.0
[1] Differs from mortality ratio for ≤ 16 yrs, p<0.05.

Italy). Note that the shifts in rates are 14-44%, indicating a short-term environmental effect which likely includes diet and other factors but is nowhere near the large between region differences seen in nonmigrants.

The population-based approaches of the past 20 yrs have focused on identifying nutrients or food classes that conferred risk or apparent protection from various cancers. The result of these efforts has been the identification of a vast array of chemical compounds and whole foods that we can liken to straws in the total diet haystack (Figure 1). Many of these are minor dietary components but their activity may be affected by the amount and type of the various macronutrients that compose the bulk of the diet haystack. Although it may be productive to investigate each of these straws separately, it is important to keep in mind that their identification from population studies arose in the midst of the consumption of different diets and individual practices, that can not be rendered neutral with statistical techniques alone. The bottom line is that diet always counts. It must always be a consideration

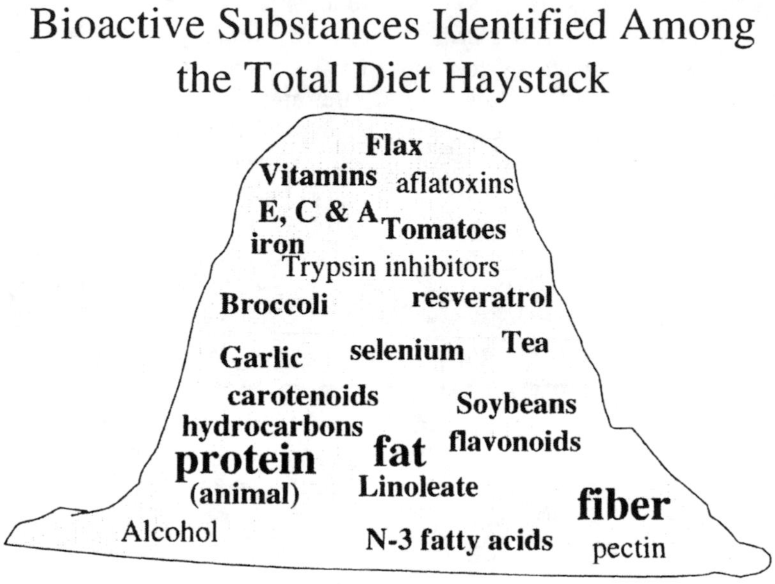

Bioactive Substances Identified Among the Total Diet Haystack

Flax
Vitamins aflatoxins
E, C & A Tomatoes
iron
Trypsin inhibitors
Broccoli   resveratrol
Garlic   selenium   Tea
carotenoids   Soybeans
hydrocarbons   fat flavonoids
protein
(animal)   Linoleate
Alcohol   N-3 fatty acids   fiber
pectin

Figure 1. Bioactive components can be likened to straws in the haystack that comprises a person's diet.

in experimental design. Not measuring it or not reporting it does not minimize its impact.

Surprisingly, few population studies have evaluated the impact of the diet pattern on cancer risk. Kune et al.[4] constructed a risk score using consumption levels of dietary fiber, vegetables, cruciferous vegetables, dietary vitamin C, beef, other meats, fat and use of vitamin supplements, all found to modulate colon cancer rates in their Australian population of 715 cases and 727 age- and gender-matched community controls. There was a linear trend (p<0.0001) for risk of colon cancer with increasing risk score, but more importantly, the relative risks rose from a protective 0.28 for a score of 2 to a high risk of 8.01 for a score of 7. These are the variances usually encountered between different countries and point to the importance of interactions between various dietary components within the total diet.

2.2.   Bioactivity is Often Greater for Whole Foods Compared to Individual Food Components

Several population studies have shown greater risk reductions with food groups compared to nutrients contained in those foods.[5] For example, the consumption of dark green and deep yellow vegetables afforded a greater reduced risk for lung cancer in smokers compared to a total carotene index calculated from a nutrient data base. The poor data base available at the time of the study, which estimated only pro-vitamin A carotenoids, could have explained the discrepancy; but also likely was the presence of other cancer preventive substances such as phenolic compounds, indoles and other carotenoids.[6] The authors attempted to rule out indoles contained in the cruciferous vegetables as important factors, by finding no risk reduction associated with their consumption. However this approach may miss the existence of important synergistic actions between a number of components contained in the same food.

How can one evaluate the possibility of these synergies in single foods and food groups? A viable approach is one used by Staack et al.,[7] who sought to characterize the role of isothiocyanates and nitriles (breakdown products of glucosinolates found in cruciferous vegetables) as cancer prevention agents. Glucosinolate breakdown products induce Phase I and Phase II detoxification enzymes, which activate and/or degrade chemical carcinogens. Rats were gavaged with 7 daily doses of one of four glucosinolate derivatives (crambene, indole-3-carbinol, iberin, and phenylethylisothiocyannate) individually, or as a mixture in the proportion found in brussels sprouts. The amounts were pegged to the threshold dose of crambene required to produce glutathione induction in rats. In an additional study the mixture at 60% and 20% of the original dose was evaluated and a control group pair-fed to the mixture group was included in each experiment. Rats continued on a semipurified, antioxidant-free diet throughout the study. The outcome measures were specific activities of a variety of liver enzymes associated with Phase I and Phase II detoxification. Phase I enzyme activity (measured as cytochrome P450 1A, associated with carcinogen activation) was increased 11-fold for the mixture and was statistically greater than the 9.4-fold increase in indole-3-carbinol, the only active derivative. Treatment with the mixture produced increases in quinone reductase (6.2 fold) and glutathione transferase (2.5 fold) activities (both Phase II enzymes associated with carcinogen deactivation) which were greater than sum of the individual responses to crambene and indole-3-carbinol, the only active derivatives.

Lowering the dose to 60% and 20% of the original mixture produced a dose response effect for these enzymes. This animal experiment demonstrated several synergistic effects of brussels sprout glucosinolate derivatives on various enzymes associated with carcinogen activation and detoxification. The study also identified doses for greatest activity in the context of the proportions found in brussels sprouts. The induction of quinone reductase activity by crambene or indole-3-carbinol alone was not impressive, and they might have been overlooked as viable anticancer compounds without the observed synergistic response of the mixture.

Animal diet studies are cost effective and allow the evaluation of individual compounds, mixtures, compared to whole foods. Inclusion of whole foods in studies opens the door to the discovery of new compounds, especially if the whole food is found to be more bioactive than the compounds being studied. Pure compounds are likely to have limited availability and are not approved for human use. Animal studies aid in evaluating the safety and proper design of subsequent human studies, especially when synergies and bi-modal dose responses for food components have been identified.

2.3.   Sound Advice to the Public is Still Likely to be Food Based

Once cancer preventive food components and nutrients are identified, there are a number of public health strategies that could be followed. Some of these are: the development of prophylactic supplements similar to multivitamins, food fortification and plant breeding programs, as well as the development of functional foods for cancer prevention. No doubt these strategies will become more prevalent than they are now but the consumer is still faced with questions of daily food choices and they face unknown risk with these strategies.

The prophylactic supplement approach does not address the risk-increasing elements in the usual diet. Diet advice will still be required for risky diet patterns. Furthermore, the supplement/fortification approach may not be appropriate for all populations of the world.

There is a tendency for the media to leap with dietary advice for the public based upon research focused on single components of the diet. The advice is then generally applied to all age groups, genotypes and conditions of chronic disease with the belief that such advice can do no harm. Issues of bioavailability, substance interactions and modifications by food preparation remain unaddressed. Clearly, the actual use of recommended diets in human studies should be the capstone research for public health recommendations.

3. DIET INTERVENTION STRATEGIES

With the case made for an investment in diet intervention studies, which should proceed simultaneously with the use of single component interventions, it must be admitted that diet interventions are fraught with difficulties in valid design, execution and interpretation of results, that are beyond those encountered with the administration of a single chemopreventive agent. Furthermore, there are several types of diet intervention strategies, and each of them present different problems in the above categories. I am going to devote most of this discussion to human intervention studies because this is what I know best, but animal studies are important as a necessary preliminary stage before expensive human studies are attempted. This is especially relevant to cancer prevention because of the multistage nature of carcinogenesis. It is imperative to know and understand the point of action in the carcinogenic process, as well as to identify appropriate dosing of the cancer preventive agent in question, before designing definitive human intervention trials where cancer, or biomarkers of cancer are used as outcome measures. These can be accomplished with animal studies, human kinetic studies, as well as small biomarker studies.

3.1   Sorting Out Anticarcinogenic Actions of Complex Food Material Using Animal Models

Animal models allow the precise control of the underlying dietary components, which also modulate different stages of carcinogenesis. One is also able to efficiently explore the actions of various fractions of the food in question. Smaller quantities of extracts and pure compounds are needed for animal studies and safety issues can be identified. As an example of this approach are the series of studies Dr. Lillian Thompson and her collaborators have conducted to characterize the anticarcinogenic properties of flaxseed. Flaxseed has many components of interest including dietary fiber, α-linolenic acid (an omega-3 fatty acid) and a lignan, secoisolariciresinol- diglycoside (SLR-G), which is converted in the human intestine to two phytoestrogens, enterodiol and enterolactone. Thompson's group used the same basic experimental design in a series of studies. Weanling rats were placed on a 20%, by weight, corn oil diet (56% of energy) and fed full-fat flaxseed or defatted flaxseed as 5% or 10% of the diet or an equivalent amount of pure SLR-G or flaxseed oil, depending upon the study. The outcomes measured were tumor incidence, number and size, as well as a number of cell proliferation indices, in response to feeding known carcinogens for breast or colon cancer at different times to control cancer staging. I will only describe two of these studies to illustrate approaches to using fractions of a whole food at different stages of the carcinogenic process.

In order to sort out the omega-3 fatty acid effect from the phytoestrogen effect of flaxseed, Serraino and Thompson[8] fed the two levels of defatted (minus α-linolenic acid) or full fatted flaxseed to rats for 4 wks and then gave each group colchicine or DMBA 24 hrs prior to killing. Table 3 presents the major results from this study. After dissecting out the breast tissue they found that the end-buds of the mammary glands, where most breast cancer starts, showed the greatest decrements in cell proliferation activity. All three indexes were significantly reduced with the 5% full-fat flaxseed diet compared to the diet containing no flaxseed and there was a trend for reduction in the defatted flaxseed but the difference was not statistically significant. The 10% flaxseed diet provided no added beneficial effect.

Table 3. Modulation of Early Markers of Breast Cancer by Components of Flaxseed in Rats: 7 animals per group were fed diets for 4 wks, then given colchicine or DMBA, killed 24 hrs later for Proliferation Index Analysis

Terminal End Bud Proliferation Indices	Basal Diet	5% Full Fat Flaxseed Diet	5% Fat Free Flaxseed Diet
Mitotic Index[1]	2.37 ± 0.32^a	1.37 ± 0.25^b	2.15 ± 0.38^{ab}
Labeling Index[2]	13.55 ± 1.89^a	8.29 ± 0.94^b	9.67 ± 1.50^{ab}
Nuclear Aberrations[3]	3.08 ± 0.86^a	1.05 ± 0.42^b	2.33 ± 0.62^{ab}

Negative correlation between urinary lignan excretion and nuclear aberrations: $r = -0.94$ ($p < 0.025$)

Means $\pm$ S.E.M. with different superscripts are significantly different ($P \leq 0.05$).
[1] number of cells arrested in metaphase/100 cells in the epithelia of the terminal end bud.
[2] number of labeled cells/100 cells in the epithelia of the terminal end bud.
[3] number of nuclear aberrations/100 cells in the epithelia of the terminal end bud.
Adapted from Serraino et al. Cancer Let 1991; 60:135-42.

It would appear from this experiment that flaxseed, in high doses, is protective at early stages of breast carcinogenesis and that both α-linoleate (ALA) and SLR are important. Flaxseed contains other nutrients such as vitamin E, which would have also been removed in the defatting process.

To evaluate the effect of flaxseed components on already established breast tumors, Thompson et al. gave a single dose of DMBA and allowed tumors to develop for 13 wks on the high corn oil diet. Then animals were randomized to each diet group, so that there were no differences in tumor incidence, diameter or volume between groups. A control group continued on the basal diet, while the experimental groups received 2.2 mmol SLR-D/day or 1.82% flaxseed oil (each equivalent to what was contained in a 5% flaxseed diet), or 2.5% or 5.0% flaxseed for an additional 7 wks. Tumor response was evaluated weekly and the major results are presented in Figure 2. All flaxseed diets and flaxseed component diets reduced the volume of existing tumors by 50% compared to the control group, while new tumor volume was significantly reduced in the SLR-D treated animals with a trend toward reduction in animals fed 2.5% or 5.0% flaxseed but not flaxseed oil.[9]

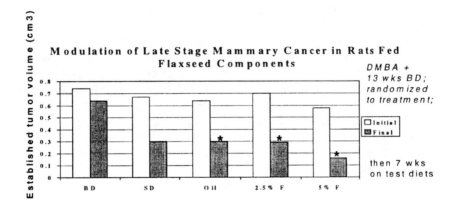

Figure 2. Effect of different fractions of flaxseed on mammary tumor volume in rats fed a basel diet for 13 wks than randomized to diets containing the various flax fractions for 7 wks. BD = basal diet; SD = secoisolariciresinol diglycoside; Oil = flaxseed oil (negligible lignans); 2.5 and 5.0% full-fatted flaxseed. * = P <0.05. Adapted from Thompson et al. Carcinogenesis 1996; 17:1373.

Flaxseed oil has a negligible lignan content whereas the flaxseed contains both ALA and SLR-D. These results exemplify the complicated issues that arise when more than one component of a food is chemopreventive at different stages of the carcinogenesis and may even be counter-productive at others.

3.2.   Diet Intervention Strategies for Research With Humans

We are pretty much confined to food, food components and diet intervention studies in humans because few compounds are approved for human use, although pure compounds with investigational drug (IND) applications will become available as part of the National Cancer Institute's Chemoprovention Program. Such studies are still problematic because of the unavailability of pure compounds in sufficient quantities. The purity of the chemopreventive compound is also an issue. Compounds are seldom pure and the type of impurities vary if the substance is chemically synthesized or extracted from botanicals. Toxicological studies may not detect the accumulation of bioactive impurities when chemopreventive agents are consumed over the course of years in clinical trials. An example of this phenomenon is the supplementation trials using β-carotene. Several of these studies reported the plasma accumulation of a compound conditionally identified as α-carotene in subjects receiving supplements.[10,11,12]

There are three types of diet intervention studies that would be useful in developing effective diets for cancer prevention and control. They are (1) controlled feeding studies, (2) single or multi-component diet modification studies and (3) food supplementation studies. I will review each of these approaches with respect to their strengths and limitations as well as issues of design, execution and interpretation.

3.3.   Human Controlled Feeding Studies

These studies involve the feeding of prepared diets of known nutrient content, generally weighed to the gram. The investigator controls the proposed chemopreventive foods and the rest of the diet. Specific age groups or even phenotypes might be recruited into such a study. A manual for the conduct of such studies has just been published.[13] Studies are labor-intensive and their conduct requires facilities, experienced investigators and staff, highly cooperative participants, and they are expensive because of food, subject honoraria and labor costs. Generally investigators can manage only 10-45 subjects (to assure precision in the study execution) on an outpatient basis, and even fewer when subjects use hospital CRC facilities. They are limited in time, with 6 months as the maximum that can be reasonably requested of both participants and study staff. Therefore cancer biomarkers or intermediate endpoints, that respond relatively rapidly, are the only outcome measures that can be used. Furthermore, since it is almost impossible to find enough high risk individuals living in the vicinity of the feeding center, the biomarkers must measure changes that happen very early in the carcinogenic process and must be commonly found in apparently healthy individuals who exhibit particular risk factors or genotypes.

The field of cancer prevention has been hampered by the lack of validated biomarkers of these early events or circumstances. Cancer prevention research would greatly benefit from a few biomarkers similar to plasma cholesterol, which has aided the discovery of diets that prevent coronary heart disease. However, new biomarkers are under active research and these need to be validated in controlled feeding studies. One class of biomarkers, that has been discussed in the literature with great enthusiasm, are DNA damage products such as the 8-hydroxy-deoxyguanosine/2-deoxyguanosine ratio in the DNA of various human tissues including circulating leukocytes.[14] A controlled feeding study using this biomarker was completed in our laboratory. It is generally supposed that the residual amount of 8-hydroxy-deoxyguanosine (8-OHdG) in DNA is a function of the balance between oxidative "hits" to the DNA and the rapidity of repair. Therefore the ratio is a steady-state measurement. We assumed that changes would be fairly rapid, so when the opportunity came to evaluate two liquid formula diets, one containing very high levels of linoleate and relatively low levels of vitamin E (putative high oxidative stress formula), and the other containing low levels of linoleate but high levels of vitamin E (putative low oxidative stress formula), we included this assay in the study. Thirty-four young healthy non-smoking men and women were fed a whole food control diet for 5 days and then randomized to either the high oxidative stress or low oxidative stress liquid formula diet for 10 days. They then consumed the control diet for 5 days and switched to the opposite liquid diet for another 10 days. Although there was

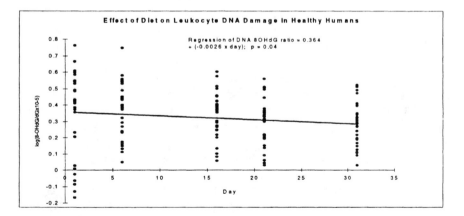

Figure 3. The downward trend of 8-OhdG/dG ratios in individual subjects' circulating leukocyte DNA over the time of the controlled feeding study. Solid line represents the Random-Effects Pattern-Mixture Model to test the downward trend. Adapted from Chen et al. Free Rad Biol Med 1999;26:695-703.

no difference in the level of DNA damage between the two diets, there was a consistent decrease in leukocyte DNA damage throughout the study (Figure 3), with a decrease in the variance of measurements as the controlled feeding progressed. The decrease was evident in both men and women, and a second study with 24 subjects using the same liquid diets with fiber produced the same 18-20% decrease by the end of the 30 day period. Although we do not know what components of the diet were effective, it points to the total diet being important. This is the first study to report such a decrease in DNA damage in healthy young subjects with a total diet intervention.[15]

Controlled feeding studies are the most appropriate design to take advantage of the new gene expression chips,[16] which may be able to identify patterns of gene expression that are cancer promoting and cancer defeating. These patterns could serve as biomarkers for the evaluation of particular dietary approaches.

3.3.1. Design Validity

Controlled feeding studies overcome problems with compliance and are especially well-suited to instances when the effect sizes are likely to be small, but they have unique problems with validity in study design. Small sample sizes and the variability of the human genome leads to a probability of conflicting results from one study to the next because of highly variable response among subjects. The early cholesterol-lowering diet studies are examples of this phenomenon. A significant portion of the population is non-responsive to fat-modified cholesterol-lowering diets and the proportion is greater for individuals with normal plasma cholesterol concentrations. The use of subjects as their own control in cross-over designs can be used for some biomarkers but carry-over effects and long response times renders this design problematic for cancer prevention studies. Another approach is to screen for a genetically homogeneous group either by phenotype expression (e.g. polyposis of the colon for colon cancer or borderline PSA levels for prostate cancer) or by phenotyping (e.g., mutations in the p53 tumor suppressor gene or BRCA1 for breast cancer[17]) and evaluate responses to diet only in high risk groups.

However, problems of small sample size remain with these approaches. For example small effects that might have enormous cancer prevention consequences may not be detected and the effectiveness of a diet strategy to be recommended for the public at-large is not addressed by studying genetically defined groups.

A novel approach to these problems using diet pattern as an intervention for hypertension has just been successfully accomplished. The Dietary Approaches to Stop Hypertension (DASH) Trial was a 5-center controlled feeding study which enrolled 459 adults with blood pressure <160 mm Hg systolic and 80-95 mm Hg diastolic. They were fed a control diet low in fruits, vegetables and dairy products but moderately high in fat for 3 weeks followed by one of three diets: (1) the control diet, (2) a diet rich in fruits and vegetables, or a (3) combination diet rich in fruits, vegetables and low-fat dairy products for 8 wks, while sodium intake and body weight were held constant. The study was able to demonstrate modest but clinically important drops in systolic and diastolic blood pressure relative to the control group for both interventions, with the greatest response in African-Americans or those with high blood pressure consuming the combination diet.[18] The DASH study and the DELTA study[19], another multi-center feeding study, have demonstrated that the difficulties of feeding the same diet at several centers can be successfully overcome and that small changes can be measured with sufficient precision. Although these studies were expensive, they are cost-effective compared to large single component or diet modification trials, where the approach or success of the intervention has been questioned. The utility of this approach to cancer prevention and control is dependent upon the validation of biomarkers by preliminary studies that firmly connect the biomarker to cancer outcome as well as its responsiveness to intervention.

The expense of this type of study mandates a commensurate investment in multi-system biomarkers, such as DNA damage, immuno-surveillance, Phase I and II detoxification as well as relevant gene expression. These multi-system approaches are often seen as having a "lack of focus", are not "hypothesis-driven", or are "fishing expeditions". However, sound hypotheses backed by scholarly scientific rationale can be developed for all these approaches because of the multi-dimensional aspects of carcinogenesis. Often lacking is the inclusion of investigators, expert in each dimension, at the design and hypothesis development stage of the project.

3.3.2. Management of Study Participants and Interpretation of Study Outcomes

The daily nature of supplying and consuming the foods provided puts a large time and effort burden on both study staff and study participants. A number of feeding strategies have been tried. These are (1) sequestration of study subjects in live-in facilities or hospital CRC's, (2) free-living subjects that consume all food in a metabolic dining room except for occasional packed food, (3) week day metabolic dining room feeding with weekend packed out food, (4) week day dining room feeding with weekend subject-selected diet consistent with the study diet and (5) completely packed-out food. Although complete sequestration might appear to provide the greatest adherence to study diets, this is often not the case, since incarceration-mentality leads to infractions for freedom's sake even in the most dedicated subject. Such studies are necessarily limited to very short times with few subjects. On the other hand, the packed-out food approach may decrease the "face time" with study staff to such a degree that the essential human relationships, that are so important to study adherence, may not be established. Instructing and expecting subjects to shop for, select and consume study diets on the weekends requires skills and food management efforts that are beyond most study participants.

The data generated from such studies are large and complicated with multiple time-points and multiple measurements provided by several laboratories. Data entry cannot be put off until the completion of the study. Additionally, management information, which is needed to evaluate the ongoing precision of the study, is being collected on a daily basis. Few investigators or reviewers recognize the need for a dedicated data and specimen manager, who is part of the management team from the start, along with the statistician. The use of multiple outcome measures brings opportunities to evaluate patterns of response, especially when large subject numbers are used, which may illuminate categories of responsiveness for physiologically or genetically identifiable subgroups.

3.4.   Single and Multi-Component Diet Modification Studies

Subjects in these studies are counseled to adhere to the diets of interest. For example, subjects are educated through multiple visits with a study dietitian, educational materials followed up by group sessions and cooking demonstrations to modify their diet to only 20% of energy from fat, or some other diet protocol. The control subjects are given a pamphlet on general diet guidelines, or a single session with a dietitian which stresses general good dietary principles. Large numbers of subjects can be managed at a number of clinical centers and interventions can be continued over several years. Studies are not limited to biomarkers or intermediate cancer endpoints, but may be able to use cancer as an endpoint in certain high-risk populations. The Polyp Prevention Trial was the first example of such a study focused on cancer prevention and control.[20] The trial sought to evaluate the effect of a self-selected diet with the goal of 20% as fat, 18 g dietary fiber /1000 kcal, and 5-8 servings of fruits and vegetables per day, on the recurrence of adenomatous colonic polyps, a precursor to colon cancer. Eight clinical sites randomized 2,079 subjects to receive extensive diet counseling[21] or continue on their usual diet for a 3 to 4 yr period. The results have not yet been published.

These studies are extremely important for evaluating the efficacy of biomarkers and intermediate endpoints because they are sufficiently large and can be carried out for a long enough time period to see a response, or even an association with a clinical outcome regardless of whether the intervention is shown to be effective. Therefore an important function of these trials is the inclusion of a number of promising biomarkers for validation and the illumination they bring to the interpretation of results, both positive and negative.

3.4.1. Diet Issues That May Attenuate Response

Although diet modification studies are essential for demonstrating the efficacy of diet approaches to cancer prevention and control, there are several diet-related reasons why a truly cancer-preventive dietary pattern may not be confirmed in a well-designed intervention trial. Eating behavior change is composed of a multiplicity of individual behaviors, including planning, shopping, food preparation and eating, that finally translate into a change in overall dietary pattern. These changes are more complicated than the better understood behaviors involved in smoking cessation.[22] Therefore, there will always be a relatively large subset of subjects who are non-adherent or partially adherent to an experimental diet. More problematic is that the investigators have only modest ability to identify non-adherers, because adherence can only be assessed by self-report and the human tendency is to report what is expected. Furthermore, since evaluation of each clinical site performance is based upon how well their subjects adhere to the dietary protocol, increased effort is often applied prior to the period of diet evaluation to encourage subjects to adhere. The effect of these two dynamics is to overestimate adherence to the experimental diet. Simultaneously, some subjects in the control group, knowing of the experimental diet because of informed consent, may have a tendency to adhere to the experimental diet. This possibility is difficult to avoid because diet modification studies cannot be masked. The solution is to demonstrate that the control group has not changed their diets even when pamphlets espousing the diet changes are given to them. Control group mean intakes from such studies generally vary little from baseline values.[23]

Finally, although the experimental group is taught to select foods that fit the putative cancer-preventive dietary pattern, there is great latitude in selecting foods. In the absence of clarity regarding specific foods, food preparation techniques, and food combinations that might be most protective, there may be subsets of diets selected which may not prevent carcinogenesis, which again will attenuate the results of the study.

Therefore, there is greater uncertainty in the application of diet interventions than in traditional drug trials, because of the difficulties in their execution. The rationale for "intent to treat" statistical analysis as the ultimate evaluation of efficacy of the proposed diet pattern should be reassessed since the assumptions that motivate this approach in drug trials may not be as relevant in diet intervention trials. The rejection of an efficacious diet may be more likely than accepting a diet that has no cancer protective effect because of intervention attenuation. This should be taken into consideration when evaluating the results of diet intervention studies.

3.5.   Food Supplement Studies

In food supplementation studies subjects are provided with food products that are consumed in addition to their regular diet. Masking of subjects and staff is often possible when equivalent foods with different ingredients are provided to the experimental and control group. Moderately large numbers of subjects can be studied in multiple centers. Past studies have been only a few months long because of the logistics of food supply and expense, but longer studies are feasible. Few have included the study of the putatively active compounds in the same study as whole foods. The most problematic issue is the use of and/or selection of the control food supplement. There are three main types of food supplementation studies and each has its own limitations.

3.5.1.   Double-masked Food Formulation Studies

These studies seek to formulate food products that contain foods with putative cancer-preventive activity, and similar products are formulated matched for energy and confounding nutrients and food components, as well as taste and appearance, so that it is difficult to identify the experimental product. Subjects are randomized to either treatment. Examples include the development of recipes for baked products with soy meal, fiber wafers, and fruit smoothies that contain hypothesized cancer preventive fruit.

This approach overcomes the difficulty of displacement of other foods in the diet to accommodate the energy supplied by the food supplement, because both the control food and experimental food will have the same energy content. It is also possible to combine several putative cancer preventive foods or food components into one formulation

The underlying diet of the subjects is generally not controlled, but must be assessed to evaluate the possibility that the diet changes or particular diet patterns confound the efficacy of the intervention. For example, what if a high fat, copious red meat diet, selected by a subset of study participants overwhelms the beneficial effect of the components contained in the supplement?

A solution to this issue is to combine the food formulation with a change in the underlying diet through diet counseling to achieve a more protective dietary pattern. This has been a standard approach for the evaluation of the effect of various dietary fibers on serum total cholesterol.[24] All subjects are counseled to select an American Heart Association-recommended diet for 2-4 wks before being randomized to the fiber-containing food product or its control. Although these studies often report good dietary compliance, all the issues related to self-selected diet modification pertain to its inclusion in food supplementation studies, in addition to the complication of changing the underlying diet during the supplementation period.

3.5.2. High Energy Food Supplements

Many of the foods proposed to have cancer preventive properties are high in energy and their distinctiveness cannot be masked by providing an equivalent-appearing control food. Published studies have used pre- and post-intervention measurements with no control group. Examples of these might be nuts, dried fruit, and (one that we just used) tomato sauce pasta dishes. Our pasta entrees delivered about 650 kcal per day, which for our older men with adenocarcinoma of the prostate constituted about 25% of their entire energy requirement.

Aside from the fact that the placebo effect becomes important when subjects know that they are in the experimental group, the issue of diet displacement of foods that had previously been in the diet also becomes prominent. Rigorous assessment of what foods and nutrients have been displaced is mandatory, and also whether energy intakes have been increased. Some increase in energy intake has been reported with nut studies as well as a larger displacement of other foods in the diet.[25] [26] The place the food holds in the diet, be it snack, entree or side dish, may make a difference in the proportion of energy added or displaced, and what class of foods are displaced.

3.5.3. Low Energy Food Supplements

Foods such as tea, broccoli and tomato juice are relatively low in energy and, aside from the selection of a control counterpart and absence of masking, do not pose the same problem of energy displacement. However, food substances vary in the amount of the putative bioactive ingredients and although these may be controlled to some extent, the longer the study and the larger the sample size the greater the difficulty in obtaining uniform material. If some of the protective substances are undetermined, the problem is magnified because of the absence of any method to standardize their intake.

Such food supplements still pose the problem of food substitution. For example, if subjects are requested to consume a cup of tomato juice a day, do they substitute this for the orange juice that they generally consume in the morning? What juice would one choose as a control since most have some interesting mix of polyphenolic compounds, which also may have some cancer protective function? If subjects consume tea, what beverage would ordinarily be used in their diet? When supplementing with a vegetable such as broccoli, is it consumed as an addition or a substitution for another vegetable? These issues must be addressed in the design of any study.

4. COMPONENTS OF EFFECTIVE DIET INTERVENTION STRATEGIES

Successful diet intervention strategies can be devised to evaluate food-based hypotheses for cancer prevention and control. Efficiency is gained if animal studies precede human studies, where possible, and controlled feeding studies precede diet modification studies. Key features of any diet based intervention strategy are: (1) Study design and population selection should be based upon a clear mechanism-based rationale. (2) Studies should include pure compounds as well as the same compounds in food matrices to enhance our understanding of food component interactions. (3) Validated biomarkers that are associated with various stages of the carcinogenic process should be included in any study so that a reasonable explanation of both negative and positive outcomes can be formulated. Several biomarkers should be included in any one study to aid in the validation process. (4) Chemical analysis of all supplements, foods, or diets used in studies should be performed not only for the substances of interest, but also other known cancer-promoting or preventing compounds, or classes of compounds, such as dietary fat. These analyses should be included in any scientific report of the study. (5) Underlying diet must always be monitored and reported with respect to the ingestion of compounds of interest and other bioactive nutrients, because inconsistencies in results from one study to another may be then understood and differences in diet among the study group may explain variances in response to the intervention. Since the inclusion of the diet assessment component of a study is costly in the collection and tedious in the analysis of the result, the tendency is to rationalize the marginal utility of the enterprise. However, weighed against the cost of repetitious studies with inconsistent results and with no viable explanation for the inconsistencies, the cost of diet assessment is minimal.

5. CONCLUSIONS

Clearly we need food and diet-based strategies for research that complement single compound studies, hopefully in the same study where possible. Progress may be more efficient if cell biologists, food chemists, nutritionists, epidemiologists and clinical researchers coordinate their research efforts by forming research interest groups which take responsibility for moving their whole particular field forward. This activity is ongoing in the field of carotenoid research, and is starting for phenolic compounds, with the formation of the Carotenoids Research Interest Group (CARIG) and the Phenolics for Health Research Interest Group (PhenHRIG), both part of the American Society for Nutrition Sciences. What distinguishes these groups is that they draw together researchers with a wide variety of training and background, and they have taken the responsibility of providing what is necessary to move the science forward.

Diet and food component intervention studies using inadequately validated approaches may produce inconsequential outcomes resulting from a multitude of unmeasured or unknown variables, leading us to prematurely discard viable diet-based cancer prevention strategies. The remedy is good study design, which includes sufficient study management measurements and mechanism-driven biomarkers to identify issues of validity, propose explanations for outcomes, and generate new hypotheses. Diet-based studies may be more difficult to execute, but the scientific pay-off for their use early in the exploration of the "dietary haystack" is likely to be large.

REFERENCES

1. U.S. Department of Health and Human Services. The Surgeon General's Report on Nutrition and Health, Public Health Service, DHHS (PHS) Publication No. 88-50210, Washington, DC, 1988, p. 180.
2. Le Marchand L, Hankin JH, Bach F, Kolonel LN, Wilkens, Stacewicz-Sapuntzakis M, Bowen PE, Beecher GR, Laudon F, Baque P, Daniel R, Seruvatu L, Henderson B. An ecological study of diet and lung cancer in the South Pacific. Int J Cancer 1995; 63:18-23.
3. McMichael AJ, McCall MG, Hartshorne JM, Woodings TL. Patterns of gastro-intestinal cancer in European migrants to Australia: the role of dietary change. Int J Cancer 1980; 25:431-37.
4. Kune S, Kune GA, Watson LF. Case-control study of dietary etiological factors: the Melbourne colorectal cancer study. Nutr Cancer 1987; 9:21-42.
5. Block G, Patterson B, Subar A. Fruit, vegetables, and cancer prevention: a review of the epidemiological evidence. Nutr Cancer 1992; 18:1-29.
6. Ziegler RG, Mason TJ, Stemhagen A, Hoover R, Schoenberg JB, Gridley G, Virgo PW, Fraumeni JG. Carotenoid intake, vegetables, and the risk of lung cancer among white men in New Jersey. Am J Epidemiol 1986; 123:1080-93.
7. Staack R, Kingston S, Wallig MA, Jeffery EH. A comparison of the individual and collective effects of four glucosinolate breakdown products from Brussel Sprouts on induction of detoxification enzymes. Toxicol Appl Pharmacol 1998; 149:17-23.
8. Serraino M, Thompson LU. The effect of flaxseed supplementation on early risk markers for mammary carcinogenesis. Cancer Lettr 1991; 60:135.
9. Thompson LU, Rickard SE, Orcheson LJ, Seidle MM. Flaxseed and its lignan and oil components reduce mammary tumor growth at a late stage of carcinogenesis. Carcinogenesis 1996; 17:1373-1376.

10. Mayne ST, Cartmel B, Silva F, Kim CS, Fallon BG, Briskin K, Zheng T, Baum M, Shor-Posner G, Goodwin WJ. Effect of supplemental beta-carotene on plasma concentrations of carotenoids, retinol, and alpha-tocopherol in humans. Am J Clin Nutr 1998; 68:642-7.

11. Albanes D, Virtamo J, Taylor PR, Rautalahti M, Pietinen P, Heinonen OP. Effects of supplemental β-carotene, cigarette smoking, and alcohol consumption on serum carotenoids in the Alpha-Tocopherol, Beta-Carotene Cancer Prevention Study. Am J Clin Nutr 1997; 66:366-72.

12. Wahlqvist M, Wattanapenpaiboon N, Macrae FA, Lambert JR, MacLennan R, Hsu-Hage BN. Changes in serum carotenoids in subjects with colorectal adenomas after 24 mo of β-carotene supplementation. Australian Polyp Prevention Investigators. Am J Clin Nutr 1994; 60:936-43.

13. Dennis BH, Ershow AG, Obarzanek E , Clevidence BA, eds. Well-Controlled Diet Studies in Humans. USA, The American Dietetic Association, 1999.

14. Halliwell B. Establishing the significance and optimal intake of dietary antioxidants: the biomarker concept. Nutr Rev 1999; 57:104-113.

15. Chen L, Bowen PE, Berzy D, Aryee F, Stacewicz-Sapuntzakis M, Riley RE. Diet modification affects DNA oxidative damage in healthy humans. Free Rad Biol Med 1999; 26:695-703.

16. Lee CK, Klopp RG, Weindruch R, Prolla TA. Gene expression profile of aging and its retardation by caloric restriction. Science 1999; 285:1390-93.

17. Hussain SP, Harris CC. Molecular epidemiology of human cancer: contribution of mutation spectra studies of tumor suppressor genes. Cancer Res 1998; 58:4023-37.

18. Harsha, DW, Lin PH, Obarzanek E, Karanja NM, Moore TJ, Caballero B, for the DASH Collaborative Research Group. Dietary approaches to stop hypertension: a summary of study results. J Am Diet Assoc 1999; 99(suppl):S35-S39.

19. Dennis BH, Stewart P, Wang C-H, Champagne C, Windhauser M, Ershow A, Karmally W, Phillips K, Stewart K, Heel NV, Farhat-Wood A, Kris-Etherton PM. Diet design for a multicenter controlled feeding trial, the DELTA program. J Am Diet Assoc 1998; 98:766-76.

20. Schatzkin A, Lanza E, Freedman LS, Tangrea J, Cooper MR, Marshall JR, Murphy PA, Selby JV, Shike M, Schade RR, Burt RW, Kikendall JW, Cahill J. The polyp prevention trial I: rationale, design, recruitment, and baseline participant characteristics. Cancer Epidemiol Biomark Prev 1996; 5:375-83.

21. Lanza E, Schatzkin A, Ballard-Barbash R, Corle D, Clifford C, Paskett E, Hayes D, Bote E, Caan B, Shike M, Weissfeld J, Slattery M, Mateski D, Daston C. The polyp prevention trial II: dietary intervention program and participant baseline dietary characteristics. Cancer Epidemiol Biomarkers Prev 1996; 5:385-92; Erratum in Cancer Epidemiol Biormarkers Prev 1996; 5:584.

22. Spring B, Pingitore R, Kessler K. Strategies to minimize weight gain after smoking cessation: psychological and pharmacological intervention with specific reference to dexfenfluramine. Int J Obes Metab Disord 1992; 16(Suppl 3): S19-23.

23. Obarzanek E, Hunsberger SA, Van Horn L, Hartmuller VV, Barton BA, Stevens VJ, Kwiterovich PO, Franklin FA, Kimm SY, Lasser NL, Simons-Morton DG, Lauer RM. Safety of fat-reduced diet: the Dietary Intervention Study in Children (DISC). Pediatrics 1997; 100:51-9.

24. Knopp RH, Superko HR, Davidson M, Insull W, Dujovne CA, Kwiterovich PO, Zavoral JH, Graham K, O'Conner RR, Edelman DA. Long-term blood cholesterol-lowering effects of a dietary fiber supplement. Am J Prev Med 1999; 17:18-23.

25. Chisholm A, Mann J, Skeaff M, Frampton C, Sutherland W, Duncan A, Tiszavari S. A diet rich in walnuts favorably influences plasma fatty acid profile in moderately hyperlipidaemic subjects. Euro J Clin Nutr 1998; 52:12-16.

26. Spiller GA, Jenkins AF, Bosello O, Gates JE, Cragen LN, Bruce B. Nuts and plasma lipids: an almond-based diet lowers LDL-C while preserving HDL-C. J Am Coll Nutr 1998; 17:285-90.

NUTRITION AND CANCER PREVENTION: NEW INSIGHTS INTO THE ROLE OF PHYTOCHEMICALS. FUTURE DIRECTIONS

Richard S. Rivlin, M.D.

Program Director, Clinical Nutrition Research Unit
GI-Nutrition Service
Memorial Sloan-Kettering Cancer Center
Professor of Medicine, Weill Medical College of Cornell
    University
Chief, Nutrition Division-Dept. of Med - Cornell Campus
    New York-Presbyterian Hospital

INTRODUCTION

A plant-based diet is important for maintaining health. Substances in fruits and vegetables, alone and in combination with one another, have been shown to have specific anticancer actions. The Ninth Annual Research Conference of the American Institute for Cancer Research has brought together leading scientists who are examining the mechanisms by means of which certain dietary agents may prevent cancer and limit its invasiveness once it has developed.

Nutrition and Cancer Prevention, edited under the auspices of AICR
Kluwer Academic / Plenum Publishers, New York, 2000.

THE SEARCH FOR ACTIVE PHYTOCHEMICALS

One of the recurring themes in cancer research today is that differences in rates of cancer prevalence among various populations around the world may relate to differences in their intake of specific dietary items. For example, the diet of Asian women has more soy and tea, with less fat, particularly saturated fat, than that of Western women. Each of these common food items may inhibit, or in the case of fat, promote the development of cancers of the breast and reproductive tract.

Populations do not, however, consume isolated nutrients; they consume food that is a combination of nutrients. Scientists are searching for combinations of nutrients that may have greater efficacy than single items in cancer prevention. For example, selenium and vitamin A may increase the ability of garlic to block activation of carcinogens, whereas linoleic acid and methionine may possibly limit garlic's efficacy.[1,2]

In our own laboratory, we have observed that zinc deficiency in rodents limits the degree to which serum levels of vitamin E can be increased after an increase in dietary intake of E. Thus, one should expect that to achieve fully the anticancer efficacy exhibited by vitamin E would require adequate dietary intake of zinc.

THE ROLE OF INTERMEDIATE BIOMARKERS

While it may be optimal to base our conclusions of efficacy of various dietary substances solely on the results of long-term, double-blind, placebo-controlled, crossover interventions to know with certainty whether any given nutrient has cancer inhibitory properties, such studies require enormous resources and prolonged duration. Interest, therefore, has turned to the search for identification and validation of intermediate biomarkers, which are biological parameters utilized to assess the progression of the neoplastic process in a given individual or animal model.

Intermediate biomarkers can also be employed to assess the efficacy of an intervention long before the development of actual cancer. Examples of such biomarkers that are currently being utilized by scientists in contemporary research include the labeling index, and proliferating zones.[4] There exists an urgent need to develop and validate intermediate biomarkers for a wide variety of human cancers.

One biomarker having increased utility is the prostate specific antigen (PSA). This laboratory test has been the subject of wide debate as a screening blood test for prostate cancer in populations of middle-aged and elderly males.

Unfortunately, it may provide a significant number of false positives in patients with benign disease, such as benign prostatic hypertrophy or prostatitis, and miss a number of smaller malignancies.[5]

Nevertheless, the value of the PSA measurement is unequivocal in monitoring the course of a given patient with prostate cancer. For example, following prostatectomy for prostate cancer the PSA titer should fall to low or undetectable levels. If in the period following prostatectomy a rapid rise in PSA titer is observed, then there is very high likelihood of recurrent disease. Thus, under certain circumstances, this test may detect prostate cancer; it does not *per se* predict grade, invasiveness or future course.

It would be enormously helpful in research studies and in patient care to have access to biomarkers that could be utilized in advance to predict the likelihood that a given individual would respond to a specific intervention. The demonstration that the new biomarker, prostate specific membrane antigen (PSM) increases in concentration rather than decreases in response to androgen deprivation[6] should be explored in this connection. PSM may prove to be a valuable marker for monitoring metastatic disease since it tends to remain within the malignant prostate cells rather than being excreted, as in the case of PSA.

THE SEARCH FOR ANIMAL MODELS

Another important need in research at present is to establish appropriate animal models that may be utilized to study mechanisms of action of phytochemicals in cancer prevention. A good friend of mine, David Perskie, has frequently chided me that "the only people interested in curing cancer in mice are doctors. The rest of us want to see cancer cured in people."

Nevertheless, the selection of appropriate animal models is highly valuable in testing activity of putative chemopreventive agents, and in gaining the necessary insights needed to pave the way for clinical trials. The area of prostate cancer research is one that has been identified as being in particular need of animal models that accurately define the progress of disease as it occurs in humans.

THE POTENTIAL OF ALTERNATIVE/COMPLEMENTARY MEDICINE

With respect to the potential of alternative/complementary medicine, sometimes called integrative medicine, in cancer prevention, we need to keep an open mind. No subject seems to polarize physicians more than this one. Many are unalterably opposed and others embrace alternative/complementary medicine perhaps too quickly and uncritically.

Let us recall that in England in the 19th century, the established treatment for dropsy, or edema, was application of leeches. Patients coming for treatment to physicians in Harley Street in London no doubt had access to leeches of the highest quality. Then word gradually spread that some ignorant midwives in rural England were claiming to cure dropsy by feeding patients with the leaves of a plant. Physicians on Harley Street had a good laugh at this outlandish idea, until it was eventually shown that the plant in question, the foxglove (Digitalis purpurea) provided digitalis, one of the central therapeutic agents for cardiac disease in modern medicine.

In similar fashion, much of value may be waiting in the wings in alternative/complementary medicine. Identification of the active principles involved and rigorous testing of efficacy and potential toxicity is urgently needed. An area of traditional Asian medicine that is undergoing validation by modern scientific techniques relates to the use of components of certain weeds and other plants for the treatment of heart disease and infections.

These weeds, as well as stems of grapes and peanuts, have been shown to contain high concentrations of resveratrol, a substance with many potentially beneficial effects on cardiovascular disease, as summarized in Table 1. Resveratrol appears to be an even more potent antioxidant that vitamin E, and is now undergoing study for its anticancer efficacy as well.[7] Subbaramaiah and his colleagues have recently shown that resveratrol inhibits transcription of cyclooxygenase-2 as well as inhibiting its basal activity in phorbol ester-treated human mammary epithelial cells, a recognized model system for the study of mammary tumorigenesis.[8]

Table 1. Effects Of Resveratrol On Coronary Heart Disease:[7]

1)   Inhibits primary platelet aggregation
2)   Blocks platelet formation of thromboxane A2
3)   Prevents synthesis of HETE
4)   Decreases hepatic synthesis of apolipoprotein A2
5)   Decreases hepatic synthesis of esterified cholesterol
6)   Blocks expression of adhesion molecules by endothelial cells in response to damage
7)   Regulates nitric oxide synthesis
8)   Has potent antioxidant effects, much greater than those of vitamin E

Similarly, the ancient use of garlic is finding scientific validation in a number of laboratories. There are accounts that garlic was fed to athletes prior to competition in the original Olympic games, constituting what appears to be documentation that garlic was one of the first "performance enhancing agents" and one that had official sanction.[9] It is of interest that garlic was believed to increase work performance and preserve health in ancient Rome, China, India, Egypt, Japan and other cultures. All of these ancient civilizations obviously had no contact with each other as they evolved independently. Yet, they arrived at many of the same conclusions about the efficacy of garlic in maintaining health, increasing work output and treating disease.

We now know that allium derivatives from garlic and also from garlic supplements have demonstrated efficacy in heart disease prevention. Furthermore, an increasing body of information from epidemiological reports, studies in animal models, in cells in culture and in cell-free systems all strongly suggest that allium derivatives from garlic have excellent potential for application to preventing and controlling cancer. At least 20 constituents derived from fresh garlic and garlic supplements have clear cancer chemopreventive and therapeutic activities.[10]

We need to submit so-called alternative/complementary therapies, particularly those already in use, to the same rigorous testing to which we subject more traditional approaches. We also must recognize the difficulties inherent in studying these therapies objectively in a double-blind fashion.

WHY STUDY MECHANISM OF ACTION OF PHYTOCHEMICALS?

Scientists are now searching for mechanisms of anticancer efficacy of common dietary items. Such efforts are not merely intellectual exercises, but rather have important practical significance. If the mechanism of action of a specific dietary substance can be elucidated, then it may be possible to utilize this knowledge to design even more effective agents.

Knowing the mechanism of action of a specific nutrient should help us decide whether to concentrate on defining its bioavailability in food or whether to restrict our efforts to the purified supplement. Studies should determine whether the concentrations necessary to achieve chempreventive efficacy can realistically be achieved from consumption of a given item as consumed ordinarily in food.

There is also the potential for genetically redesigning foods to contain larger amounts of active ingredients. Examples of genetic engineering of foods to enhance efficacy would include selenium-enriched garlic and beef containing higher amounts of conjugated linoleic acid (CLA).

Knowledge of mechanism should also help to explain the organ-specificity of some chemoprevention initiatives. Thus, while B-carotene has previously been shown to have benefit in protection against oral cancer, it has no apparent efficacy against colon polyps or melanoma skin cancer, and may actually cause harm in heavy smokers with lung cancer.[11,12] An important gap in knowledge is the need to elucidate interactions among nutrients, drugs and phytochemicals. Some of the reasons why studying mechanisms of action of phytochemicals are important are summarized in Table 2.

Table 2. Why Study Mechanism Of Action Of Phytochemicals?

1)   To definitively confirm anti-cancer efficacy
2)   To explain organ specificity of response
3)   To establish precise concentrations needed to achieve efficacy
4)   To enable study of interactions among other phytochemicals, drugs or nutrients
5)   To learn whether efficacy can be achieved by amounts in food or whether supplements are needed
6)   To design even more effective agents

Another emerging theme is that the age at which an intervention is initiated may be crucial to its success. One hypothesis is that the most important effects of soy products are exerted on the pre-pubertal breast and may provide protection against breast cancer by encouraging early evolution of the breast tissue in much the same way as early pregnancy has been shown to be protective against breast cancer. So while it probably is never too late to begin to take appropriate action on diet and lifestyle, the earlier one intervenes, the more likely will success be obtained.

WHAT SHALL WE TELL PATIENTS WHEN KNOWLEDGE IS UNCERTAIN?

Finally, patients with cancer, individuals at increased risk of developing cancer, as well as the general public all want to know what steps they should take now to minimize their chances of getting cancer and how to limit its spread once cancer has occurred. In my opinion we cannot abdicate our responsibility to inform the public about the current status of our research.

Even though many of the findings are preliminary and preclinical, I believe that we need to advise the public based on the knowledge acquired so far. Patients who have just been diagnosed with cancer, or healthy individuals at risk because of the finding of cancer in close relatives, are often desperate and want to act immediately. They do not want to wait until results are available from future clinical intervention trials many years from now.

It is my philosophy that we should guide patients based upon what has been shown to a reasonable certainty and then inform them about which are "promising lines of research". For example, we are learning that soy products, low-fat diets, garlic, tomato products and possibly tea, selenium and vitamin E may have promising potential in prevention of cancer of the prostate. Similarly, soy, tea, fiber and selenium, as well as calcium and vitamin D, possibly may be useful agents in prevention of cancer of the colon.

If we shirk our responsibilities as scientists to inform the public, vulnerable individuals will turn – and have already turned in many instances – to less informed sources for their information and guidance. Such advice may be misleading and even dangerous.

We must all join forces – scientists, government, industry, and the general public – to support major scientific and public health initiatives in disease prevention. The recommendations that we are currently giving to prevent cancer based on present knowledge should also be suitable for the prevention of heart disease, still the number one killer in the United States. It is of interest in this connection that two compounds widely being examined for their anticancer efficacy, namely S-allylmercaptocysteine from garlic and resveratrol from grapes, have specific activity against atherosclerosis. Thus, preventing one disease should help to prevent others. There is a remarkable convergence of dietary goals with respect to prevention of cancer, heart disease, as well as obesity and diabetes.

Much of medicine today is focused on "putting out fires", i.e., treating acute disease, such as the heart attack, stroke or cancer, without really pausing to consider the origin or prevention of these diseases. The late Ernst Wynder used to remind us that when Walter Mitty dreamed of becoming a doctor, he dreamed of becoming a neurosurgeon, not a practitioner of public health and preventive medicine. More attention must be paid to the slower, less dramatic aspects of disease prevention if we are going to succeed in the long run in reducing death and suffering from cancer.

FUTURE GOALS

Our goal should be to bring molecular biology and molecular genetics into nutrition research and to increase first class clinical investigation. We hope eventually to be able to utilize knowledge of a given individual's family history, genetic constitution and risks for disease to prescribe specific foods and perhaps supplements to reduce significantly that individual's risk for developing disease later in life.

ACKNOWLEDGMENTS

This work was supported in part by the Clinical Nutrition Research Unit grant (CA-29502) from the National Institutes of Health. Partial funding was also provided by grants from Wakunaga of America Co., Ltd., The Frank J. Scallon Medical Research Foundation, The Ronald and Susan Lynch Foundation, The Sunny and Abe Rosenberg Foundation, The Rosenfeld Heart Foundation, Now Natural Foods and The Allen Foundation.

REFERENCES

1. Ip C, Lisk DJ. Modulation of phase I and phase II xenobiotic-metabolizing enzymes by selenium-enriched garlic in rats. Nutr Cancer 1997; 28:184-188
2. Milner JA. Garlic: its anticarcinogenic and antitumorigenic properties. Nutr Rev. 1996; 54:S82-86
3. Bunk MJ, Dnistrian AM, Schwartz MK, Rivlin RS. Regulation of plasma concentrations of vitamin E by dietary zinc. Proc Soc Exp Biol Med. 1988;190:379-384
4. Richter F, Newmark HL, Richter A, et al. Inhibition of Western diet-induced hyperproliferation and hyperplasia in mouse colon by two sources of calcium. Carcinogenesis 1995;16:2685-2689
5. Catalona WJ, Richie JP, Ahmann FR, et al. Comparison of digital rectal examination and serum prostate-specific antigen in the early detection of prostate cancer: Results of a multicenter clinical trial of 6,630 men. J Urol. 1994;151:1283-1290
6. Pinto JT, Heston WDW. Prostate specific membrane antigen: A unique folate hydrolase. A review of recent findings. Prostate 1999;1:15-26
7. Jang M, Cai L, Udeani GO, et al. Cancer chemopreventive activity of resveratrol, a natural product derived from grapes. Science 1997; 275:218-220
8. Subbaramaiah K, Chung WJ, Michaluart P, et al. Resveratrol inhibits cyclooxygenase-2 transcription and activity in phorbol ester-treated human mammary epithelial cells. J Biol Chem. 1998;273:21875-21882
9. Rivlin RS. Historical perspective on the use of garlic. J Nutr, 1999 In press
10. Pinto JT, Rivlin RS. Garlic and other allicin vegetables in cancer prevention. In *Nutritional Oncology,* Heber D, Blackburn GL, Go VLM, eds. San Diego: Academic Press, 1999 pp. 393-403
11. Omenn, Goodman GE, Thornquist MD, et al. Effects of a combination of beta carotene and vitamin A on lung cancer and cardiovascular disease. N Engl J Med. 1996;334:1150-1155
12. Redlich CA, Chung JS, Cullen MR, et al. Effect of long-term beta-carotene and vitamin A on serum cholesterol and triglyceride levels among participants in the carotene and retinol efficacy trial. Atherosclerosis 1999;145:425-432

CHEMOPREVENTION: PROGRESS AND OPPORTUNITY

Elizabeth C. Miller, Zhiming Liao, Yanping Guo
Swati M. Shah and Steven K. Clinton

Division of Hematology and Oncology
Department of Internal Medicine
The Ohio State University College of Medicine
and Public Health
B402 Starling Loving Hall
320 West 10th Avenue
Columbus, Ohio 43210-1228

1. INTRODUCTION

A generally accepted definition of chemoprevention is the administration of purified chemical agents for the prevention of clinical cancer. This concept is commonly thought to have emerged a little over two decades ago and is attributed to cancer biologists who were elucidating the role of various natural substances and pharmacologic agents on the stepwise progression of cancer.[26] However, a brief review of public health and medical advances over the twentieth century will reveal that the concept and application of chemoprevention for various disease processes evolved directly from the great successes of nutritional scientists in the early decades of this century. Regardless of the conceptual origins of cancer chemoprevention, the progress in identifying agents, testing them in preclinical models, followed by human intervention studies, has rapidly accelerated in recent years. The century ends with the success of the Breast Cancer Prevention Trial (BCPT) illustrating the ability of the anti-estrogen Tamoxifen to prevent breast cancer in a cohort of women at high-risk.[10] Indeed, it is our opinion that chemoprevention, tobacco control, and the application of early detection strategies provide the opportunity to reduce cancer mortality by at least 50% within a generation.[11] The objective of this review is to provide the broad audience of cancer prevention investigators with a brief overview of the progress and future promise of cancer chemoprevention.

2. NUTRITION AND THE CHEMOPREVENTION OF DISEASE: HISTORICAL PERSPECTIVES

At the beginning of the twentieth century, Americans suffered from a number of diseases that today have been virtually eliminated and are a clinical rarity if seen on the wards of modern hospitals. Diseases such as rickets, goiter, beriberi, and pellegra were prevalent in the early 1900's and of uncertain etiology. Many of these diseases were thought to be of infectious etiology. Research in the nutritional sciences was still in its infancy and limited to the knowledge that protein, fat, and carbohydrates were the basic chemical components of foods. The meticulous work of nutritional biochemists lead to the purification and identification of compounds derived from foods that would reverse disease processes in rodent models that mimicked the signs and symptoms of human disease. The concept that foods contained small quantities of "vital amines" (vitamins) emerged. From this rigorous research, the concept of essential nutrients to prevent or reverse specific deficiency syndromes became firmly established. This knowledge provided the framework for medical and public health initiatives that rapidly impacted upon disease incidence and morbidity. Several examples of highly effective and low cost chemopreventive strategies for the prevention of nutritional diseases provide hope that history may be repeated with similar approaches targeting cancer.

In the 1800's and early 1900's, goiter was a widespread problem in Appalachia and the areas surrounding the Great Lakes. Sea salt (which contains several minerals including iodine) was recommended as a treatment of goiter for years before iodine was reported to be the element effective in goiter treatment.[2] Between 1910 and 1920, Kendall and Marine conducted iodine experiments on Ohio schoolgirls and concluded that goiter could be prevented with sodium iodide.[17] We now appreciate that the iodine content of the soil is poor in certain geographic areas and incorporation into crops and foods is thus insufficient to provide dietary needs. In 1922, iodized salt was introduced into the food supply of Michigan, which resulted in a marked reduction in goiter and subsequently led to widespread fortification of salt that continues today.[18] This example illustrates how easily the alteration of a staple food can serve as a vehicle for a chemopreventive agent and may dramatically influence the incidence and morbidity of a common disease process.

Much like today's cancer epidemiology literature, clues to identification of disease preventive nutrients were derived from human studies. In the 1930's, investigators reported that higher levels of fluoride were found in the water of populations experiencing a lower incidence of dental caries but a higher incidence of mottled teeth (a sign of excessive fluoride).[21] Over the next ten years, investigators were able determine the essential role for fluoride and define the optimal amount of fluoride in water to promote healthy teeth without mottling. Today, over half of the United States population consumes fluoridated water while many more obtain supplemental fluoride via toothpaste and multivitamin supplements resulting in a significant improvement in dental health.[21]

Once relatively common, pellegra, beriberi, and ariboflavinosis are nutrient deficiency diseases that are now only found in specific malnourished subpopulations such as alcoholics and those living in severe poverty. Indeed, the pellegra syndrome includes psychiatric disorders that contributed significantly to the number of institutionalized patients 100 years ago under deplorable conditions. Pellegra was considered a disease of infectious etiology following its characterization in the decades following the Civil War and was known as the disease of the four D's: diarrhea, dermatitis, dementia, and death. From 1906 to 1940, it was estimated that over 3 million cases and over 100,000 deaths were attributed to pellegra. The elucidation of niacin (vitamin B3) as an essential dietary factor rapidly lead to chemoprevention strategies and the virtual eradication of pellegra from the United States. Flour, rice, pasta and other bakery products have been fortified with niacin, thiamin, and riboflavin since the early 1940's. More recently, folic acid has been added to cereals, along with the other B vitamins, based upon recent data documenting its critical role for normal neurologic development of a fetus *in utero*. [6] Nutritional epidemiology studies have documented that average American women of childbearing age consume only half of the 400 microgram folic acid Recommended Dietary Allowance (RDA). As mandated by the Food and Drug Administration (FDA), beginning in January 1998, all enriched grain products must also be fortified with folic acid. [5] It is estimated that fortification of grains with folic acid may reduce the incidence of neural tube defects by 50% to 70%.[3] Public health approaches for the chemoprevention of B vitamin deficiency have been particularly effective since little or no risk is involved with intakes commonly derived from a fortified diet.

When addressing cancer chemoprevention strategies for a large population, iron deficiency anemia illustrates some potential obstacles. Current levels of iron fortification (in enriched grains and cereals) have significantly reduced the overall incidence and severity of iron deficiency anemia, although menstruating women still have excessive losses not addressed by standard fortification levels. Efforts to further increase the amount of iron in fortified foods and further reduce the risk of iron deficiency anemia for the highest risk groups is not favored due to a potential and serious risk to another population subgroup. Individuals with a disease known as hemochromatosis, which is associated with excessive iron accumulation, would be adversely affected with an increase in the amount of iron derived from iron-fortified foods. Therefore, efforts to further reduce iron deficiency anemia focus upon the identification of high-risk subgroups (such as growing teenagers and menstruating women), using medical approaches and public education. Health caregivers who are trained to identify high-risk groups for individual supplementation and public education have heightened awareness of iron deficiency.[21] Indeed, many cancer chemopreventive agents will not be incorporated into foods due to risk of toxicity. High-risk groups should be identified and treated under a physician's care.

Rickets was a devastating and widespread disease of American children at the turn of the century, primarily in impoverished city communities. Although the skeletal defects such as bowed-legs are recognizable to nutritional scientists from historical photos in textbooks, additional deformities in growing children also contributed to significant mortality. For example, chest deformities and impaired ventilation enhanced susceptibility to lethal pulmonary infections. It was estimated that over half of all child hospitalizations 80 years ago involved complications of rickets. Identification of vitamin D in the 1920's and clinical use rapidly led to the near elimination of rickets in American children within a decade. Although the Vitamin D requirement can be met through a diverse diet and exposure to sunlight, it was the supplementation of pure vitamin D to dairy products and margarine that has assured that nearly all Americans consume amounts that prevent deficiency symptoms.[14]

Vitamin A deficiency is the leading cause of blindness and visual impairment in the world.[24] Although vitamin A deficiency is rarely seen in modern Americans, it is widespread in developing countries. In addition to the greater availability of food sources of vitamin A (due to our diverse food supply), most Americans are assured of meeting their vitamin A requirements through the supplementation of margarine and dairy products with vitamin A. Additional efforts are underway worldwide to provide improved vitamin A nutrition into diets of diverse populations for the chemoprevention of visual defects. Since many populations in different cultures consume few dairy products, other foods may serve as vehicles for the consumption of supplemental vitamin A or provitamin A carotenoids, such as beta-carotene.[25,28]

Each of the above examples illustrate how a disease process of poorly understood etiology at the turn of the century was nearly eliminated in the American population using many of the same principles that we currently discuss in the emerging field of cancer chemoprevention. The challenge of eliminating these diseases may have seemed nearly impossible to clinicians, public health specialists, and scientists 100 years ago, just as many now view cancer as an inevitable consequence of aging. The successes of nutritional sciences should provide optimism that our current efforts in cancer chemoprevention will also prevail.

3. AGENTS FOR CANCER CHEMOPREVENTION

Development of agents for cancer chemoprevention has traditionally focused upon purified agents. Indeed, many investigators are now broadening their interpretation in recognition that a continuum exists between pure chemicals and complex foods (Figure 1). We are now in an era where horticultural techniques and food processing technology can alter the natural composition of food to enhance the profile of potential anti-cancer substances. Furthermore, selective breeding and genetic engineering offers opportunities to manipulate animal and plant products and develop new foods to foster cancer preventive properties. For example, health food stores now offer lycopene enriched extracts developed from of new strains of tomatoes selected for high concentrations of the ruby red carotenoid. Unfortunately, benefits of lycopene supplementation have yet to be clearly defined. [7] Proponents of soy products can now purchase isoflavone rich extracts of soy concentrations of genistein that far exceed what could be achieved from traditional soy based foods. Many of these new products, extracts, concentrates, and functional foods have blurred the previously clear definitions between nutrition and chemoprevention. Regardless of how we define these substances in the future, the opportunities to develop new agents and products for cancer prevention have never been greater. What is clearly needed from the government is improved regulatory definitions and empowerment of federal agencies to monitor efficacy, labeling, and safety of these products.

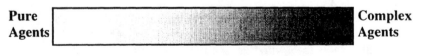

Pure Agents		Complex Agents
Drugs	Functional Foods	Diet
Vitamins	Genetically Enhanced Foods	
Minerals	Food Extracts	
Hormones	Herbs	
Phytochemicals	Phytopharmaceuticals	

Figure 1. The expanding continuum of chemopreventive approaches.

The development of effective chemopreventive agents typically proceeds through several key steps prior to human studies. The preclinical phase requires basic research for agent identification and discovery followed by evaluation of efficacy in several rodent models. A promising new agent then requires toxicology assessment, scale-up synthesis, formulation, the validation of surrogate endpoints in laboratory models that can be used in subsequent clinical studies, and finally a thorough regulatory review. Primary cell cultures, human orthotopic transplants, and animal models of early tissue dysplasia are being developed for screening of compounds. New model systems based upon specific molecular defects developed through gene knock-out and transgenic techniques offer characteristics that are hopefully more relevant to specific human cancers.

Agents for human chemopreventive efforts may be derived from an increasingly vast array of sources including: (a) hormones and anti-hormones, (b) modulators of carcinogen metabolism, (c) antioxidants, (d) modulators of prostatglandin and leukotriene metabolism, (e) synthetic retinoids and other ligands or inhibitors for the steroid receptor superfamily, (f) vitamins, (g) essential minerals, (h) vaccines and antibiotics, (i) inhibitors of intracellular signal transduction, (j) anti-angiogenic agents, (k) inhibitors of matrix metalloproteinases, (l) inhibitors of polyamine biosynthesis, (m) inhibitors of cell cycle control such as cyclin-dependent kinases, (n) monoclonal antibodies, and (o) gene therapy.

In addition to agent identification, future efforts will also focus upon novel methods of delivery. For example, high local concentrations of an agent may be achieved with limited systemic toxicity if methods for delivery to target mucosal surfaces can be developed. New techniques employing aerosols to expose the oral pharynx, larynx, and lung tissue of high-risk smokers to chemopreventive agents may prove effective due to greater local concentrations with less systemic toxicity. Other tissues likely to benefit for targeted local administration of chemopreventive agents include the cervix, bladder, colon, and skin.

A concept that has yet to be significantly developed for cancer prevention is combination chemoprevention. This approach is the basis for the dramatic success of curative chemotherapy in childhood leukemia, and adult testicular cancer.[13] The combination of several chemopreventive agents with different cellular targets, unique mechanisms of action, and non-additive toxicity offers enormous potential benefits. In addition, combining dietary and nutritional interventions with active chemopreventive agents may significantly potentiate the activity of purified agents.

A critical component of agent development is the precise characterization of toxicity profiles. Unlike chemotherapy for advanced cancer where very high toxicity is accepted in face of a lethal disease, those participating in most cancer chemoprevention studies are generally healthy and acceptance of toxicity will be much lower. It is critical that efforts continue in the evaluation and quantification of more subtle quality of life side effects that may be more common with cancer chemopreventive agents.

For example, an agent that increases frequency of loose stools or a decline in sexual function will quickly be discontinued by many patients unless the perceived risk of cancer and potential benefit of the agent is very high. Low tolerance for side-effects will influence compliance and research on new approaches for insuring that individuals consume the chemopreventive agent are necessary.

4. BIOMARKERS

Well-characterized biomarkers are critical for the cost effective and rapid clinical evaluation of cancer chemopreventive agents. Biomarkers can fall into several different conceptual categories. For example, we desperately need biomarkers that are indicators of biological effects of the chemopreventive agents. One of the major obstacles to the development of the class of agents called antioxidants is the lack of biomarkers of oxidative damage that are sensitive and specific indicators of effects mediated by agents such as vitamin C, tocopherols, carotenoids, selenium and other phytochemicals. Although progress continues in these areas, there is currently no consensus among investigators concerning which biomarkers may be most useful as short term indicators of an anticancer biological effect for most antioxidants. The importance of biomarkers specific for the action of a putative chemopreventive agent cannot be under-emphasized. If every putative chemopreventive agent requires testing in long term and costly studies with cancer as an endpoint our progress will be slow. Short-term studies employing surrogate biomarkers as endpoints in order to better define the appropriate dose and schedule of administration of an agent are critical. The short-term studies allow investigators to maximize the ability of long term studies to address the issue of efficacy.

Another class of biomarkers often employed in chemoprevention studies includes the variety of cellular changes which can be detected by genetic, histological and biochemical analysis and are specific for the disease process that is being targeted for intervention. For example, a growing number of histologic precursors to cancer have been identified based on morphologic and cytological criteria. The ability of a chemopreventive regimen to reverse premalignant lesions can be undertaken as a prelude to longer cancer prevention studies. These lesions include oral leukoplakia, carcinoma *in situ* of the cervix, colonic adenomatous polyps, prostatic intraepithelial neoplasia (PIN), Barrett's esophagus, actinic keratoses, dysplastic nevi, and dysplastic bronchial metaplasia.[16]

Another conceptual approach to biomarkers involves a focus upon cellular and molecular targets involved in the cancer process that may be altered by a putative chemopreventive agent. These include nuclear morphology, proliferation rates, apoptosis rates, oncogene or tumor suppression gene expression, growth factor expression, tumor angiogenesis, expression of matrix metalloproteinases, mutations in specific genes, and chromosomal alterations. The ability to accurately quantitate biomarkers has been greatly enhanced by computerized image analysis and laser capture microdissection of tissue.[19,22] The application of new technology will allow investigators to measure the expression of biomarkers with high sensitivity and reproducibility and minimize the variation associated with human observation.

5. STUDY POPULATIONS AND COHORTS

Large Populations

In some situations, future cancer chemoprevention efforts may focus upon large populations or cohorts. An intervention targeting large populations must be relatively inexpensive, highly effective, and exhibit little risk for toxicity. An important example of how this approach may be applied is the use of the hepatitis vaccine to prevent liver cancer and liver failure in high-risk geographic areas such as China.[20] Cancer vaccines have not traditionally been considered chemopreventive agents, but clearly the principles of prevention are the same. There are several chemoprevention trials currently underway that are investigating the role of selenium in cancer prevention. Indeed, if selenium proves to have cancer chemopreventive activity in humans, one approach is to incorporate modest concentrations of selenium into fertilizers that are used in areas of the world where soil concentrations are low. The subsequent incorporation into biomolecules in the food products would increase selenium intake for a broad population.

High-Risk Cohorts

It is likely that most chemopreventive efforts will focus on populations at highest risk. Targeting high-risk groups offers several advantages for clinical studies. The overall greater frequency of cancer incidence allows agents to be tested in studies with fewer participants over shorter duration, thus providing significant cost savings that can be invested in additional research. An elegant example is the recent Breast Cancer Prevention Trial with tamoxifen (BCPT).[10] The trial was limited to women identified to be at high-risk for breast cancer based upon several factors such as family history and age. The study was able to reach a definitive conclusion and was terminated early in part because the breast cancer outcomes were more common in this high-risk group than would occur in a cross section of the entire population. The benefits of tamoxifen for breast cancer prevention provide a stimulus to proceed with newer agents and combinations in high-risk cohorts.

High-Risk Lifestyles

The successes of cancer epidemiology have helped to characterize high-risk cohorts by identifying high-risk lifestyles, exposure to occupational and environmental carcinogens, premalignant markers and familial and genetic risk factors. Lifestyles that are likely associated with a greater risk of certain cancers include: tobacco use (many different cancers), alcohol (oral cavity, possibly breast), affluent dietary patterns (colon, breast, and prostate), obesity (distal esophagus), and a sedentary lifestyle (colon).[1] Chemopreventive agents in conjunction with alterations in high-risk behaviors offer important opportunities for clinical studies.

Occupational Exposure to Carcinogens

Some of the earliest and most convincing evidence of chemical carcinogenesis in humans has come from occupational exposures. Prominent examples include lung cancer and mesothelioma in asbestos workers (especially among workers who smoke cigarettes), hepatic angiosarcomas in vinyl chloride polymerization workers, and myeloid leukemias in workers exposed to benzene used as a solvent in the rubber industry.[23] Specific groups for chemopreventive studies can be identified through unions and professional organizations.

Environmental Carcinogens

Exposure to chemical carcinogens in the environment continues to be a subject of great concern. Examples include various carcinogenic materials in air pollution, halogenated hydrocarbons in drinking water, chemicals such as polychlorinated biphenyls and dibenzodioxins from chemical plant emissions or inadequate waste chemical disposal, and pesticide residues in various food products.[4,12] New approaches to define exposure to specific carcinogens in populations and perhaps the quantitation of residues in human tissues will help define high-risk cohorts for prevention studies.

Premalignant Lesions

The presence of a premalignant lesion (also called a precancerous lesion) identifies another high-risk population for chemoprevention studies. Premalignant lesions are generally found by physicians, dentists, nurses or by self-examination. These lesions do not always develop into cancer, but they are known to be associated with increased cancer risk (Table 2). More importantly, in many cases, premalignant lesions have been demonstrated to be reversible.[23] Identification of these lesions provides an opportunity to define high-risk groups for chemopreventitive intervention.

Prior Cancer Diagnosis / Treatment

Survivors of an initial malignancy are often at high-risk of future primary cancers and serve as an ideal source of participants in chemoprevention trials. For example, those treated with cyclophosphamide (Cytoxan) for childhood cancers are at greater risk of bladder cancer decades later. [13,15] Many cancer therapeutic agents are mutagens, and secondary leukemia has been a common finding in some clinical studies.[15] Female children treated with mediastinal radiation for lymphoma or other thoracic cancers may subsequently experience a greater rate of breast cancer. [13,27] However, other factors may contribute to high-risk following successful therapy of cancer. Smokers who are fortunate enough to detect a tobacco-related cancer of the oral mucosa or lung and undergo successful therapy are at significant risk of developing a second primary cancer of the same tissues due to the previous carcinogenic insult. Similarly, resection of a superficial bladder tumor is likely to be followed by recurrent superficial tumors over the next few years.

Genetics

Perhaps the most important future progress in the identification of a high-risk group will emerge from the field of cancer genetics. The cloning of the human genome is soon to be accomplished and the genetic blueprint will allow clinical geneticists to rapidly identify and characterize specific inherited defects or polymorphisms of genes that influence cancer risk. Some of the best examples thus far identified include the high-risk breast cancer genes (BRCA) and colon cancer genes (HNPCC). [8,9] The opportunities for chemoprevention are indeed exciting, since the mechanisms of action of the genes will be defined and specific animal models characterized for the identification of agents targeting the specific defects will be developed. The precision of targeting specific agents for defined genetic lesions should greatly enhance efforts to define highly effective chemoprevention studies.

6. DESIGN OF CHEMOPREVENTION TRIALS

A step-wise process is typically employed in establishing chemopreventive strategies. Pre-clinical studies in cell culture and animal models continue to provide an important screen for effective agents, characterization of mechanisms of action, and identification of potential biomarkers or toxic outcomes. Once a chemopreventive compound has been found to be effective in cell culture and experiment animals, the compound is tested in human clinical trials. There are three phases of clinical trials, which must be completed before a chemopreventive substance can be made available for general use. The first step is a phase I trial. A phase I trial is limited in participants and short-term with the purpose to determine dose-related tolerability and safety. Since the major goal of chemoprevention is to apply cancer prevention agents to large numbers of healthy people, only a minimal amount of toxicity will be tolerated.   Different doses of the test agent are given to healthy subjects for a short period of time, and side effects are monitored. In addition to determining safety, phase I trials also evaluate target-tissue levels, drug interactions, and patient adherence.

Once the toxicity profile and pharmacology of the investigational agent is determined, phase II trials are implemented, with the goal of determining the biologic activity and the maximum dose of the agent that does not produce unwanted side effects in larger studies. Phase IIA chemoprevention trials are typically small scale, short-term studies designed to assess a series of intermediate endpoints and define biomarkers that may be relevant for future studies. The phase IIB studies focus on a narrower dose-range and establish a dose that will specifically modify an intermediate endpoint response.

Phase III trials have a larger number of participants and frequently last many years. The goal is to definitively determine if a proposed agent actually prevents cancer. The major end point of phase III trials is cancer incidence, but other factors, such as long-term toxicity and biomarker modulation, are also studied. Because of the length of phase III trials, several obstacles arise: long-term patient compliance can be difficult, the trials become very expensive, and usually these trials require thousands of participants in order to achieve statistical significance. Nonetheless, phase III trials are important and necessary to support chemoprevention claims.[11] Promising results have emerged from many phase III studies, including the use of retinoids for the chemoprevention of squamous cell cancer of the head and neck, as well as the use of anti-estrogens for the prevention of breast cancer.

REFERENCES

1. American Institute for Cancer Research. *Food, Nutrition and the Prevention of Cancer: a Global Perspective*, Washington, DC: American Institute for Cancer Research 1997.
2. Anonymous. Iodine fortification and thyrotoxicosis. Nutr Rev 1970;28:212-214.
3. Anonymous. Recommendations for the use of folic acid to reduce the number of cases of spina bifida and other neural tube defects. MMWR Morb Mortal Wkly Rep 1992; 41:1-7.
4. Austin H, Keil JE, Cole P. A prospective follow-up study of cancer mortality in relation to serum DDT. Am J Public Health 1989; 79:43-46.
5. Bentley JR, Ferrini RL, Hill LL. American College of Preventive Medicine Public Policy Statement: Folic acid fortification of grain products in the U.S. to prevent neural tube defects. Am J Prev Med 1999;16:264-267.
6. Berry Rj, Li Z, Erickson JD, Li S, et al. Prevention of neural-tube defects with folic acid in China. China-U.S. Collaborative Project for Neural Tube Defect Prevention. N Engl J Med 1999;341:1485-1490.

7. Clinton SK. Lycopene: chemistry, biology, and implications for human health and disease. Nutr Rev 1998;56: 35-51.

8. de la Chapelle A, Peltomaki P. Genetics of hereditary colon cancer. Annu Rev Genet 1995;29:329-348.

9. de la Chapelle A, Peltomaki P. The genetics of hereditary common cancers. Curr Opin Genet Dev 1998;8:298-303.

10. Fisher B, Costantino JP, Wickerham DL, Redmond CK, et al. Tamoxifen for prevention of breast cancer: report of the National Surgical Adjuvant Breast and Bowel Project P-1 Study. J Natl Cancer Inst 1998;90:1371-1388.

11. Greenwald P, Kramer BS, Weed DL, eds. *Cancer Prevention and Control.* New York, NY: Marcel Dekker, 1995.

12. Hoar SK, Blair A, Holmes FF, Boysen CD, et al. Agricultural herbicide use and risk of lymphoma and soft-tissue sarcoma. JAMA 1986;256:1141-1147.

13. Holland JF, Bast RC, Morton DL, Frei E, et al. *Cancer Medicine, 4ᵗʰ edition,* Baltimore, MD: Williams and Wilkins, 1997.

14. Hollick MF, Shao Q, Liu WW, Chen TC. The vitamin D content of fortified milk and infant formula. N Engl J Med 1992; 326:1178-1181.

15. Johansson SL, Cohen SM. Epidemiology and etiology of bladder cancer. Semin Surg Oncol 1997; 13:291-298.

16. Kelloff GJ, Malone WF, Boone CW, Steele VE, Doody LA. Intermediate biomarkers of precancer and their application in chemoprevention. J Cell Biochem - Supplement 1992;16G:15-21.

17. Kimball OP, Marine D. The prevention of simple goiter in man. Arch Inst Med 1918; 22:41.

18. Lee K, Bradley R, Dwyer J, Lee SL. Too much versus too little: the implications of current iodine intake in the United States. Nutr Rev 1999;57:177-181.

19. Liotta LA. Probing the depths of degradation: matrix metaloproteinase-2 and endometrial menstrual breakdown. J Clin Invest 1996;97:273-274.

20. Mahoney FJ. Update on diagnosis, management, and prevention of hepatitis B virus infection. Clin Microbiol Rev 1999;12:351-366.

21. Mertz W. Food fortification in the United States. Nutr Rev 1997; 55:44-49.

22. Mukherjee P, Sotnikov AV, Mangian HJ, Zhou J. Energy intake and prostate tumor growth, angiogenesis, and vascular endothelial growth factor expression. J Natl Cancer Inst 1999;91:512-523.

23. Schottenfield D, Fraumeni Jr. JF. *Cancer Epidemiology and Prevention,* New York, NY: Oxford University Press, 1996.

24. Sizer FS, Whitney EN. "The Vitamins" In: *Nutrition Concepts and Controversies, 7ᵗʰ edition,* Belmont, CA: West Wadsworth, 1997.

25. Solon FS, Fernandez TL, Latham MC, Popkin BM. Planning, implementation , and evaluation of a fortification program. Control of vitamin A deficiency in the Philippines. J Am Diet Assoc 1979;74:112-118.

26. Sporn MB. Combination chemoprevention of cancer. Nature 1980;287:107-108.

27. Tinger A, Wasserman TH, Klein EE, Miller EA, et al. The incidence of breast cancer following mantle field radiation therapy as a function of dose and technique. Int J Radiat Oncol Biol Phys 1997; 37:865-870.

28. Toro O, de Pablo S, Aguayo M, Gattan V, et al. Prevention of vitamin A deficiency by fortification of sugar. A field study. Arch Latinoam Nutr 1977;27:169-179.

ABSTRACTS

Poster Abstract # 1

Sphingolipids in Foods and Differential Sensitivity of Human Colon Cancer Cells to Sphingoid Bases and Ceramides

Eun-Hyun Ahn and Joseph J. Schroeder
Department of Food Science & Human Nutrition
Michigan State University
East Lansing, MI 48824-1224

Complex dietary sphingolipids have been shown to protect against development of colon cancer (Schmelz et al., Cancer Res. 56: 4936, 1996). The amounts of sphingolipids in foods are poorly defined and the mechanism by which complex sphingolipids protect against colon cancer is not known. The purpose of the present study was to quantitate sphingolipids in dairy products and soy fractions and to investigate the effects of the bioactive sphingolipid metabolites, sphingoid bases and ceramides, on growth and death of HT-29 and HCT-116 human colon cancer cells. The concentrations of total sphingolipids and free sphingoid bases (nmol/g of dry weight) in foods were: nonfat dry milk (203 + 75; 146 + 78); yogurt (138 + 55; 1.2 + 0.3); Swiss cheese (167 + 45; 6.5 + 7.6); full fat soy flakes (609 + 627; 2.6 + 1.1); soy flour (610 + 509; 1.6 + 0.3); isolated soy protein (210 + 112; 2.8 + 1.7) (mean + SD, n=4). Most sphingolipids in foods were present as complex sphingolipids with sphingosine as the predominant sphingoid base backbone. Both exogenous free sphingosine and sphinganine inhibited growth and caused death of HT-29 and HCT-116 cells; whereas, only C2-ceramide and not C2-dihydroceramide inhibited growth and caused death of the colon cancer cells suggesting that the 4,5-trans double bond was necessary for the inhibitory effect of ceramide. DNA gel electrophoresis and morphologic observation using fluorescent dyes suggest that sphingosine, sphinganine, and C2-ceramide killed cells by inducing apoptosis. The results demonstrate that sphingolipids are significant constituents of dairy products as well as soy fractions and suggest that the protective effects of complex dietary sphingolipids may be mediated by their metabolic break-down products, sphingoid bases and/or ceramide, which inhibit growth and induce apoptosis in human colon cancer cells

Supported by the Michigan Agricultural Experiment Station.

Poster Abstract # 2

Prevention of Papillomavirus Initiated Cancer By the Phytochemical Indole-3-Carbinol

F Yuan[1], D-Z Chen[1], L Jin[1], M Qi[1], J Arbeit[2], K Liu[1], D Sepkovic[3], HL Bradlow[3], K Auborn[1]

[1]Dept Otolaryngology, Long Island Jewish Medical Center, New Hyde Park, NY
[2]Dept Surgery, UCSF, San Francisco, CA
[3]Strang Cancer Center, New York, NY

The E6 and E7 proteins of highly oncogenic types of papillomaviruses, such as HPV16, are cofactors for cervical cancer. Circumstantial and direct evidence indicates that estrogen promotes this cancer. This study investigated whether indole-3-carbinol (I3C) could prevent cervical cancer. I3C (from broccoli, cabbage, Brussels sprouts, cauliflower) is an active chemopreventative and anti-estrogen. Mice with the transgenes for HPV16 E6 and E7 under a keratin 14 promoter develop cervical cancer when given estradiol chronically. Slow release 17-beta-estradiol pellets (0.125mg/60days) were implanted in female mice fed an AIN diet or an AIN diet supplemented with 2000 ppm I3C. More than 70% of mice on the AIN diet developed cervical cancer whereas< 4% of mouse receiving dietary I3C developed cervical cancer or high-grade dysplasia. We further investigated anti-estrogenic activities of I3C in cervical cells using CaSki cells, which have integrated HPV16 sequences. While estradiol increased HPV16 expression in CaSki cells, both I3C and 2-hydroxyestrone (a metabolite considered anti-estrogenic) decreased HPV16 expression. Using quantitative RT-PCR, we determined that I3C increased expression of CYP1A1 and CYP1A2, enzymes that catalyze 2-hydroxylation of estradiol. I3C reduced CYP1B1, an enzyme responsible for the carcinogenic metabolite, 4-hydroxyestrone. GC-MS analysis confirmed a large amount of estradiol was converted to 2-hydroxyestrone after treatment of CaSki cells with I3C. Therefore, I3C promotes favorable estrogen metabolism in cervical cells. Whereas estrogen increases proliferation of cervical cells, I3C induces apoptosis. Using both CaSki and C33A cells, the amount of apoptosis was dependent on the relative amounts of estrogen and I3C. Therefore, both estrogen and I3C influence the balance between proliferation and apoptosis. With the mouse model, we provide direct evidence that I3C should be a useful preventative for cervical cancer. In vitro, we provide mechanisms whereby I3C can influence the development of cervical cancer.

(This work was supported by CA3385 from the National Cancer Institute.)

Poster Abstract # 3

Enhancement of Mitomycin C Antitumor Activity in Human Tumor Cell Lines by Dietary Inducers of DT-Diaphorase

Asher Begleiter[1,2,3,4] Xiaowei Wang[1,2,3] Geoffrey P. Doherty[1,2,3] Marsha K. Leith[1,4] and Thomas J. Curphey[5]

[1]Manitoba Institute of Cell Biology, [2]Manitoba Cancer Treatment and Research Foundation, [3]Departments of Pharmacology and Therapeutics and [4]Internal Medicine University of Manitoba, Winnipeg, CANADA
[5]Department of Pathology, Dartmouth College, Hanover, NH

DT-diaphorase is a two-electron reducing enzyme that activated the bioreductive antitumor agent, mitomycin C (MMC). Cell lines having elevated levels of DT-diaphorase are generally more sensitive to MMC. We have shown that DT-diaphorase can be induced in human tumor cells by a number of compounds including dietary components like 1,2-diathiole-3-thiones. In this study, we investigated whether induction of DT-diaphorase could enhance the cytotoxic activity of MMC in six human tumor cell lines representing four tumor cell types in vitro. DT-diaphorase was induced by many dietary inducers, including propyl gallate, dimethyl maleate, dimethyl fumarate, and sulforaphane. The cytotoxicity of MMC was significantly increased in four tumor lines with the increase ranging from 1.4- 1.3-fold. In contrast, MMC activity was not increased in two human tumor cell lines that had high base levels of DT-diaphorase activity. There was a small increase in toxicity to normal human marrow cells when MMC was combined with 1,2-diothiole-3-thione, but this increase was minor in comparison with the 3-fold increase in cytotoxicity to tumor cells. This study demonstrates that induction of DT-diaphorase can increase the cytotoxic activity of MMC in human tumor cell lines, and suggests that it may be possible to use dietary inducers of DT-diaphorase to enhance the efficacy of bioreductive antitumor agents.

(Supported by the Medical Research Council of Canada and the American Institute for Cancer Research.)

Poster Abstract # 4

Inhibition of azoxymethane induced colon cancer by orange juice

Y. Miyagi[1], A.S. Om[1], K.M. Chee[2], and <u>M.R. Bennink</u>[1]
[1]Michigan State University, East Lansing, MI
[2]Korea University, Seoul, KOREA

Certain flavonones, limonoids, and cumarins present in citrus foods inhibit chemically induced cancer in animal models. In these studies, purified citrus phytochemicals were used to inhibit carcinogenesis. It would be inappropriate to extrapolate from these results that consuming a citrus product will inhibit cancer. There has been only one study (Se et al., Nutr Cancer 26:167, 1996) showing that feeding a citrus product (double strength orange juice) delays onset of mammary cancer in rats. The objective of this study was to determine if feeding single strength, pasteurized orange juice would inhibit azoxymethane (AOM) induced colon cancer in male Fisher 344 rats.

Colon cancer was initiated by injecting 15mg AOM/kg of weight at 22 and 29 days of age. One week after the second AOM injection, orange juice replaced drinking water for the experimental group (N=30). Growth during the 28-week 'post initiation' feeding experiment was similar for both dietary treatments and there was no difference ($P>0.05$) in weight gain. Feeding orange juice reduced tumor incidence by 22% ($P<$ or $= 0.05$). The average number of colon tumors was similar (0.97 vs. 1.2) for both groups, but, there was a strong trend ($P=0.13$) towards a smaller average tumor burden (mg tumor per rat) for the group drinking orange juice (118 vs. 210). Decreased tumor incidence was associated with a decreased labeling index and proliferation zone in the colon mucosa. Hesperidin, limonin glucoside, and chymotrypsin inhibitor are chemopreventive agents in orange juice that most likely account for the decreased colon tumorigenesis associated with feeding orange juice.

(Tropicana Products, Inc. provided Tropicana Pure Premium orange juice and financial support for this study.)

Poster Abstract # 5

Optimal Ratio of n-3/n-6 Fatty Acids for Maximum Inhibition of Human Breast Cancer Cell Growth in vitro

Hilda Chamras, Ani Ardashian and John A. Glaspy
Division of Hematology/Oncology
UCLA, School of Medicine
Los Angeles, CA

There is evidence from both epidemiological and experimental studies that dietary fatty acids (FA) influence the development and subsequent progression of breast cancer. Moreover, specific FAs may exert opposing effects so that the net result is dependent on their relative concentration in the diet. It has been suggested that the n-3/n-6 FA ratio in the diet may negatively be correlated with the risk of breast cancer mortality, however the optimal ratio of n-3 to n-6 FA that minimizes the human breast cancer cell growth has not been established. We investigated the effect of different ratios (0.1 to 10) of decosahexaenoic acid (DHA) to linoleic acid (LA) on MCF-7 and MDA-MB-231 breast cancer cells, and HMEC normal human mammary epithelial cell growth in vitro. Due to variation in sensitivity of cells to FAs, different ranges of FA concentrations were used. In a FA concentration range of 1 to 10M, MCF-7 cell growth was inhibited 30% at a DHA/LA ratio of 0.1 and no significant change was seen up to FA ratio of 10. However, MDA-MB-231 cell growth was stimulated at ratios of 0.1 to 0.5 and the optimal ratio of DHA/LA for minimum growth was 1.0. At higher concentrations of Fas (10-100M), MCF-7 cell growth was inhibited 30% and 90% at ratios of 0.1 and 10, respectively. MDA-MB-231 cell growth stimulation was 40% at a ratio of 0.1 and 20% at a ratio of 5.0. The optimal ratio for maximum inhibition was observed at a ratio of 10. HMEC cell growth was not affected at low FA concentrations. At higher concentrations, only 25% inhibition was observed at DHA/LA ratio of 10. These results suggest that there is a difference in the sensitivity to FAs between MCF-7 and MDA-MB-231 cells, and the increase in the DHA/LA ratio can suppress the MCF-7 and MDA-MB-231 cell growth in vitro. This study provide an important contribution to a better understanding of the effects of varying concentrations and ratios of exogenous FAs on breast cancer cell growth, which could have significant implications for breast cancer prevention and treatment.

Poster Abstract # 6

Molecular Effects of Indole-3-Carbinol on PC3 Prostate Cancer Cells

Sreenivasa R. Chinni, Yiwei Li, and Fazlul H. Sarkar
Department of Pathology
Karmanos Cancer Institute
Wayne State University School of Medicine
Detroit, MI 48201

Prostate cancer is one of the most common cancers in men and it is the second leading cause of male cancer death in the United States. Many studies have shown that the consumption of fruits and vegetables, which provides several classes of compounds, including indole-3-carbinol (I3C), may have a protective effect against the development of prostate and other human malignancies. Since the mortality and morbidity due to prostate cancer will likely increase because of a rise in longevity and since no optimally effective cure is available, there is a renewed interest in developing preventive strategies for this disease. Since I3C appears to have significant biological activity, and no molecular mechanism has been established in prostate cancer cells, we hypothesize that I3C may have significant effect on prostate cancer cells in cell growth inhibition and apoptosis. Here, we report the results of our preliminary studies, which showed that I3C is a potent inhibitor of PC3 prostate cancer cell growth. Induction of apoptosis was also observed in this cell line when treated with I3C, as measured by DNA laddering and PARP cleavage. We also found an up-regulation of p21WAF1 and Bax, and down-regulation of Bcl-2 and CDK6 in I3C treated cells. In addition, we investigated the role of DNA binding activity of a transcription factor, NF-kB, which was shown to be inhibited in I3C treated PC3 cells. Moreover, I3C abrogated the NF-kB activation by two known inducers, such as H_2O_2 and TNF-α. From these results, we conclude that I3C inhibits the growth of PC3 prostate cancer cells, protect cells from oxidative stress, induces G1 cell cycle arrest and apoptosis, and regulate the expression of apoptosis-related genes. These findings suggest that I3C may be an effective chemopreventive or therapeutic agent against prostate cancers.

Poster Abstract # 7

Regulation of Enzyme Activity and Selenoprotein Gene Expression in Rat Prostate by Selenium

M.J. Christensen, A.B. Rand, K. Ames, W.E. Spencer, L.E. Bertrand
Department of Food Science and Nutrition
Brigham Young University
Provo, UT 84602.

Reports of a protective effect of selenium (Se) supplementation against prostate cancer in humans have focused attention on the metabolism of this nutrient in this tissue. To examine Se metabolism in prostate weanling male Sprague-Dawley rats were fed a Torula yeast-based Se-deficient diet or the same diet supplemented with 0.15 or 2.0 ppm Se as sodium selenite for 9 weeks. Activity of cellular glutathione peroxidase (EC 1.11.1.9) (GPX1), glutathione S-transferase (EC 2.5.1.18) (GST), and estrogen sulfotransferase (EST) were measured in liver and prostate cytosol. Expression of the genes for the selenoproteins GPX1, iodothyronine 5'-monodeiodinase, Type 1 (ID), and selenoprotein P (SeP) was assayed in prostate using RT-PCR. As expected, activity of GPX1 in Se-deficient liver was less than 1% of control or high Se values. Se-deficient prostate GPX1 activity averaged 32% of the control value and 27% of the high Se average. Compared to the control, activity of GST (using CDNB as substrate) was 22% and 21% higher in Se-deficient and high Se rat liver, respectively. In prostate there was no significant effect of Se on GST activity. In liver, activity of EST toward estrone was unaffected by dietary Se while activity toward estradiol was increased with each increase in Se intake. Activity of EST was not detected in rat prostate. Steady state levels of mRNA for GPX1 were 4-fold higher in Se-adequate than in Se-deficient prostate. Differences in expression of SeP were even larger than for GPX1. Expression of ID was not detected. Thus, in rat prostate the effects of Se deficiency on enzyme activity and gene expression for these species are less dramatic than those observed in liver. The exception is SeP, for which differences in gene expression between Se deficiency and Se adequacy were markedly higher in prostate than those previously observed in liver.

Poster Abstract # 8

Suppression of Breast Cancer Cell Growth in Athymic Nude Mice by Docosahexaenoic Acid by a Mechanism which includes Antiangiogenesis

David P. Rose and Jeanne M. Connolly
Division of Nutrition and Endocrinology
American Health Foundation
Valhalla, NY 10595

Diets rich in linoleic acid (LA), an omega-6 fatty acid, stimulate the progression of human breast cancer cell solid tumors in athymic nude mice, whereas docosahexaenoic acid (DHA) and eicosapentaenoic acid long chain omega-3 fatty acids, exert suppressive effects. In the present study we used DHA derived from marine microalgae to determine the effects of feeding low levels of the fatty acid on the growth of MDA-MB-231 cells injected into the thoracic mammary fat pads of female nude mice without altering the level of dietary LA. Four different isocaloric diets were used; all of which provided 20% (wt/wt) total fat. The control diets contained either 8% (20 mice) or 4% (50 mice) LA; the omega-3 fatty acid-supplemented groups of 50 mice were fed 4% LA-containing diets plus 2% or 4% DHA. The tumor growth rates were reduced significantly in mice fed the 4% LA, compared with the 8% LA, diet; the addition of 4% DHA to the 4% LA-containing diet produced a further reduction in tumor growth rate (p=0.003 at and after week 6). The final tumor weights were also reduced in the DHA-fed mice compared with the 8% LA dietary group (2% DHA, p=0.02; 4% DHA, p=0.01), and in the 4% DHA-fed mice compared with the 4% LA dietary group (p=0.02); a similar trend for mice fed the lower level of DHA did not achieve statistical significance. Tumor prostaglandin E2 concentrations were reduced by feeding the lower LA level; further dose-dependent decreases occurred in the DHA dietary groups, and were accompanied by reduced levels of 12- and 15-hydroxyeicosatetraenoic acids. These changes in eicosanoid biosynthesis may have been responsible for the observed decreases in cell proliferation, indicated by the suppressed Ki-67 expression, increases in apoptotic activity, as reflected in TUNEL immunohistochemical staining, and reduced tumor microvessel density, indicated by CD-31 immunohistochemistry. Microvessel count correlates with cell proliferation (p<0.001), both of which are lowest in the 4% DHA-fed tumors, suggesting that dietary n-3 fatty acid may reduce tumor growth by mechanisms which include suppression of angiogenesis.

Poster Abstract # 9

Modulation of Bak and BCL-XL expression in hamster pancreatic neoplasms by the diet-derived isoprenoids perillyl alcohol and farnesol

Pamela Crowell, A. Siar Ayoubi, Bryan McFarland, Yvette Burke, and Bruce Ruggeri
Department of Biology
Indiana University-Purdue University
Indianapolis, IN 46202

Previous studies from our lab have shown that the diet-derived isoprenoids perillyl alcohol and farnesol induce apoptosis and increase the expression of the proapoptotic protein Bak in cultured pancreatic tumor cells. Here, we tested the hypothesis that these isoprenoids would increase Bak expression and apoptosis in pancreatic neoplasms in vivo. At time 0, 90 male Syrian golden hamsters were given the first of 3 weekly 20-mg/kg i.p. injections of N-nitrosobis(2-oxopropyl)amine (BOP). From weeks 5-42, animals received control, 2% (w/w) perillyl alcohol, or 1-% farnesol diets. At week 42, pancreatic lesions were evaluated. Pancreatic carcinoma incidence was 46% in control animals, 37% in those fed perillyl alcohol, and 32% in the farnesol group. The average number of tumors per animal in hamsters fed control, perillyl alcohol, and farnesol diets was 0.54 ± 0.12, 0.37 ± 0.09, and 0.39 ± 0.12, respectively (mean $\pm$ SEM, n=28). In hyperplastic pancreatic lesions, perillyl alcohol and farnesol doubled the percentage of apoptotic cells and increased Bak protein expression ($P<0.05$). At the same time, expression of BCL-XL, an antiapoptotic protein that antagonizes Bak, was decreased by the isoprenoids. Thus, perillyl alcohol and farnesol can increase Bak expression in vivo, and this effect may contribute toward their antitumorigenic effects.

(Support: American Institute for Cancer Research 96A053 to PLC.)

Poster Abstract # 10

The dietary antioxidants, lycopene and carnosic acid, synergize with retinoic acid and 1,25-dihydroxyvitamin D_3 in the inhibition of growth and induction of differentiation in leukemic cells

Michael Danilenko, Hadar Amir, Michael Shteiner, Irene Priel, Judith Giat, Joseph Levy and Yoav Sharoni
Department of Clinical Biochemistry
Faculty of Health Sciences
Ben-Gurion University and Soroka Medical Center
Beer-Sheva, ISRAEL

Consumption of diets rich in vegetables and fruit has been found to inversely correlate with cancer incidence. The anti-cancer activities of the tomato carotenoid, lycopene, and the rosemary diterpene, carnosic acid, were recently described in experimental models. In this study, we show that incubation of myeloid leukemia cells (HL-60 and U937) with micromolar concentrations of these agents causes a substantial time-dependent inhibition of cell growth (IC_{50}=1-2 µM). The inhibitory effect of lycopene and carnosic acid in HL-60 cells was associated with a delay in the cell cycle progression manifested by the accumulation of cells in the G0-G1 phase and a decrease in the percentage of cells in the S phase. Lycopene alone induced a moderate cell differentiation as evidenced by an increase in CD14 expression, phorbol ester-activated generation of superoxide radicals and the appearance of the functionally active receptors for the chemotactic peptide, N-formyl-Met-Leu-Phe. In contrast, carnosic acid alone had no effect on cell differentiation. However, both lycopene and, to an even higher extent carnosic acid, synergistically augmented (100-1000-fold) the differentiating effects of low concentrations (0.1–1 nM) of all-trans retinoic acid (atRA) and 1,25-dihydroxyvitamin D_3 ($1,25(OH)_2D_3$). This action was detected as early as 20-24 h following drug addition. At longer incubations (= 5 days), enhancement of the anti-proliferative effects of atRA and $1,25(OH)_2D_3$ by the antioxidants could be observed as well. Both atRA and $1,25(OH)_2D_3$ are potent differentiation agents that have potential implication for chemoprevention and leukemia therapy. However, their major clinical limitation is a pronounced toxicity at therapeutic concentrations. Thus, the potentiation of the response of leukemic cells to these differentiation inducers may endorse the use of lycopene and carnosic acid in combination differentiation therapy that would permit lower doses of atRA and $1,25(OH)_2D_3$.

Poster Abstract # 11

Pyridoxal Treatment of Estrogen Receptor-Positive Breast Cancer Cells In Vitro Results in Decreased Cell Number and DNA Synthesis

Barbara A. Davis and Brandy E. Cowing
Human Nutrition, Foods and Exercise Department
Virginia Tech
Blacksburg, VA 24061

Vitamin B_6, in its active form pyridoxal 5'-phosphate (PLP), has been repeatedly demonstrated to modulate steroid hormone action. However, the effect of this vitamin on estrogen action in mammary tissue has not been investigated. In these preliminary studies, pyridoxal (PL) was used to study the effect of Vitamin B_6 on estrogen-dependent breast cancer cell growth in vitro. T-47D cells (HTB 133, ATCC) were maintained in minimal essential medium (MEM) supplemented with L-glutamine, sodium pyruvate, non-essential amino acids, bovine insulin and 10% fetal bovine serum (FBS). For counting and proliferation experiments, cells were seeded at 2-3 x 10^4 cells/well in a 6-well plate. Twenty-four hours later, medium was changed to phenol-red free MEM with supplements as above and charcoal-stripped FBS, plus or minus 17β-estradiol ($0.01\mu M$) and PL. After 9d, cells were trypsinized and counted in Trypan Blue using a hemocytometer. DNA synthesis was determined by measuring ^{3}H-thymidine incorporation in cells following a 3h incubation with $2\mu Ci$ ^{3}H-thymidine. Total cell numbers in experimental media (EM) containing estradiol (E) and 1mM or 3mM PL were, respectively, 40% and 10% that of control cells maintained in EM + E. Similarly, incorporation of ^{3}H-thymidine in cells maintained in EM+E+PL (1mM and 3 mM) was reduced to 69% and 15% that of cells maintained in EM+E. Furthermore, in cells maintained in media devoid of estradiol, PL supplementation at either concentration resulted in similar decreases in cell number and ^{3}H-thymidine incorporation. These data suggest that vitamin B_6 may be affecting growth of estrogen-dependent breast cancer cells via both steroid-dependent and independent mechanisms.

Poster Abstract # 12

Whole Almonds, but not Almond Oil or Almond Meal in the Diet Decrease Both Colonic Aberrant Crypt Foci and Cell Turnover in a Rat Colon Cancer Model

P.A. Davis and C.K. Iwahashi
Departments of Internal Medicine and Nutrition
University of California, Davis
Davis, California

Diet plays a significant role in colon cancer, a leading cause of US cancer deaths. To investigate the effect of nut (almonds and almond components) consumption on colon cancer, their effects on the colon cancer marker aberrant crypt cell foci (ACF) and labeling indices (LI) in azoxymethane injected (2x 15mg/kg) Fisher 344 rats were assessed. Almonds were added either as ground up whole almonds (WA), as ground up partially defatted almond meal (AM) or as almond oil (AO) alone to a high risk (53% energy as fat), 8% total dietary fiber semi-purified diet that was equalized for nutrient content. Ten animals/group consumed (ad lib) either cellulose -C-, raw wheat bran (RWB) or the almond containing diets for 24 weeks. No differences in overall weight gain or feed intake was seen. Animals were injected with BrdU (100mg/kg) one hour prior to being killed by CO_2. Colons were removed and processed with ACF and BrdU positive cells enumerated by methylene blue staining and immunohistochemistry, respectively. ACF in RWB did not differ statistically (ANOVA) from C while WA ACF were 33% and 40% lower ($p < 0.03$ Fisher's LSD) compared to RWB or C, respectively. Cell turnover as assessed by LI showed a similar pattern with WA LI being 28% and 38% lower ($p < 0.04$ Fisher's LSD) compared to RWB and C, respectively. The results indicate that whole almonds reduce colon cancer in an animal model and suggest that whole almonds might reduce colon cancer risk in human diets as well.

(Funded by the Almond Board of California.)

Poster Abstract # 13

The use of the estrogen receptor-alpha knockout (ERaKO) mouse as a model to study the effects of phytoestrogens in reducing cancer through an ERa dependent mechanism

J. Kevin Day[1,2] Ruth S. MacDonald[1,2,3] Cindy Besch Williford[4] and Dennis B. Lubahn[1,2,5]
[1]Genetics Area Program, [2]Departments of Biochemistry, [3]Nutritional Sciences,
[4]Veterinary Pathobiology, and [5]Child Health
University of Missouri, Columbia, MO 65211

Epidemiologically, the consumption of soy foods is associated with a reduced incidence of hormonally influenced ailments such as heart disease and cancer. Principle concerns in the use of soy foods to prevent and reduce the incidence of cancer are the mechanistic pathways by which they exert their protective effect. Present in soy are several common phytoestrogens. These compounds have long been suspected of acting through an estrogen receptor-dependent pathway. The objective of this study was to examine the effect of the phytoestrogen genistein on DMBA-induced mammary tumor development in estrogen receptor-alpha knockout (ERaKO) mice. The design was a 2 X 2 factorial with wild type (ER-WT) and ERaKO mice fed either a casein based control diet (without genistein), or a casein based diet with genistein (1 gm genistein/kg diet). Mice were fed the semi-purified diets ad libitum from weaning. Mammary tumors were induced by subcutaneously implanting two medroxyprogesterone acetate pellets (20 mg each) on week 7, followed by oral DMBA (1 mg/dose) administration on weeks 9, 10, 12 and 13. Mice were continued on the experimental diets and monitored for tumor development. Mammary tumors of several classifications developed in 75% of WT and 0% of ERaKO mice. No statistically significant differences in tumor number, weight, histology or latency was observed in the WT mice due to dietary genistein intake. Mice fed genistein consumed less food, and weighed significantly less than mice fed the control diet. No differences in serum IGF-I or IGFBP-3 were observed due to the dietary treatment or genotype. However, serum estrogen concentrations tended to be higher in the ERaKO compared to the WT mice, and genistein tended to decrease the concentration in both groups. This study demonstrates no protective effect of a high dietary genistein intake on DMBA-induced mammary tumors. It also suggests that DMBA-induced mammary tumors do not arise from cells present in the rudimentary ductal structures of ERaKO mice.

Poster Abstract # 14

Effect of short-term flaxseed supplementation and fat modification in men with prostate cancer

Wendy Demark-Wahnefried, David T. Price, Thomas Polascik, E. Everett Anderson, Robin Vollmer
Duke University Medical Center
Durham, NC

Previous research in both animals and humans suggests that dietary fat and fiber affect the hormonal and eicosanoid milieu, and therefore may influence the progression of hormonally-linked cancers. We undertook a pilot study to explore whether a flaxseed supplemented (30 g/day), fat restricted ($\leq$ 20% of energy) diet could affect indices related to prostatic neoplasia among men diagnosed with early stage prostate cancer. Diets were imposed short-term, during a 3-4 week period prior to prostatectomy.

Preliminary data on 13 subjects suggest that this dietary regimen is associateed with significant decreases in free testosterone (28.9 ± 18.2 to 21.7 ± 13.3 ng/dl; p=.022) and total cholesterol (195 ± 37 to 163 ± 25 mg/dl; p<.001), with a trend toward lower testosterone levels (391 ± 115 to 329 ± 120 ng/dl; p=.057). While no overall differences were observed in prostate specific antigen (PSA) from baseline to follow-up, when men with Gleason sums ≥ 7 (N=5) were excluded from the analysis, a trend toward lower PSA was noted (8.9 ± 4.5 to 7.9 ± 4.5 ng/dl; p=0.10). Histologic sections from treated patients compared to historic controls [matched on age ($\pm$ 3 years), race, biopsy Gleason sum, disease laterality, % positive biopsy cores/total biopsy cores, and PSA at diagnosis ($\pm$ 10%)] exhibited decreased proliferation rates (MIB-1 staining) among men with Gleason sums < 7, but not among those with high grade disease. No differences were observed with regard to p53 and bcl-2 (apoptotic incides). These data provide evidence that a flaxseed supplemented, fat restricted diet may have a biological effect on established prostate cancer which may be mediated through a hormonal mechanism. Thus, these data suggest that dietary alterations may have a direct effect on malignant prostate cancer cells and also suggest a need for larger study to determine the benefit of this dietary regimen as either a complementary or preventive therapy.

Poster Abstract # 15

Women are able to consume eleven servings of fruits and vegetables daily with or without lowering dietary fat intake

J. B. Depper , K. M. Poore, V.E. Uhley, V. Maranci, S. Lababidi, L. K. Heilbrun, and Z. Djuric.
Barbara Ann Karmanos Cancer Institute
Detroit, MI. 48201, U.S.A.

Consumption of fruits, vegetables and fat has been suggested to influence breast cancer risk. In this ongoing research study, the independent and interactive effects of high fruit/ vegetable intake and low fat intake on markers of cancer risk are being examined. Subjects are premenopausal women, aged 21-50, who have first degree relatives with breast cancer. Subjects were randomized to one of four dietary plans for one year: control (C), low-fat (LF), high fruit-vegetable (HFV), or combination (LFHFV). We used a modified version of the American Dietetic Association exchange lists to increase fruit and vegetable consumption with a goal of nine servings/day in a specified variety. The women on low-fat diets also counted grams of fat eaten with a goal of 15% of calories from fat. Four day food records were collected from all groups at baseline, 3, 6, 9, and 12 months. Preliminary data on 48 women indicates excellent compliance. The percent calories from fat in the LF group went from 30% at baseline to 13% by 12 months, and their fruit and vegetable intake remained fairly constant. The percent calories from fat in the LFHFV group went from 33% to 16%, and fruit and vegetable intake went from 3.9 to 11.0 servings/day. Fruit and vegetable intake in the HFV group increased from 3.8 to 11.6 servings, while keeping their fat intake relatively constant. These data indicate that it is possible to selectively manipulate dietary fat and fruit and vegetable intake over a 12-month period, which makes research on the relative effects of these nutrients on biomarkers of cancer risk feasible in humans.

(This study was supported by grants CA72292 and CA22453 from NCI.)

Poster Abstract # 16

Oncolyn Causes Regression of Breast Carcinoma and Other Solid Tumors in Mouse and Man

Arthur H.K. Djang[1], Sun Hui[2], M. Bud Nelson[3]

[1]Sante' International, Jamestown, NY

[2]Division of Experimental Pathology and Clinical Therapeutics, Tinajin Cancer Hospital, CHINA

[3]Division of Surgical Oncology, The Arthur G. James Cancer Hospital and Research Institute, The Ohio State University, Columbus, OH

Plants are considered a valuable resource for the discovery and development of novel, naturally derived agents to treat cancer. To date, six plant-derived anticancer drugs have received FDA approval for commercial production (taxol, vinblastine, vincristine, topotecan, etoposide, and teniposide) with others being evaluated in clinical trials worldwide, such as camptothecin. Oncolyn, a formulated combination of extracts from three edible plants, was evaluated by itself, or in combination with cytoxan/adriamycin/cysplatin, 5_FU and methotrexate, for anticancer activity in a mouse subrenal capsule assay and subsequent clinical application for various tumors.

The mouse subrenal capsule assay technique is a well accepted model in which potential antitumor agents are tested for efficacy in inhibiting growth of human tumor xenografts. The subrenal capsule assay has been used to determine anti-cancer activity of various agents against one or more human tumors including renal cell carcinoma, colorectal cancer, breast cancer, liver cancer, choriocarcinoma, ovarian adenocarcinoma, lung cancer, esophageal cancer, prostate carcinoma, and urinary bladder carcinoma. The use of the subrenal capsule human tumor xenograft assay has also been validated as a model that can accurately evaluate chemotherapeutic agents for clinical efficacy with concordance rate ranges from 77-90%.

The mouse subrenal capsule assay with human tumor xenografts was performed with surgically removed tumor tissues, according to the technique of Bogden and Griffin. Small tumor explant fragment circa 1mm size was implanted below the transparent mouse renal capsule. After abdominal wall closure, mice (105 for each experiment) were observes for the effect of Oncolyn and standard chemotherapeutic agents. On day 5, tumor fragment size, vascularity and tumor cellular changes were recorded. Oncolyn causes reduction of tumor size, inhibited vascularity on the surface and in the periphery of implanted tumor fragment and other morphological changes such as karyopyknosis and karyorrhexis consistent with apoptosis.

In summary, Oncolyn alone or in combination with other chemotherapeutic agents synergistically inhibited the growth of implanted human breast carcinoma, squamous cell carcinoma of the lung and adenocarcinoma of the rectum in mouse.

Results of clinical application of Oncolyn for chemoprevention and therapy for patients with breast carcinoma, prostate carcinoma, colon carcinoma, lung carcinoma, breast intraductal papilloma, melanoma, and lymphoma will be on display. Oncolyn showed no known side effects.

Four (4) tables, six (6) photomicrographs with references.

Poster Abstract # 17

Prostate Cancer Progression in a Transgenic Mouse Model: Dietary Intervention

Janice G. Dodd, Ph.D., Jacquie Schwartz and Patricia Sheppard
Department of Physiology
University of Manitoba
Winnipeg, Manitoba
CANADA

Mortality from advanced prostate cancer (CaP) is low in Asia compared to North America despite similar incidences of latent, non-invasive prostatic lesions. Diet has been implicated in this striking difference in cancer progression, in particular the consumption of soya products. An abundant soya isoflavonoid has been identified as a potential preventive agent. Genistein inhibits protein tyrosine kinases (PTKs) in multiple cellular signaling pathways. Growth of prostate cancer cells is inhibited by genistein at high doses (higher than available by diet); however, assessment of dietary genistein in preventing cancer progression has been hampered by a lack of suitable in vivo models. We have established a transgenic mouse model for CaP, which demonstrates progression from epithelial dysplasia to carcinoma in a reproducible sequence. The transgenic mice develop prostatic intraepithelial neoplasia (PIN) similar to human precursor lesions, and the tumors are androgen-dependent. Most importantly, receptor PTKs (EGF-R, c-met, erbB2, and erbB3) which are key biomarkers in human CaP are also elevated in the mouse model. We are using this novel in vivo model to test the ability of genistein, an inhibitor of PTKs, to delay or prevent the progression of prostate cancer.

Pilot study data confirms that genistein does influence tumor progression in the transgenic mice. In transgenic (tumor-forming) and non-transgenic (control) males receiving dietary genistein (0gm/kg or 25mg/kg) from weaning and monitored for incidence, latency and histology of prostate neoplasia, genistein delayed tumor progression. In addition, genistein reduced significantly the expression of receptor PTK, and altered the profile and level of tyrosine phosphorylated proteins in the prostate.

The relatively slow growth rate of human CaP provides a window for therapeutic intervention; even modest changes in the rate of tumor progression through dietary intervention could result in substantial reductions in the incidence of clinically relevant cancers.

Poster Abstract # 18

Chemoprevention of renal cell carcinoma with active vitamin D3

Tomoaki Fujioka, Nozomi Mastushita, Yasushi Suzuki, Toshiki Kato, Hideo Tokunaga,
Masaya Ogata and So Omori
Department of Urology
Iwato Medical University School of Medicine
Morioka 020
JAPAN

We studied the influence of 1,25(OH)2D3 (act VD3) on gap junctional intercellular communication (GJIC) and renal carcinogenesis. Using the MIT assay, non-cytotoxic concentrations of act VD3 and a tumor promoter (EHEN) were determined for cultured human renal proximal tubular cells (HRPTC). GJIC function was assayed by the scrape-loading dye transfer technique. Connexin 43 (Cx43) mRNA expression was examined by the RT-PCR method. A chemoprevention study was conducted to evaluate the efficacy of act VD3 as an inhibitor of renal carcinogenesis in a male Wistar rat model created by co-administration of EHEN and uracil.

Non-cytotoxic concentrations act VD3 enhanced the GJIC function of HRPTC, while EHEN suppressed this function. When the cells were treated with EHEN and act VD3 simultaneously, the GJIC function remained at the pretreatment level. We also demonstrated Cx43 mRNA expression of HRPTC treated with EHEN and act VD3 simultaneously. Intraperitoneal administration of act VD3 reduced the incidence of cancer in the rat carcinogenesis model.

These data suggest that act VD3 has a potent anticarcinogenic effect on the kidneys by preserving the GJIC function of proximal tubular cells.

Poster Abstract # 19

Resveratrol Inhibits Phase II Activation of the Food Mutagen N-Hydroxy-Phip by Human Mammary Epithelial Cells and Enzymes.

J.G. Dubuisson, R. Southard, D. L. Dyess, and J. W. Gaubatz
Department of Biochemistry and Molecular Biology
University of South Alabama
Mobile, AL 36688-0002

Heterocyclic amines are present in the diets of many individuals who regularly consume cooked meats and fish. Some of these compounds are carcinogenic in animal models. The most abundant heterocyclic amine found in the American diet is 2-amino-1-methyl-6-phenylimidazo[4,5-b]pyridine (PhIP) which induces mammary gland tumors in rats. However, PhIP must be metabolically converted to DNA reactive derivatives to become carcinogenic. Phase I activation of PhIP occurs in the liver by hydroxylation of the amino group in the 2 position, forming 2-hydroxyamino-PhIP (N-OH-PhIP) an intermediate carcinogen. N-OH-PhIP must be metabolized further by phase II esterification in target tissues thereby generating PhIP-DNA adducts.

We have shown that human mammary epithelial cells exhibit low capacity of phase I activation of PhIP but may be potent phase II activators of N-OH-PhIP. Four pathways of phase II activation have been described in homogenates of human mammary cells. Acetyltransferase, kinase, and sulfotransferase activation were observed with cytosolic enzymes from breast tissue, whereas prostaglandin H synthetase was associated with the microsomal fractions. Although the relative activity of each pathway differed between individuals, acetyltransferase and kinase activities appeared to be major activators of N-OH-PhIP.

We discovered that the anti-tumor compound resveratrol inhibited the formation of PhIP-DNA adducts in primary human mammary epithelial cell cultures. Therefore, resveratrol might have chemopreventive properties in dietary modification of human breast cancer incidence. To determine possible sources of DNA damage inhibition, each phase II activation enzyme was assayed in the presence and absence of resveratrol. The results showed that resveratrol consistently inhibited acetyltransferase and sulfotransferase activation. In contrast, cytosolic kinase activity was mostly stimulated by resveratrol. Thus. the mechanism of resveratrol inhibition on carcinogen processing in human mammary cells remains to be determined.

(Research supported by DOD grant DAMD17-96-1-6121 and NCI grant CA78510)

Poster Abstract # 20

Role of Dietary Fats and Estrogens in the Etiology of Prostate Cancer: A Rat Model

Jan Geliebter[1,3], Christina Zeoli[1], Niradiz Reyes[1], Ted Lai[1], Janet Piscitelli[6], Joan Pillitteri[1], Bandaru Reddy[4], Michael Iatropoulos[2], Geoffrey Kabat[5], Jacob Steinberg[6] and Abraham Mittelman[3].

Dept. of [1]Microbiology & Immunology, [2]Pathology and [3]Medicine,
New York Medical College, Valhalla, NY;
[4]American Health Foundation, Valhalla, NY;
[5]Dept. Preventative Medicine, SUNY at Stony Brook, Stony Brook, NY;
[6]Dept. of Pathology, Albert Einstein College of Medicine/Montefiore Medical Center, Bronx, NY

Prostate cancer is the most common malignancy of men in America and the second leading cause of cancer deaths. The American Cancer Society estimates that in 1999 over 179,000 American men will be diagnosed with prostate cancer and 37,000 deaths will be attributed to the disease. A more complete understanding of the risk factors for prostate cancer is essential for the design of rational programs for disease prevention. Epidemiological studies suggest that a diet high in animal fat, for more than one generation, is associated with an increased risk of prostate cancer. This may reflect the requirement for a combination of two events for the development of prostate cancer; the initiation of carcinogenesis and the progression of the neoplastic process. Further, estrogen has been found to be growth factor for the prostate. Our aim is to more fully develop the ACI rat model to investigate the role of dietary fats and estrogens in the etiology of prostate cancer. We have maintained ACI rats for two generations (mothers and pups), on high fat and control diets for 6, 12 and 18 months (high fat diet #1 - 23.52% corn oil; high fat diet #2 - 22.52% beef fat/1% corn oil; control diet 5% corn oil, by weight). We are currently analyzing prostate hyperplasia/cancer, testosterone and estrogen levels, prostatic aromatase mRNA levels, and plasma triglyceride levels in these rats. Results from these studies will lead to a better understanding of the contribution of dietary fats and estrogens to the etiology of prostate cancer and facilitate the rational design and assessment of potential dietary programs (such as phytochemicals) for prostate cancer prevention.

Poster Abstract # 21

Oxygen Radical Absorbance Capacity (ORAC) of Fruits and Vegetables and their Flavonoid Content

Susanne M. Henning, Fathy M. Hassan, David Heber and Vay Liang W. Go.
UCLA, Center for Human Nutrition
Los Angeles, CA 90095.

The flavonoid content of fruits and vegetables contribute considerably to their antioxidant capacity and health benefits. Flavonoids (>4000) constitute the largest group of plant phenols and are mostly esterified with various sugars forming more water soluble glycosides. Their antioxidant capacity depends mainly on their chemical structure - amount of hydroxyl groups.

AIM: The aim of this study was to compare the ORAC value of water and water/methanol (20:80 v/v) extracts of 25 fruits and vegetables to their flavonoid content determined by HPLC. The ORAC assay was performed using a Perkin Elmer fluorescent plate reader (HTS 7000 Plus Bio Assay Reader) and the method by Cao and Prior (Methods in Enz. 299:50, 1999). The HPLC method to detect 12 flavonoids (catechin, epicatechin, epicatechin gallate (ECG), gallocatechin gallate (GCG), rutin, quercetrin, quercetin, naringenin, hesperitin, kaempherol, cyanidin, malvidin) and 2 isoflavones (genistein and daidzein) is based on UV/VIS detection with gradient elution (mobile phase A: methanol/acitonitrile (2:1) and B: acetic acid (0.1%)).

RESULT: The ORAC value ranged from 0 to 179 µmol Trolox equivalent per 100 g food with cucumber without peel, lettuce and fresh tomato being among the lowest (<15) and frozen raspberries, fresh cherries, garlic and spinach among the highest (>75). The ORAC values for water and water: methanol extracts were highly correlated (R=0.94). Rutin, quercetrin and quercetin were the most commonly occurring flavonoids in these fruits and vegetables. The peak area of rutin, however, was poorly correlated to the ORAC value (R=0.68), as was the total area for all peaks (R=0.44).

CONCLUSION: The ORAC value reflects the total antioxidant capacity. To improve the correlation between the ORAC value and the antioxidant components of fruits and vegetables other antioxidants such as carotenoids and ascorbic acid need to be evaluated.

Poster Abstract # 22

Pharmacodynamic Effects and Mechanisms of Action of Perillyl Alcohol in Humans

R.J. Hohl and K. Lewis
University of Iowa College of Medicine
Iowa City, IA

Perillyl alcohol is a naturally occurring monoterpene that has shown antitumor and cancer preventative activity in preclinical studies. Because of these properties and that it is a dietary constituent there is intensive interest in defining the underlying mechanism(s) for its anticancer effects. We have previously demonstrated that perillyl alcohol in vitro in high concentrations may inhibit farnesyl protein transferase (FPTase), which is the enzyme that catalyzes RAS post-translational processing, and in lower concentrations will reduce RAS levels. We have hypothesized that these effects may contribute to perillyl alcohol's anticancer activity. To investigate whether these in vitro effects are observed in vivo we have completed a phase I trial of perillyl alcohol. Perillyl alcohol is given four times daily for two weeks followed by two weeks off. The main toxicities have been have been gastrointestinal (nausea and vomiting, satiety and gastroesophageal reflux) and fatigue. Pharmacokinetic data demonstrate that sufficiently high plasma levels of perillyl alcohol that are needed to display biologically active can be accomplished with tolerable doses of 1200 mg/m2 four times per day. Correlative laboratory studies demonstrated that mononuclear cell RAS levels varied after perillyl alcohol treatment and decreased in 3 of the first 7 patients analyzed with the most dramatic decrease being to 30% of control. Further in vitro studies have suggested that the down-regulation of RAS in some cell types was not a consequence of a reduction in RAS mRNA indicating that a decrease in RAS mRNA transcription or increase in RAS protein degradation may underlie these observations.

(Supported by the NIH and the AICR.)

Poster Abstract # 23

Resveratrol Suppress TNF-a Activation of the Transcription Factor, NFxB and the Degradation of its Regulatory Protein IxBa

Minnie Holmes-McNary and Albert S. Baldwin, Jr.
Lineberger Comprehensive Cancer Center
University of North Carolina at Chapel Hill
Chapel Hill, NC 27599-2795

Increasing evidence indicates that dietary constituents can suppress the onset or progression of certain human diseases. For example, resveratrol, a phytoalexin found in grapes, has been shown to function by blocking inflammation and oncogenesis in certain animal models. Resveratrol has been shown to have antioxidant properties as well as antiproliferative properties of some cancer cells in vitro. The transcription factor NFxB is strongly linked to inflammatory diseases and is associated with oncogenesis. Since NFxB activation is associated with inflammatory and oncogenic diseases, we asked whether resveratrol inhibited NFxB activation. We used to human macrophage THP-1 cell line, since it is well characterized regarding the activation of NFxB and the induction of NFxB regulated gene expression. Our data indicate that resveratrol is a potent inhibitor of NFxB activation in response to both TNFa and LPS stimulation in THP-1 cells. Consistent with the ability to block NFxB activation, resveratrol inhibited IxBa degradative response in THP-1 cells after 15 minutes. Consistent with its cancer chemopreventive properties, resveratrol induced apoptosis in Rat-1 fibroblasts undergoing transformation following the induced expression of oncogenic H-Ras. Thus, resveratrol is likely to function by inhibiting inflammatory and oncogenic diseases, at least partly, through the inhibition of NFxB activation by blocking IxBa degradation. Thus, the data may explain aspects of the so-called "French paradox" and may provide a molecular rationale for the role of this potent chemopreventive compound in blocking the initiation of oncogenesis.

Poster Abstract # 24

Pinto Bean Phytochemicals Reduce Colon Cancer Incidence in Rats

J.S. Hughes[1], S. Wilson-Sanders[2] and C. Ganthavorn[3]

[1]Foods and Nutrition, California State University, San Bernardino, CA

[2]University of Arizona, Animal Care Diagnostic Laboratory, Tuscon, AZ

[3]UC Cooperative Extension, Riverside County, Moreno Valley, CA

Beans (*Phaseolus vulgaris*) are the most widely consumed legume in the world and are a rich source of several phytochemicals including polyphenols. Epidemiological studies show a low incidence of colon cancer in many Latin American countries where the consumption of pinto beans is high. The purpose of this research was to obtain experimental data on the anticarcinogenic properties of pinto beans by evaluating their ability beans to inhibit colon cancer in rats. Male F344 rats were exposed to the carcinogen azoxymethane (AOM), and then fed either a pinto bean or casein diet. Incidence of colonic tumors was used as the primary endpoint in the study. Animals on the casein and bean diets were treated with AOM once weekly for two weeks. All diets were isocaloric. The protein content of the diets was adjusted to 18% with casein, and the fat content was adjusted to 5% with corn oil.

The rats on the pinto bean diet had considerably fewer colon adenocarcinomas than rats on the casein diet (5 vs. 22 tumors), and significantly fewer rats on the bean diet ($p<0.05$) had colonic tumors (24% vs. 50%). Tumor multiplicity was also lower for the bean fed rats, and significantly fewer ($p<0.05$) tumors per tumor bearing rat were observed in bean fed rats (1.00 ± 0.0 vs. 2.50 ± 0.58). This study demonstrates that pinto beans contain potent anticarcinogens capable of inhibiting AOM-induced colon cancer in rats. However, the specific anticarcinogen phytochemical components within pinto beans have not been identified. Additional research is needed to clarify the role of various pinto bean phytochemicals in inhibiting colon carcinogenesis.

(Supported by the American Institute for Cancer Research Grant No. 91SG05)

Poster Abstract # 25

Arachidonic Acid induces gene expression and growth of Human Prostate Cancer PC-3 Cells

Millie Hughes-Fulford and Vicki Gilbertson
Laboratory of Cell Growth (151F), Veterans Affairs Medical Center-San Francisco
Department of Medicine, University of California-San Francisco

Although a high fat diet has been linked with an increased incidence of prostate cancer, little information is available on which fatty acids are responsible for growth induction and their mechanism of action. This abstract reports that arachidonic acid (AA), an essential fatty acid, induces immediate early gene expression and stimulates growth of prostate cancer cells. Linoleic acid (LA) and its metabolites AA and PGE2 increased growth of PC-3 cells. In contrast, two fatty acids, oleic acid (OA), a major constituent of olive oil and eicosapentaenoic acid, (EPA), found in fish oil, inhibited growth of prostate cancer cells. AA upregulated c-fos and cox-2 message within minutes in a dose dependent manner. Enzymatic activity of COX-2 was also increased in a dose dependent manner after 3 hours of exposure. AA gene regulation of c-fos and cox-2 is probably not acting through a PPRE since neither promoter region has this sequence. Functional uptake of AA was studied using fluorescent microscopy. Within the first 3 hours of incubation with exogenous AA, uptake was apparent at the cell membrane. After 24 hours of AA exposure, the fatty acid was localized to the perinuclear region: COX-2 has also been found in the perinuclear region during growth stimulation. Taken together, these data show, for the first time, that the essential fatty acid AA accumulates in the perinuclear region and promotes immediate early gene expression in prostate cancer cells. Finally, we found that AA promotes prostate tumor growth while EPA and OA, fatty acids that are found predominately in fish and olive oils inhibit growth of the PC-3 cells.

Poster Abstract # 26

Calorie Restriction and Indomethacin Suppress p-Cresidine-Induced Bladder Carcinogenesis in p53-Deficient Mice.

Stephen Hursting, Monica Liebert, Lawrence Baum, Jian-cheng Shen, Houston, TX; Claudio Conti, John DiGiovanni, Susan Fischer, Smithville, TX;
John French, Research Triangle Park, NC

INTRODUCTION AND OBJECTIVES: Heterozygous p53-deficient (p53+/-) mice, relative to wild-type mice, are highly susceptible to bladder carcinogenesis induced by chronic dietary exposure to the aromatic amine p-cresidine, a suspected human carcinogen. We previously observed that p-cresidine increases bladder cyclooxygenase (COX)-1 and 2 mRNA expression and that bladder tumors lose the expression of prostaglandin dehydrogenase. We also observed that bladder p-cresidine-DNA adducts are detectable in COX-1 wild-type mice but not in COX-1 knockout mice, suggesting the CoX pathway may be a prevention target in this model. The purpose of this study was to evaluate the effects of calorie restriction (CR), fenretinide (a synthetic retinoid) and indomethacin (a non-steroidal anti-inflammatory drug) on p-cresidine-induced bladder tumor development.

METHODS: One hundred male p53+/- mice (6-8 weeks of age) were randomized to receive: i) control diet (AIN-76A diet with 0.5% w/w p-cresidine, administered ad libitum); ii) 20% CR regimen (modified AIN-76A diet with 0.625% p-cresidine, administered in daily aliquots equivalent to 80% of the control group's daily intake); iii) fenretinide diet (AIN-76A diet with 0.5% p-cresidine plus 0.004% fenretinide); or iv) indomethacin diet (AIN-76A diet with 0.5% p-cresidine plus 0.0075% indomethacin, administered ad libitum). Following 12 weeks (5 mice/treatment) or 26 weeks (20 mice per treatment) on their respective diet regimens, the mice w re killed and their bladders and other tissues excised and analyzed histopathologically.

RESULTS: All control and fenretinide-treated mice developed bladder tumors, primarily transitional cell carcinomas. In contrast, CR and indomethacin reduced bladder tumor incidence (relative to controls) by 30% (p<0.05) and 60% (p<0.01), respectively.

CONCLUSIONS: The p-cresidine induced bladder cancer model in p53+/- mice is responsive to preventive interventions, specifically to indomethacin and moderate CR. In addition, the activity of these interventions may involve modulation of the COX pathway, suggesting that this pathway is a target for bladder cancer prevention strategies.

AICR 97A052 and NIEHS P30ES07784.

Poster Abstract # 27

Use of Nutritional Supplementation and Dietary Changes Among Children with Cancer

D.D. Kennedy, K. M. Kelly, J. S. Jacobson, S.M. Braudt and M. A. Weiner.
Columbia University College of Physicians and Surgeons
New York, NY 10032

Complementary/alternative medical therapies (CAM), including nutritional supplements, are increasingly used by adult cancer patients; very few surveys have focused on children with cancer. We interviewed 75 patients and their family members at our medical center. We asked about efforts made since the cancer diagnosis to improve health using agents or procedures not prescribed by physicians, reasons for such use, and whether the respondents had discussed them with their physicians. Of the 75 participants 65% had made a nutritional change; 47% changed their diet, 36% took a nutritional supplement, 27% tried herbs and 7% ingested another substance (e.g. shark cartilage). The major reasons for making the dietary and nutritional changes were to improve overall health, to boost the immune system, to decrease side effects of conventional therapy and to remove toxins from the body. Only 4 (5%) stated that they hoped it would help reduce the tumor. Of the 75 participants, 55 were enrolled on clinical trials for the treatment of cancer. Of these 55, over 50% made dietary changes, 33% were taking nutritional supplements, 27% were supplementing with herbs and another 8% were ingesting other substances orally. Since herbs and nutritional supplements have biological activities that could interfere with the chemotherapy being given, it is imperative that the patient know of the possible consequences and that their oncologist be aware of what they are ingesting. In this study, only 50% of the dietary changes, ingestion of herbs and other substances were mentioned to the physician, while most of those taking nutritional supplements told their doctor. Our results suggest that many children with cancer are taking nutritional/herbal supplements and that the physician is not always aware of it. Further study is needed to determine the safety, efficacy, and favorable and unfavorable interactions of these substances with conventional therapies.

Poster Abstract # 28

DNA Integration site of a murine retrovirus associated with leukemogenesis during folate deficiency

Don J. Park and Mark J. Koury
Division of Hematology/Oncology
Vanderbilt and Veterans Administration Medical Centers
Nashville, TN

Folate deficiency in mice at the time of infection with the anemia-inducing strain of the Friend leukemia virus complex results in an increased incidence of leukemia. Analysis of clonal leukemia cell lines from normal and folate deficient mice showed that the incidence of the two most common genetic changes, insertional retrovirus promoter activation of the Spi-1 oncogene and mutation/disruption of the p53 tumor suppressor gene, did not account for the increased incidence of leukemia in the folate deficient mice. We have attempted to determine whether the folate deficient state with its impaired DNA synthesis and repair capacities leads to a site-specific retroviral integration that could explain the increased incidence of leukemia in these Friend virus-infected mice. If such a specific site increased the expression of an oncogene or disrupted the expression of a tumor suppressor gene, then the increased incidence of Friend virus-induced leukemia in folate deficiency could be explained. To avoid confusion related to cross-hybridization with the many endogenous retrovirus-like elements in the murine genome, we used two dimensional Southern blotting in our screening with a probe corresponding to the F-MuLV helper virus component of the Friend leukemia virus complex. Leukemia cell lines derived from folate deficient mice had an increased number of viral integrations. Furthermore, we identified potential folate-sensitive integration sites from leukemia cell lines derived from folate deficient mice. In order to clone these sites, we screened a genomic library from a folate deficient leukemia cell line that had intact Spi-1 and p53 genes. One DNA close isolated from this screening was used to subclone a murine genomic DNA sequence flanking the specific viral integration site. Our preliminary results using both cell lines derived from leukemic mice and primary leukemias from the spleens of the leukemic mice showed rearrangement on Southern blot of this DNA sequence in 30% (6/20) of leukemias from folate deficient mice and only 10% (1/10) leukemias from control mice. Whether this DNA sequence is related to known folate-fragile sites, oncogenes, or tumor suppressor genes has not yet been determined.

Poster Abstract # 29

Variation Analysis in Plasma (-Sitosterol and Campesterol Measurements in Premenopausal Women

Jiang Hong Li[1], Atif B. Awad[2], Carol S. Fink[2], Yow-Wu Bill Wu[3], Lyn Hill[1], Maurizio Trevisian[1], Paola Muti[1]

[1]Dept.of Social and Preventive Medicine, [2]Nutrition Program, [3]Nursing School, State University of New York at Buffalo, Buffalo, NY

Phytosterols are plant sterols that are structurally similar to cholesterol and characterized by their anti-carcinogenic and anti-atherogenic properties. (-Sitosterol and campesterol are the predominant phytosterols in the blood. The present study aimed to examine the technical and biological variability of plasma (-sitosterol and campesterol measurements in premenopausal women. The intra-class correlation coefficient (ICC) was used to estimate these two sources of variability. To study reproducibility of the measurement (technical variability), three healthy premenopausal women were recruited. Each of them provided a single blood sample that was subdivided into six aliquots and analyzed within the same run by the same laboratory technician. The ICCs of the assay for plasma (-sitosterol and campesterol were 0.88 and 0.94 (95% Confidence Interval low bounds [95% CIlow] were 0.66 and 0.82), respectively. To study the reliability of sitosterol and campesterol measurement over time (biological variability), seven premenopausal women were recruited. Over a six-month period, each woman provided once a month a fasting blood sample at the same time of day, and the same numerical day of her menstrual cycle. Plasma was prepared immediately after blood draw and stored at 80 °C. All plasma samples from the same individual were processed at the same time by the same technician at the end of the six month period. The ICCs of plasma (-sitosterol and campesterol over time were 0.91 (95% CIlow 0.49) and 0.58 (95% CIlow 0.31), respectively. The high reproducibility of the two plasma phytosterol measurements, and the good reliability of the two plasma phytosterol measurements over time showed that they are suitable for epidemiological studies.

Poster Abstract # 30

Studies on Tyrosine Phosphorylation and Apoptosis in Lymphocytes Isolated from Healthy Women After Single Dose Treatment with Genistein

Wlodek Lopaczynski, LeAnne Tyndall, Craig Albright, and Steven Zeisel
Department of Nutrition
University of North Carolina
Chapel Hill, North Carolina 27599-7400

It is well established that exposure to genistein can result in the inhibition of cell proliferation in cancer cell lines. Studies in vitro show that genistein is a competitive inhibitor of tyrosine kinases and an inducer of apoptosis in cultured cells. The objectives of the single dose administration study of genistein were to determine the parameters and characteristics of genistein toxicity in humans, the safely delivered dose, a recommended dose for the multiple dose phase, and analysis of tissue levels to determine efficacy in chemoprevention or cancer treatment. 24 healthy postmenopausal female subjects were treated with a single dose of one of two genistein preparations (PTI G-2535, 70% unconjugated isoflavones containing 43% genistein; PTI G-4660, 100% unconjugated isoflavones containing 90% genistein provided by Protein Technologies International). We delivered a determined dose of genistein (2, 4, 8 or 16 mg/kg body weight). We observed no changes in behavior or on physical examination that related to the treatment. Lymphocytes were obtained from blood samples taken at various times after genistein ingestion. We did not observe an increase in apoptosis in lymphocytes harvested after 24 hr treatment with either 8 or 16 mg/kg doses of G 4660. However, we observed increased activity of AKT kinase (protein kinase B) in samples 3 h after genistein administration. Activated AKT is implicated in survival signaling in a wide variety of cells. Western blot analysis with a phosphotyrosine antibody showed a large decrease in protein tyrosine phosphorylation at 3 and 5 h post dose in lymphocyte lysates isolated from three female subjects treated with 8 or 16 mg/kg doses of G4660. We conclude that high doses of genistein (8-16 mg/kg) inhibit protein tyrosine phosphorylation in human lymphocytes isolated from treated patients, but these doses do not result in increased lymphocyte apoptosis.

(Supported by NCI - Contract Number NCI-N01-CN-75035)

Poster Abstract # 31

Capsaicin consumption, Helicobacter pylori infection and Gastric Cancer

López-Carrillo L[1], López-Cervantes M[1], Ramírez-Espitia A[1], Robles-Díaz G[1], Mohar-Betancourt A[1], Meneses-García A[3], López-Vidal Y[1].

[1] Mexico National Institute of Public health,

[2] Mexico National Institute of Nutrition,

[3] Mexico National Cancer Institute,

[4] Mexico National Autonomous University

Capsaicin (trans-8-metil-vanillyl-6-nonenamida) is the main natural pungent compound of chili peppers. So far, experimental studies yielded conflicting results regarding the potential of Capsaicin to be a carcinogen1. In humans, there is some evidence indicating that chili pepper consumption increases the risk for GC incidence, yet it is still scarce.

To date only one published epidemiological study was specifically designed to evaluate the relationship between chili pepper consumption and gastric cancer, and it yielded positive results2. In two other studies the authors were able to assess this same question. One of those was performed in India 3 and the other in Korea, 4 and both found that the consumption of foods prepared with chili peppers was related with an excess risk for GC. However, a common feature of all these studies was a rough assessment of the exposure, because none of them had a direct measurement of the actual Capsaicin intake, as a function of the types and amounts of chili peppers being consumed. 1

On the other hand, Helicobcater pylori (Hp) has also been considered to be a human carcinogen,5 in view of the results reported by several prospective studies in the earlier 90's.6-9 although a strong direct association is not yet widely accepted10. Anyhow, a situation of great scientific interest is to study the potential interactions between Hp infection and dietary factors in regard to gastric cancer incidence; at this time only a few studies have focused on such questions but yielded inconclusive results.11-12
In this paper we report on the results of a case-control study spanning three geographical areas of Mexico, and it was aimed at evaluating the independent as well as the combined effects of Capsaicin intake and Helicobacter pylori infection on gastric cancer risk.

This study was supported by the American Institute of Cancer Research (Grant No. 96A137), the Pan-American Health Organization (Grant AMR941086975-01), and the US National Cancer Institute and, the Mexico Ministry of Health.

Poster Abstract # 32

Methylseleninic acid induces apoptosis and inhibits matrix metalloproteinases of vascular endothelial cells

Cheng Jiang[1], Howard Ganther[2] and <u>Junxuan Lu</u>[1]
[1]AMC Cancer Research Center, Denver, CO 80214
[2]University of Wisconsin, Madison, WI 53706

Earlier work by Ip and Ganther had indicated that a monomethyl selenium (Se) species such as methylselenol may be an, if not the, active cancer chemopreventive Se metabolite in vivo. Methylseleninic acid (MSeA) was synthesized to provide a proximal precursor for methylselenol generation in vitro. Its effects on the proliferation/survival and the matrix metalloproteinase (MMP) activities of human umbilical vein endothelial cells (HUVEC) were examined in cell culture to explore the hypothesis that the cancer chemopreventive activity of Se may in part be mediated through an antiangiogenic effect. Both endothelial cell proliferation and certain MMPs are required for angiogenesis. In growth assays, MSeA at serum achievable levels concentration-dependently decreased cell number predominantly by inducing apoptosis. On an equimolar basis, MSeA was 4 fold more efficacious than the inorganic reference compound sodium selenite for the cyticidal activity. A brief MSeA treatment (6hr) of HUVEC decreased both the secreted (conditioned medium) and cell-associated (lysate) gelatinolytic activity at 72 kD corresponding to gelatinase A/MMP-2 in a concentration dependent manner with 50% inhibition at ~2μM. A 53 kD gelatinolytic activity in the conditioned medium was inhibited by MSeA treatment in the same fashion. However, incubation of the conditioned medium from the control cells with MSeA directly in the test tube for 6hrs did not inhibit these gelatinolytic activities. This observation indicates that the inhibitory effect required cellular metabolism/activation of MSeA. In contrast to MSeA, selenite at a level that exerted cytocidal effects did not inhibit these MMPs. Taken together, the data are consistent with the Se anti-angiogenesis hypothesis and point to a direct endothelial apoptogenic activity and an anti-matrilytic activity as likely mediating processes for the active Se metabolite (methylselenol or related Se species) to achieve an anti-angiogenic effect.

(Supported by grants from AICR 97A083, DOD BC980909 and NCI CA45164)

Poster Abstract # 33

Plasma Lycopene and Carotenoid Profiles in Prostate Cancer Patients Supplemented with Mixed Vegetable Juice

Heber D, Yip I, , Go VLWG, Liu W, Elashoff RM, Lu Q
UCLA Center for Human Nutrition.
UCLA School of Medicine
Los Angeles, CA

Introduction: Increased plasma lycopene has been associated with a reduced risk of prostate cancer, but there is little information on whether dietary intervention can change lycopene levels.

Aim: This study was done to determine whether juice supplementation and dietary intervention would lead to an increase in bioavailable lycopene and other carotenoids in prostate cancer patients.

Patients and Methods: Thirty-eight patients (ages 52 to 79) with prostate cancer stages T1C to T2C not under active treatment were studied over a three month period. Patients were instructed in a very low fat (15% energy from fat) and high fiber (18 g/1000 kcal) diet emphasizing fruits, vegetables, soy protein and whole grains. In addition to diet instruction, patients received 6 ounces per day of a mixed vegetable juice (V-8, Campbell's Soup Company, NJ) and 200 mcg selenium supplement. Plasma carotenoids and food intake were assessed at baseline and 3 months of follow-up.

Results: Diet instruction did not result in an increased intake of beta carotene from the diet over the three month intervention as determined by food frequency questionnaire. After 3 months supplementation, plasma concentrations of lycopene increased by 43% (p=0.002), alpha-carotene by 46% (p=0.0109), beta-carotene by 30% (p=0.0268), and beta-cryptoxanthin by 36% (p=0.0391) compared to baseline.

Conclusion: A highly significant increase of carotenoids and lycopene was observed in prostate cancer patients given dietary instruction and a mixed vegetable juice supplement suggesting that a juice supplement can increase bioavailable lycopene and carotenoids in prostate cancer patients.

Supported by CaPCure (The Association for the Cure of Prostate Cancer) and the National Cancer Institute (Grant No. CA 42710)

Poster Abstract # 34

Folic Acid: Regulation of Growth of Colon and Gastric Cancer Cell Lines

A. Khan, R. Jaszewski, F.H. Sarkar, O. Kucuk, and A.P.N. Majumdar.
John D. Dingell VA Medical Center and
Departments of Medicine and Pathology
Wayne State University School of Medicine
Detroit, MI

Results from several laboratories, including our own, suggest that folic acid may be chemopreventive against colon cancer. However, little is known about the regulation of this process. We hypothesize that folic acid exerts its chemopreventive effect of the colon by inhibiting proliferation and enhancing differentiation and/or apoptosis. To test this hypothesis, we examined the changes in proliferation and protein levels of bax (whose expression is positively related to apoptosis) and connexcin (C-43; involved in cell-cell communication; an indicator of differentiation) in two colon cancer cell lines (HCT-116 and CaCo-2). These parameters were also measured in a gastric cancer line (Kato-III) to determine whether folic acid may also be chemopreventive against gastric cancer. In each of these cell lines, bax and Cx-34 levels, as assessed by Western-immunoblot, was increased significantly by 30-50% after 48 h of exposure to folic acid (625 ng/ml). We further hypothesize that EGF-receptor (EGFR) may play a role in regulating folic acid-induced changes in proliferation, differentiation and apoptotic processes. Indeed, we found folic acid (625 ng/mg) to significantly inhibit (40-60%) EGFR tyrosine kinase activity and tyrosine phosphorylation of EGFR as well as the relative concentration of the 14kDa precursor form of TGF-α (one of the ligands of EGFR) in membranes of Kato-III as well as HCT-116 and CaCo-2 cells. Our data suggest a chemopreventive role for folic acid in colon and gastric cancers, as evidenced by the inhibition of proliferation and stimulation of differentiation and apoptotic processes in colon and gastric cancer cell lines. We also suggest that diminished activation of EGFR tyrosine kinase resulting from decreased membrane accumulation of TGF-α may partly be involved in regulating these processes.

(Supported by grants from the Department of Veteran Affairs)

Poster Abstract # 35

Role of dimethylglycine (DMG) in melanoma inhibition

Mani S[1], Whitesides JF[2] and Lawson JW[1]

[1]Department of Microbiology & Molecular Medicine, Clemson University, Clemson, SC

[2]Department of Animal & Veterinary Science, Clemson University, Clemson, SC

The natural product dimethylglycine (DMG), a metabolite in the choline degradation pathway, has been shown to modulate immune responses. In our laboratory mice, pretreated with DMG followed by injection with B16 melanoma cells, survived and displayed no metastasis. Control mice exhibited rapid extensive metastasis and death. In cell culture studies using cytokine bioassays, we found that DMG increased the production of the inflammatory cytokines TNF-α, IL-1 and IL-2. In addition, both stimulated and unstimulated lymphocytes exhibited enhanced ability to kill melanoma cells in co-culture systems in the presence of DMG. Melanoma cells primed with DMG were more susceptible to lymphocyte killing. Also, MHC-I expression in peripheral blood lymphocytes was elevated upon treatment with DMG. There was a 50-60% increase in cells expressing MHC-I with a 20 channel increase in mean fluorescence for MHC-I. Finally, in chick embryos DMG reduced the B16 melanoma tumor formation on the chorioallantoic membrane by over 50%.

The effect of dimethylglycine (DMG) on melanoma can be summarized as a three front attack on the tumor in which: (1) DMG enhances Th1 (inflammatory) cytokine production of stimulated lymphocytes, (2) DMG leads to an increased MHC-I expression in stimulated lymphocytes, and possibly (3) DMG directly acts on the melanoma cells preventing tumor formation. Thus, DMG may play a role in the prevention and treatment of malignant melanoma and other cancers.

Poster Abstract # 36

Whole Grain Breakfast Cereals, Antioxidants and Health

Miller G, Rigelhof F, Marquart L, Prakash A and Kanter M.
General Mills
Minneapolis, MN.

Considerable scientific evidence suggests that whole grains, as commonly consumed in the United States and Europe, reduce risk for chronic disease including cancer and heart disease. Whole grains provide a wide range of nutrients and phytochemicals that may work synergistically to optimize human health. A majority of the fiber, B-vitamins, total minerals, lignans, phytoestrogens, phenolic acids and phytate are found in the bran. The germ is rich in oil and vitamin E while the tocotrienols, plant sterols and oryzanol are associated with the germ and bran. Increased consumption of fruits and vegetables has been associated with protection against age-related disease. It is believed that antioxidant content, including vitamin C, vitamin E and (-carotene provides this protection. Whole grain cereals also contain a wide range of common and unique antioxidants. Ronald Prior (USDA) reports on studies using the oxygen radical absorbance capacity (ORAC) method, and determined that one serving of breakfast cereal provides antioxidants essentially equal to the amount in a whole day's intake of fruits or vegetables. We find similar results, using 2,2-diphenyl-1-picrylhydrazyl (DPPH) to determine antioxidant content, for breakfast cereals, fruits and vegetables. Whole grain cereals ranged from 2500-3600 (moles Trolox equivalents/100 grams (TE); high bran cereals contain up to 5300 TE while whole grain or bran cereals with raisins had 3300-4700 TE. By comparison, berries (raspberries, blackberries, blueberries or strawberries) contained from 3300-5500 TE. Other fruits were as high as 2000 TE for plums but generally ranged from 600-1500 TE. Melons were very low having 100-200 TE. The highest vegetable analyzed was red cabbage at 1400 TE, followed by garlic at 1300 TE. Otherwise, vegetables ranged from beets at 800 TE to cucumbers at 100 TE and celery at 60 TE. Cooking or peeling reduces antioxidant content by10 to 50%. These results clearly show that whole grain breakfast cereals are among the very best sources of dietary antioxidants with a consistently high content. Chronic diseases are initiated from a multitude of complex interactions. It is reasonable to speculate that multiple factors, including a wide range of antioxidants such as those found in grains, are important protective agents.

Poster Abstract # 37

Phytoestrogens and Western Diseases: What a Clinician Should Know

W. Mazur, S. Heinonen, K. Lusa, T. Nurmi, M. Uehara and H. Adlercreutz
Department of Clinical Chemistry
University of Helsinki
Folkhälsan Institute for Preventive Medicine, Nutrition and Cancer
P.O. Box 60
FIN-00014   Helsinki
FINLAND

The practice of medicine often involves the prescription of specific plant foods or their potent derivatives, to treat a wide spectrum of illnesses. Two important pathways for the biological actions of plant-derived chemicals involve binding either to hormone receptors or to enzymes that metabolize hormones. Edible plants contain a number of natural compounds, which mimic the biological effects of estrogens by virtue of their ability to bind to and activate the nuclear estrogen receptors. These hormone-like diphenolic phyto-estrogens of dietary origin include isoflavonoids, coumestans and lignans. Our interest in these 'plant oestrogens' derives from the results of epidemiological studies on diet and Western diseases including hormone-dependent cancers (breast, prostate), colon cancer as well as CHD. Incidences of the diseases in question are lower in peoples of Asia compared to their counterparts in Western countries. Consequently we have carried out, or have been involved in, prospective studies on cancer, menopause studies in women, dietary intervention and cross-sectional studies, pharmacokinetic and bioavailability studies of phyto-oestrogens, studies on lipids and CHD, as well as *in vitro* studies on cancer, angiogenesis and apoptosis. Several lines of evidence, including epidemiological, clinical trial data, and basic science, suggest that both lignans and isoflavonoids, with potential estrogenic, antiestrogenic, antioxidative, antiviral, antiproliferative, anticarcinogenic and antiatherogenic properties, are among the dietary factors affording protection against cancer and atherosclerosis. Herein we report our achievements and results of interest for the clinical practice.

Poster Abstract # 38

Phytoestrogens: The Case of Lignans. Occurrence in Foods, and Pharmacokinetic Study in Humans

Witold Mazur[1], Mariko Uehara[2] and Herman Adlercreutz[1]

[1]Department of Clinical Chemistry, University of Helsinki, and Folkhälsan Institute for Preventive Medicine, Nutrition and Cancer, P.O. Box 60, FIN-00014 Helsinki, FINLAND

[2]Department of Nutritional Science, Faculty of Applied Bio-Science, Tokyo University of Agriculture, Tokyo, JAPAN

Plants abound in essential phytochemicals produced for their various vital functions. The same compounds seem to be crucial for human health and disease. Recent human epidemiologic and laboratory animal and cell studies on cancer and heart disease brought into light the phyto-oestrogens - naturally occurring principles, which share with steroidal estrogens an ability to activate the oestrogen receptors. The best known non-steroidal phyto-oestrogens include the isoflavones daidzein, genistein, formononetin, and biochanin A, and the coumestan coumestrol, and the lignans secoisolariciresinol and matairesinol. Acknowledging the potentially chemoprotective role of these non-nutrients we have quantified all biologically important isoflavonoids and lignans in cereals, oilseeds and nuts, legumes, vegetables, fruits, berries and beverages such as tea, coffee and wine. Herein we present a review of our studies on staple plant foods indicating that plants, besides a large diversity of chemicals with a number of biological properties, contain biologically active phyto-oestrogens - precursors of hormone-like compounds in mammalian systems.

One of the fundamental issues in the field of phyto-oestrogens deals with screenings of the most commonly consumed plants and plant-derived foods. Our ID-GC-MS-SIM method has allowed a specific, quantitative, reproducible, and sensitive determination of the biologically most important phyto-oestrogens in food samples. The method has been applied successfully to a wide-spectrum of edible plants from these devoid of phyto-oestrogens to those containing high concentrations of the chemicals. Although the isoflavones are restricted within the Leguminosae, the lignans, particularly SECO, are wide-spread in plant foods. It should be kept in mind, however, that lignan concentrations in cereals and grains are underestimated due to unknown reasons.

A diversity has been described for naturally occurring phytoestrogens, which share with steroidal estrogens an ability to activate the estrogen receptors. The major known non-steroidal phytoestrogens are the isoflavones daidzein, genistein, formononetin, and biochanin A, and the coumestan coumestrol, and the lignans secoisolariciresinol and matairesinol. Phytoestrogens have been demonstrated to possess a broad spectrum of biological properties making them potential to influence human health and disease. Considering the potentially chemoprotective role of these non-nutrients it is of importance to know more about their presence in the human diet. Therefore we measured isoflavonoids and lignans in nine edible berries using an isotope dilution gas chromatography-mass spectrometry method for foods and found substantial concentrations of lignan secoisolariciresinol (1·39-37·18 mg/kg; dry weight), and low amounts of matairesinol (0-0·78 mg/kg; dry weight), and no isoflavones.

Poster Abstract # 39

Diallylsulfide inhibition of methylamylnitrosamine metabolism by P450s and diallyldisulfide clearance from rat blood

CR Morris, D. Yao and SS Mirvish
Eppley Institute for Research in Cancer
Department of Pharmaceutical Sciences
University of Nebraska Medical Center
Omaha, NE 68198

Garlic/garlic oil are promising chemopreventive agents against cancer. Of garlic oil, 26% is diallyldisulfide (DADS) and 2-3% is diallylsulfide (DAS). Methylamylnitrosamine (MNAN), a rat esophageal carcinogen, is activated by 1-hydroxylation, which produces pentaldehyde and DNA methylating agents. We investigated inhibition of MNAN metabolism by DAS. $[^3H]$-Pentaldehyde formation from $[^3H$-pentyl$]$-MNAN was measured by HPLC of its dinitrophenylhydrazone (Chen, Cancer Res. 59:91-98, 1999). Incubations used 20-150 µM MNAN, 0.25-8.0 µM DAS and 10-20 pmol cytochrome P450/tube. Maximum inhibition required preincubation of DAS for 15 min with the P450. DAS inhibited MNAN metabolism by rat CYP2E1, rat CYP2B1 and human CYP2E1 with K_i values of 2.0, 0.1, and 0.2 µM, respectively. These low values suggest normal intakes of garlic would inhibit nitrosamine metabolism.

We measured DADS clearance rate from blood of adult male MRC-Wistar rats fed commercial diet. DADS was recovered from 0.25 ml heparinized rat blood by addition of 2 ml acetonitrile, centrifugation, concentration and HPLC with UV detection. DADS recovery: $90 \pm 4\%$ (mean $\pm$ SD, n = 6). Detection limit: 2 µg/ml blood. We injected DADS solutions in polyethylene glycol-400 into femoral vein of anesthetized rats and withdrew blood samples from femoral artery. Rats given 20 and 50 mg DADS/kg showed steady decreases in DADS concentration, with complete clearance after 20-30 min. Hence, if DADS but not its metabolite allylmercaptan (Egen-Schwind, Planta Med. 58:301-305, 1992) inhibited nitrosamine activation, inhibition would occur for only short times after garlic ingestion.

(Support: American Institute for Cancer Research grant, Univ. Neb. Toxicology Program fellowship to C.R.M., NCI core grant P30-CA-36727.)

Poster Abstract # 40

Blood lycopene concentrations increase in healthy adults consuming standard servings of processed tomato products daily.

C Moxley, S Schwartz, N Craft, V DeGroff, E Giovannucci, S Clinton.
The Ohio State University Cancer Center, Dept of Food Science and Technology
Craft Technologies, Inc.
The Harvard School of Public Health
The consumption of tomato products is associated with a reduced risk of several cancers. Overall, human studies suggest that benefits may be achieved with approximately one serving of tomato products per day. Lycopene, the predominant carotenoid in tomatoes, is hypothesized to be one component contributing to the health benefits of tomato products. High plasma lycopene concentrations are associated with a reduced risk of prostate cancer in the Physicians' Health Study (Gann, et.al, 1999.). The present study was designed to determine plasma lycopene concentrations in healthy adults (n=36, ages 18 to 65) consuming standard daily servings of three processed tomato products: Prego[TM] Spaghetti Sauce (SS), Campbell's Tomato Soup (TS), or V8[TM] vegetable juice (J). All 36 subjects consumed a lycopene-free diet for the first two weeks (washout period) in order to determine lycopene clearance rates from the blood. Participants were assigned to one of three (n=12) intervention groups consuming single standard servings of SS (21 mg lycopene/1/2 cup), TS (12 mg lycopene/1cup), or J (17 mg lycopene/8 oz) daily for 4 wk without any other sources of lycopene. Blood samples were obtained at enrollment and weekly thereafter for HPLC analysis of carotenoids. Total plasma lycopene concentrations (Mean ± SE) decreased from 1.05 ± 0.07 to 0.54 ± 0.05 umoles/L (p<0.0001) during the washout period. In all intervention groups, plasma lycopene concentrations increased and plateaued between 2-4 wk. Plasma lycopene levels for those consuming SS, TS, and J increased to 2.08 (192% p < 0.0001), 0.91 (122%, p<0.0001), and 0.99 (92%, p<0.0001) umoles/L, respectively. This study demonstrates that lycopene is cleared from the plasma with a $T^{1/2}$ of approximately 14 days. Lycopene is readily absorbed from SS, TS, and J although bioavailability differs for each product. The study demonstrates that a single daily serving of processed tomato products can significantly increase blood lycopene.

(Supported by NIH-NCI R0172482, NIH-NCI R01CA74666, NIH-NCI P30 CA16058 to the OSU Comprehensive Cancer Center, OARDC Competitive Grants Program and The Campbell's Soup Co.)

Poster Abstract # 41

Modulation of growth factor-induced cell cycle progression by the tomato carotenoid, lycopene, in MCF-7 mammary cancer cells.

Nahum A, Amir H, Danilenko M, Karas M, Giat Y, Levy J, and Sharoni Y.
Department of Clinical Biochemistry
Faculty of Health Sciences
Ben-Gurion University and Soroka Medical Center
Beer-Sheva, ISRAEL

The anticancer activity of lycopene, the major tomato carotenoid, has been suggested from in vitro, in vivo and epidemiological studies. We have previously shown that lycopene inhibits basal and IGF-I induced growth of mammary and endometrial cancer cells. In IGF-I or serum stimulated MCF-7 mammary cancer cells, lycopene treatment slowed down cell cycle progression through G1-S phases. Thus, we aimed to determine the changes in the amount and activity of the molecular components of the cell cycle machinery associated with the lycopene effect. Lycopene treatment caused hypophosphorylation of the retinoblastoma protein and related pocket proteins. This effect resulted from reduced cyclin-dependent kinase (Cdk4 and Cdk2) activities observed in the carotenoid-treated cells. Since the inhibition of kinase activities was not due to a decrease in Cdk protein amount, we determined whether it resulted from changes in the levels of cyclins D and E and the CDK inhibitor p27. A lower abundance of cyclins D1 and D3 was found in the lycopene-treated cells, which can account for the reduction of Cdk4 activity. However, the cyclin E level did not change, implying a different mechanism for Cdk2 inhibition. As the total level of p27 was not altered either, the p27/cyclin E ratio was examined in the protein complex immunopercipatated by an anti-cyclin E antibody. Indeed, a significant increase in this ratio was found in the lycopene-treated cells as compared to the control cells. In summary, these results suggest that lycopene slows down cell cycle progression primarily via reduction of the level of cyclin D, the "growth factor sensor," and an increase in the p27/cyclin E ratio that inhibits the activity of G1/S Cdks and pRb phosphorylation.

Poster Abstract # 42

Dietary Factors That Induce Detoxification Enzymes Also Inhibit Proliferation in Human HT29 Colon Carcinoma Cells

R.Y. Odom, Y.G. Wirsky and W.G. Kirlin
Morehouse School of Medicine
Atlanta, GA

Epidemiologic data has shown dietary components to be both causative and preventative factors in the development of cancer. It has been suggested that diets with a high vegetable, fruit and fiber content, in particular, reduce the risk of colon cancer. A variety of mechanisms have been proposed to explain how these dietary components function in a cancer preventative role. One proposed mechanism involves an increase in the expression of the detoxification enzymes glutathione S-transferase (GST) and NAD(P)H:quinone oxidoreductase (NQO1). In HT29 colon carcinoma cells, we have found that dimethyl fumarate (DMF) and benzyl isothiocyanate (BIT), found in fruits and cruciferous vegetables, respectively, and butyrate, a by-product of the fermentation of dietary fiber by colonic bacteria, all increase the activity of GST and NQO1. Butyrate is also a differentiating agent for HT29 cells. To determine whether BIT and DMF, which induce GST and NQO1 activity, also affect carcinoma cell proliferation, HT29 cells were treated with 5 to 25 mM benzyl thiocyanate (BIT) and 20 to 100 mM dimethyl fumarate (DMF). In a concentration-dependent manner, BIT and DMF decreased thymidine incorporation to less than 25% of controls. These decreases in cell proliferation were reversible by pretreatment with 1 to 5 mM N-acetyl cysteine (NAC). In contrast, the NaB-mediated decreases in cell proliferation to less than 25% of controls were not reversible by NAC. These results indicate that a decrease in cell proliferation may be another mechanism by which dietary factors may protect against colon cancer.

(Support: MBRS/GM-028248).

Poster Abstract # 43

Glutathione (GSH) Depletion and the Effects of Nutritional Repletion of GSH (All-Immune() on Immunologic Function in Malignancy.

R.H. Keller, M.D.; X. Wen, M.D. ; S. Luck, RN, HNC and C.W. Patrick, Ph.D.
Immune Balance Technologies (IBT) and VitImmune, Hollywood, Florida
University of Miami School of Medicine, Miami, Florida.

Intracellular glutathione (GSH) is a requisite for normal lymphocyte activation as well as T cell and NK cytotoxicity. In various cancers, however, it has been suggested that the tumors co-opts GSH, resulting in elevated tumor cell GSH, depleted immune cell GSH, and compromised immunologic function. We examined T cell glutathione levels in patients with various malignancies and the effects of repletion of GSH with a patented nutritional preparation (All-Immune) on immunologic numbers and function.

Nine patients with various malignancies have been studied longitudinally using a patented test (IBT) to measure intralymphocyte GSH levels and a patented (VitImmune) nutritional replacement formula (All-Immune). The malignancies examined include Breast (N=7), Prostate (N=2) and enrollment is ongoing. No patients had received systemic chemotherapy before evaluation, but all were on hormonal therapy. Parameters evaluated included: CD4, CD8 and NK function using flow cytometry; sIL2-R levels and HHV-6 IgG (ELISA); and T cell glutathione levels. The initial mean T cell GSH level was 292 (96 ng/1X106 (NL 515 (165) (p< .05). After an average of 90 days of replacement with All-Immune, the mean T cell GSH level was 755 (101ng/1X106 (p=.005). The mean initial CD4 T cell number was 790 (125, while post-therapy the mean CD4 number was 1054 (217 (p=.03). In addition, HHV-6 reactivation (associated with immune compromise) had an initial mean of 18.2(2.2 and was 8.7 (1.4 (p=.003) after All-Immune. SIL-2R, an indicator of immune activity, had an initial mean of 625 (118 U/ml), while post therapy it was increased at 1016 (435 U/ml (NS). NK activity, however, remained statistically unchanged and in the low normal range even after treatment.

These preliminary data suggest that depleted T cell GSH levels in patients with malignancies are associated with immunologic compromise and that T cell GSH levels and immunologic parameters are, at least in part, corrected with All-Immune

Poster Abstract # 44

Induction of apoptosis in cultured lymphoid cells by genistein, resveratrol, curcumin and ascorbic acid.

Myron Wentz, Alexander Malugin and Sergey Preobrazhensky.
Apoptosis Research Laboratory, USANA
Salt Lake City, Utah

Numerous studies indicate that natural phytochemicals, genistein (GS), resveratrol (RS), curcumin (CU), as well as ascorbic acid (AsA), can be cytotoxic and induce apoptosis in cultured malignant cells. Using a new flow cytometric assay, we have compared the induction of apoptosis in cultured lymphoid (CEM-C7) cells by these compounds and have studied the effect of cell density on this process. Fluorescence microscopy was used to study morphological changes of cells during the induction of necrosis and apoptosis. GS and RS induced apoptosis in cultured lymphoid cells in a rather wide range of concentrations, while the effective range of concentrations of CU and AsA is relatively narrow. Most of the cells in the presence of AsA and CU were killed via the necrotic pathway. Cytotoxicity and induction of apoptosis by GS and CU were not affected by cell density, while cytotoxicity of RS and AsA was increased with a decrease of cell density. At cell densities lower than 30,000 cells/ml, AsA was able to kill tumor cells at concentrations lower than a normal average concentration of AsA in blood. Based on the results of this study, two different patterns of the induction of apoptosis by natural compounds can be suggested. Some compounds induce apoptosis in a wide range of concentrations, while others do so only in a relatively narrow range. The results of experiments with various cell densities allow us also to suggest that GS and CU can efficiently kill tumor cells in vivo even at high cell densities, while AsA at physiological concentration in blood can be potentially effective in preventing the dissemination of single tumor cells.

Poster Abstract # 45

Multiple Herbal Therapy: A New Approach Into Cancer Treatment

Luay J. Rashan[1] and Farid J. Rashan[2]

[1]Department of Pharmacology and Therapeutics, Faculty of Pharmacy, Applied Science University, Amman 11931, Jordan

[2]University of Mosul, Mosul, Iraq

Purpose: The purpose of this study was to evaluate the toxicity and to determine the appropriate dose of the intramuscular injection of the novel water-soluble extract (WSE)1,2,3.

Patients and Methods: Between March 1988 to January 1990, 25 consecutive, eligible patients with advanced breast cancer (ABC) and 15 patients with resected colon cancer (RCC) were treated by the authors. All patients had received palliative chemotherapy and / radiotherapy. Intramuscular injection of the active material of the WSE (30-60 mg) was administered once/daily for two to four months.

Results: The limiting non-cumulative toxicity was a sharp increase in body temperature (38.5(C), vomiting and nausea. The toxicity was otherwise predictable and manageable. The maximum tolerated dose (MTD) established at 50-70 mg of the active material, the recommended dose was 55 mg daily. There was no treatment related deaths. Ten patients with ABC achieved complete response (CR) and the other fifteen patients showed a partial response (PR). The fifteen RCC patients; five had Duck's C and ten had Duke's D(M1) resected tumors. The five patients with Duke's C showed complete response with no peritoneal recurrences (with a median duration of follow up of 18 months). The other ten Dukes D patients achieved partial response. However, four patients had recurrence of 18 months.

Conclusions: This trial confirm the activity of the water soluble extract in both ABC and RCC tumors. Although, the follow-up is short, however, the complete remissions achieved and the lack of recurrent peritoneal metastasis is very encouraging. Additional trials with this approach are in progress especially on carcinoids and prostate tumors since the present results confirm the activity of the extract both in vitro and in vivo.

References:
Rashan, L.J. and Al-Allaf, T.A.K: Multiple Herbal Therapy: A new approach into cancer treatment. 1. Some in vitro and in vivo studies. Phytomedicine . Vol. 3. Suppl.1.pp.43. 1996/97.

Rashan, L.J.: Multiple Herbal Therapy: A new Approach into cancer treatment. 2. Some preclinical results. Phytomedicine. Vol.3. Supple. 1. PP. 44. 1996/97.

Rashan, L. J.: Multiple Herbal Therapy: A new approach into antiviral treatment. Some in vitro and in vivo results. 12th world AIDS Conference. Geneva-Switzerland June 28th- July 3rd 1998. Monduzzi Editore S.p.A.-Bologna (Italy): 459-462.

Poster Abstract # 46

Effects of selenite plus endonuclease inhibitors and antioxidants on cytotoxicity and generation of 8-hydrodeoxyguanosine in normal human keratinocytes.

C.-L. Shen, B. C. Pence, and W. Song
Department of Pathology
Texas Tech University Health Sciences Center
Lubbock, TX 79430.

We previously reported that high doses of selenite (SeL) supplementation resulted in cytotoxicity and induction of 8-hydrodeoxyguanosine (8-OHdG) in DNA of primary human keratinocytes (NHK). The present study focused on the effects of selenite (SeL) plus endonuclease inhibitors (copper sulfate, CuSO4; zinc sulfate, ZnSO4; and aurintricarboxylic acid, ATA) and antioxidant (vitamin C, Vit C) on viability and 8-OHdG formation in DNA of NHK. NHK were treated with SeL at 0 and 10 Se (g/ml medium doses plus each of CuSO4 (0, 7.85, and 15.7 (M), ZnSO4 (0, 39, and 78 (M), ATA (0, 250, and 500 (M), or Vit C (0, 0.4, and 0.8 (g/ml) for 24 hours. In the absence of SeL treatment, only CuSO4 and ATA significantly decreased cell viabilities ($P<0.05$). Protection of NHK against cytotoxicity by high dose of SeL (10 (g/ml medium) plus endonuclease inhibitors or antioxidant occurred in the following order of magnitude of effects: SeL+CuSO4 > SeL+ATA > SeL+Vit C. In addition, the synergetic effects of SeL and ZnSO4 were observed in induction of cytotoxicity. Without SeL supplementation, only ZnSO4 and ATA elevated 8-OHdG formation in a dose-dependent manner. When NHK cells were co-incubated with SeL at 10 (g Se/ml medium and each of endonuclease inhibitors or antioxidant, ZnSO4, CuSO4, and Vit C protected NHK from SeL-induced DNA damage with the reduction of 8-OHdG formation. However, SeL+ATA treatment increased 8-OHdG adducts. These data demonstrate that the use of CuSO4 and VitC protected NHK from high dose SeL-induced cytotoxicity and DNA damage.

(This research was supported by NIH, CA 76675.)

Poster Abstract # 47

Polyunsaturated Fats From Corn and Fish Oil Inhibit the Growth of H. Pylori

Duane T. Smoot[1], Beverly Teter[2], Cornell R. Allen[1], Hassan Ashktorab[1], Joseph Sampugna[2].
[1]Dept. of Medicine and Cancer Center, Howard University, Washington, D.C.;
[2]Dept. of Chemistry & Biochemistry, University of Maryland, College Park, MD

H. Pylori only colonizes gastric mucosa and is felt to be responsible for 50 - 60% of all stomach cancers. Polyunsaturated fats have been shown to inhibit growth of H. pylori. Since, fat is digested in the duodenum, the stomach contents will contain mostly triglycerides (TG) and phospholipids (PL). H. pylori elaborates lipase, which digests fat. Therefore, we evaluated the ability of oils to inhibit the growth of H. pylori and measured the ability of H. pylori to obtain free fatty acids from these oils. H. pylori was grown on trypticase soy agar (TSA) with 5% sheep blood for 48 hrs prior to each experiment. H. pylori (5x16 bacteria/ml) was placed for 1 hr in media containing fatty acid free bovine serum albumin (BSA) complexed to corn, fish or olive oil at different concentrations.

Afterwards, H. pylori was plated onto TSA plates for 72 hours and growth was assessed by optical density using a spectrophotometer. Fish oil was the most bacteriostatic oil, totally inhibiting growth at a concentration of 1.0% (v/v). Corn oil almost completely inhibited bacterial growth (>90%) at a concentration of 10% (v/v). Olive oil showed a slight growth inhibition (15%) at higher concentrations (10 - 20%). H. pylori was exposed to fish, corn or olive oil for 3 or 6 hours, following which the media lipids were extracted and lipid classes were determined using thin layer chromatography. Evidence of TG hydrolysis was judged by release of FFA and presence of partial glycerides. After 6 hr of incubation there were more FFA present than at 3 hrs. The elaboration of free fatty acids correlated with the ability of these oils to inhibit growth of H. pylori. Diets high in polyunsaturated fat are likely to inhibit bacterial growth, and thereby, may limit the risk of stomach cancer from this bacterial infection.

Poster Abstract # 48

Can An Essential Fat Reduce The Cancer-Producing Potential Of Cancer-Causing Chemicals?

Paul Stitt, President
ENRECO, INC.
800-962-9593

Fats are generally considered to be a contributory cause of cancer. Scientific evidence is now showing that although it is true that several types of fats increase the incidence and growth rate of tumors in rats, there is one class of fats that can actually reduce the incidence and growth rate of tumors. Omega-3 is an essential nutrient for all mammals, since mammals cannot manufacture it. In 1993, the American Institute of Nutrition increased the recommended level of Omega-3 in the diet of rodents fur-fold because of immune disorders in the rats fed the AIN-76 diet for the longer term. Nineteen research papers on carcinogenesis have been published showing that whenOmega-3 (perilla oil, flax oil, or purified fish oil(is added to the diet of test animals, fewer and smaller tumors have been observed after various mutagenic chemicals (methynitrosourea, benzopyrene, dimethyl benzanthracene, etc.(have been added to the diet. When using whole ground flaxseed as a source for Omega-3, established tumors in rats have actually shrunk in size within six weeks. The same general effects have been observed when Omega-3 is present in the test diet. Fewer tumors are initiated. Tumors grow slower. Tumors are less lethal. Chemotherapy is more effective. Omega-3 has been found to prevent excess inflammatory reaction and has been found to counteract the effect of PGE2 made from Omega-6.

Poster Abstract # 49

Effect of Soy Flakes, Flour, Genistein and Calcium on Rat Colonic PCNA Levels After Induction of Colon Cancer with Azoxymethane (AOM)

D. Thiagarajan, M.R. Bennink, L.D. Bourquin, F.A. Kavas
Department of Food Science and Human Nutrition
Michigan State University
East Lansing, MI 48824

Proliferating Cellular Nuclear Antigen (PCNA), a delta polymerase accessory protein is present in all cells capable of cell division. The quantity of PCNA represents a potentially useful marker for the study of mucosal proliferative activity and, therefore, colon cancer risk. A study was designed to investigate the chemopreventive abilities of different soy products on colon carcinogenesis as reflected by changes in nuclear and total PCNA. Total PCNA was measured by immunoquantification using a slot-blot method and nuclear PCNA by immunohistochemical detection (IHC). Colon cancer was initiated in rats by injecting 15mg/kg body weight AOM subcutaneously at 21 and 28 days of age. At 35 days of age they were placed on the dietary treatments (n=9 or 10/treatment) soy concentrate: SC (very low in isoflavone content) as the control diet, full fat soy flakes: SFK, defatted soy flour: SF, genistein: GEN (150 ppm), calcium: CAL (SC diet with 0.5% calcium, the rest of the diets had 0.1% calcium), and a low-fiber diet for a period of 12 weeks. At the end of this period, the animals were sacrificed, entire colons were removed, and sections were scraped for mucosa to perform slot-blot quantification of PCNA. One cm sections from the distal end of each colon was processed for IHC detection of PCNA for proliferation analses and the remaining colon were stained for aberrant crypt foci analysis. Rats fed SFL and SFK had the lowest levels of the quantified PCNA (slot-blot method) when compared to SC, GEN, CAL and the low-fiber fed rats, at $P<0.05$. Furthermore, these results positively correlate with the differences in the LI ($r=0.81$, $P<0.0001$) and PZ ($r=0.65$, $P<0.0001$) analyses of PCNA by IHC, demonstrating that the slot-blot quantification of PCNA may serve as an easy and accurrate assay to test candidate compounds in dietary intervention and clinical studies of colon carcinogenesis. These results indicate that one or more phytochemicals present in soy is responsible for the antiproliferative effect (as reflected by chanfes in slot-blot quantified PCNA levels as well as in the PCNA mitotic indices) observed after initiation of colon cancer.

Poster Abstract # 50

In Vitro Anti-Proliferative and Pro-Communicative Properties of DADS

Veronique Robert, Carine Huard, Catherine Chaumontet, Frederic Veran, Muriel Thomas,
Francois Blachier and Paule Martel
Laboratoire de Nutrition et Securite Alimentaire
INRA, Jouy en Josas
FRANCE

Our team develops in vitro strategies to study molecular mechanisms accounting for protective effects of micronutrients toward cancer. As part of this program, we have recently investigate the effects of Diallyl Disulfid (DADS, a major oil-soluble component of garlic) on rat liver epithelial cells (REL) and human tumoral colonic cells (HT29 G-/+). We have antipromoting phase of carcinogenesis:
Cell proliferation by means of cell counting and flow cytometric analysis
Cell communication through gap junctions measured by a dye transfer assay
DADS 100mM, which is a non cytotoxic concentration, blocks the proliferation of REL and HT29 cells after a 24 hour treatment. So, DADS has anti-proliferative effects on these two cell types; however molecular mechanisms involved in this growth arrest appear to be cell specific. The growth arrest of REL cells was DADS-concentration dependent and was not accompanied by a modification of cell cycle phases. On the contrary, the inhibition of HT29 proliferation was observed only at 100mM DADS (50 or 75 mM did not modify cell density) and this growth arrest reflected a cell accumulation in G2/M phases.

Since our laboratory has observed that anti-proliferative properties of natural compounds are often associated with an increase of intercellular communication, we have studied modulation of communication in the presence of DADS. At 10mM DADS, we obtained a 1.8 fold stimulation of REL cell communication. HT29 did not communicate; consequently, they were not further tested in the dye transfer assay.

In conclusion, the anti-carcinogenic properties of DADS could be relevant to its anti-proliferative effects and to its capacity of increasing intercellular communication.

Poster Abstract # 51

Tabebuia Avellanedae Ext. "Taheebo" : A New useful Tea as Cancer Chemoprevention

Harukuni Tokuda[1], Eiichiro Ichiishi[1], Toshikazu Yoshikawa[1], Hoyoku Nishino[1] and Shinichi Ueda[2]
[1]Kyoto Prefectoral University of Medicine   Kyoto 602-0841, JAPAN
[2]Kyoto University, 606, Kyoto, JAPAN

Studies in Brazil are reviewed on the treatment of several important disease of *Tabebuia avellanedae* aqueous extract by traditional folk medicinal reports. Oral administration of aqueous extracts of this powder (inner bark, provided by Tabeebo Japan Co, Ltd.) inhibited promotion stage of carcinogenesis in mouse skin (carcinogen/promoter: DMBA/TPA, DMBA/UVB light), in mouse lung (4 NQO/8% glucerol). The role of this materials as biologica, antioxidants may be an important mechanism for the physiological activity of these abnormal conditions. Recently, we found that *Tabebuia avellanedae* constituents including lapachol and its derivative 5-hydroxy-2 (1 hydroxyethyl) -naphtho [2, 3-b] furan-4, 9-dione (NFD) were examined for inhibitory effects in vitro on Raji cells of activation by TPA combined with n-butyric acid and in vivo on mouse skin of DMBA as initiator and TPA as promoter. These observations seem that this material is more extensively as one of the agents for the purpose of cancer prevention.

Poster Abstract # 52

Anti-oxidative and anti-tumor promoting Activity of Okinawan naturally occurring plants

Eiichiro Ichiishi[1], Harukuni Tokuda[1], Yoko Aniya[2], Yoko Okuda[1], Toshikazu Yoshikawa[1] and Hoyoku Nishino[1]

[1]Kyoto Prefectoral University of Medicine   Kyoto 602-0841, JAPAN
[2]Ryukyu University, Okinawa 903-0129, JAPAN

As part of our study of natural materials as chemopreventive and therapeutic agents, we have investigated several naturally occurring plants all over the world and anti-oxidative or anti-tumor promoting activity has been evaluated based on superoxide scavenging and a short term in vitro assay involving Epstein-Barr virus early antigen activation promoted by phorbol ester. An epidemiological study showed a lower risk of various cancer types among people who consume native Okinawan plants in Okinawa prefecture, JAPAN. In search for candidate materials, herbal and edible plants collected from Okinawa prefecture and we tested in vitro and in vivo experimental systems for cancer chemopreventive agents. Of these materials, some crude samples exhibited potent anti-oxidative and anti-tumor promoting activity. The data accumulated in experimental studies will be presented suggesting that usable samples are promising candidates as chemopreventive agent.

Poster Abstract # 53

Chemopreventive Activities of Resveratrol Against Nitric Oxide Induced Carcinogenesis

Harukuni Tokuda[1], Eiichiro Ichiishi[1], Throu Mukainaka[1], Masato Okuda[2], Takao Konoshima[2], Govind Kapadia[3], Toshikazu Yoshikawa[1] and Hoyoku Nishino

[1] Kyoto Prefectoral University of Medicine Kyoto 602-0841, JAPAN
[2] Kyoto Pharmaceutical University, 607-8414, Kyoto, JAPAN
[3] Howard University, Washington DC 20059, USA

Nitric oxide (NO) plays an important role in number of physiological functions. Hence donor of NO may be useful for treatment of several diseases. But NO is also a mutagen and can cause mutations in both microorganisms and mammalian cells. In the course of the survey of the possible role of NO, we found that synthetic NO donor, NOR1 (this can release NO spontaneously at a steady rate and also confirmed that they byproducts do not possess any significant bioactivities) induced papillomas on two stage mouse skin carcinogenesis test as tumor initiator. This presentation focus how various preparations experimentally inhibited NO induced carcinogenesis. We previously showed that including materials in wines are potent chemopreventor implicated in chemical carcinogenesis. We now tested the anti-initiating activity of wine constituents resveratrol against NOR1 induced carcinogenesis. These studies are being carried out to guide the development of new classes tumor initiator and to evaluate their potential chemopreventor for inhibiting NO induced tumor.

Poster Abstract # 54

Meta-Analysis of Soy Intake and Breast Cancer Risk

Bruce Trock[1], Leslie White Butler[1], Robert Clarke[3], Leena Hilakivi-Clarke[2]

Departments of Human Oncology, Psychiatry[2], and Physiology and Biophysics[3].
Lombardi Cancer Center
Georgetown University Medical Center
Washington, DC 20007.

Background: High soy intake in Asian countries has been proposed as a factor contributing to the low breast cancer risk among Asian women. However, soy is being marketed and recommended to the public as if a clear protective effect has been established, when in fact the epidemiologic data are rather limited. Because in vivo and in vitro data show estrogenic effects for genistein, the major component of soy, it is important that associations between soy and breast cancer risk be evaluated before recommendations can safely be made. Therefore, we performed a meta-analysis of epidemiologic studies examining soy and breast cancer risk. Methods: A literature search based on keywords associated with soy, specific isoflavones, phytoestrogens, and breast cancer. An Internet search was also conducted to identify unpublished data. We analyzed data using the measures of soy intake provided in the studies, and also normalized intake to daily grams of soy protein. Odds ratios (ORs) were pooled using Mantel-Haenszel methods, and random effects models were used in the presence of significant heterogeneity of ORs across studies.

Results: Nine studies were included in the analysis (five in Asian women living in Asian countries; one in the West, and two in non-Asian populations). The size of ORs varied considerably , as did the level of soy defined as high intake. A modest statistically significant reduction in risk was associated with high soy intake over all studies, OR = 0.87 (95% CI: 0.80, 0.96). However, this effect was confined to premenopausal women, OR = 0.80 (95% CI: 0.71, 0.90). There was no protective effect at all in postmenopausal women, OR = 1.01 (95% CI: 0.86, 1.19). There was also no significant effect of soy among women in Asia, OR = 0.95 (95% CI: 0.83, 1.09).

Conclusions: Although there is some evidence of a small reduction in premenopausal breast cancer risk associated with soy intake, no association was observed for postmenopausal women, or women in Asia. Interpretation of these results is complicated by the small number of studies, crude measurement of soy intake, inconsistent control of confounding factors, and the low percentage of non-Asian subjects consuming soy. Coupled with the fact that some studies suggest potentially adverse effects of soy, these data suggest that recommendations for women to increase their soy intake to prevent breast cancer or prevent its recurrence are premature, and that larger, more rigorously controlled studies are needed.

Poster Abstract # 55

Dietary Inositol Hexaphosphate Reduces Aberrant Crypt Formation in the Colon of Azoxymethane-Injected Rats

April D. Carney, Nancy D. Turner, Robert S. Chapkin and Joanne R. Lupton
Department of Animal Science and the Faculty of Nutrition
Texas A&M University
College Station, TX

Colon cancer is the second leading cause of health from cancer in the United States. Aberrant crypt foci (ACF) are thought to be premalignant lesions from which colon cancer develops, and the number of crypts within a foci is believed to be predictive of tumor development. Inositol hexaphosphate (IP6, phytate), is abundant in many plant foods, especially wheat bran. Epidemiological and experimental studies indicate IP6 is protective against colon cancer development, yet exact mechanisms remain unknown. To determine if IP6 affects ACF development, we incorporated one of three levels of IP6 (0.0, 0.6 or 1.2 g/kg) into the diet of 21-day-old Sprague Dawley rats (n=60). After the first and second week of consuming the experimental diets, 30 rats received carcinogen injections (AOM) and 30 received saline. After 4 weeks of consuming the diets, rats were terminated, the colon removed, cut in half longitudinally, and fixed before staining in 0.5% methylene blue to count ACF. ACF are characterized by darker staining, enlarged crypts and elongated lumens, and are found as single crypts (ACI) or multiples (ACF2, ACF3, etc.) Data were analyzed using SAS with the main effect of IP6 level. Only AOM-injected rats developed aberrant crypts. The number of ACI decreased ($P<0.003$) from 52.1 for the 0.0 IP6 level to 33.8 and 31.4 for the 0.6 and 1.2 levels, respectively. The 1.2 IP6 level produced the fewest ACF2 relative to the 0.0 ($P<0.0001$) or 0.6 ($P<0.03$) levels. ACF3 and foci with 3 or more ACF were reduced ($P<0.04$) by the 1.2 IP6 level. Total AC were reduced by the 1.2 ($P<0.0004$) and 0.6 ($P<0.01$) levels relative to the 0.0 level. These data demonstrate that IP6 within the diet can reduce both the number and multiplicity of ACF, supporting the hypothesis that IP6 may protect against colon cancer development.

Poster Abstract # 56

Diindolylmethane Reduces HT-29 Colon Cancer Cell Number by Decreasing Proliferation and Increasing Apoptosis

N.D. Turner[1], J. Zhang[1], L.A. Davidson[1], R.S. Chapkin[1], S. Safe[2], and J.R. Lupton[1]

Faculty of [1]Nutrition and [2]Toxicology, Texas A&M University, College Station, TX

Diindolymethane (DIM) is a dimer formed from indole-3-carbinol (in cruciferous vegetables) that has anticancer properties. To determine how DIM might protect against colon cancer, we examined the effect of DIM and a chlorinated analog, 4-CI-DIM, on cell number, proliferation (BrdU labeling) and apoptosis (histone-based ELISA) in HT-29 colon cancer cells. Cells were incubated with 7% serum in DMEM media for 2 d, serum-free media for 1 d, followed by an incubation with DIM or 4-CI-DIM in 3% serum media. After 72 h of treatment, cell number decreased ($P<0.0001$) by 76 or 95% with 25μM DIM or 4-CI-DIM, respectively, compared to 3% serum control. The decrease resulted from a 73 and 92% reduction ($P<0.003$) in proliferation by DIM and 4-CI-DIM, respectively, and a 490% increase ($P<0.0001$) in apoptosis with 4-CI-DIM. We also performed a dose-response study using 5, 10 or 25 μM DIM and 4-CI-DIM after 24, 48, or 72 h of treatment. After 24 h, 25μM DIM and 4-CI-DIM reduced ($P<0.03$) proliferation by 550 and 61%, respectively, but only 25μM 4-CI-DIM increased ($P<0.0001$) apoptosis (96% more than controls). By 48 h, both the 10 and the 25μM concentrations of each molecular reduced ($P<0.04$) proliferation and increased ($P<0.005$) apoptosis. After 72 h, proliferation was reduced by 10 and 25μM 4-CI-DIM ($P<0.0002$) and by 10 ($P<0.04$) and 25μM DIM . We conclude that dietary DIM is a strong proliferation inhibitor and apoptosis inducer, but that the synthetic analog, 4-CI-DIM, has even greater biopotency. Therefore, these compounds may protect against colon cancer by decreasing cell cycle progression and by increasing apoptosis.

(Supported by a grant from NIEHS Center for Environmental and Rural Health (P30-ES09106).

Poster Abstract # 57

Fructooligosaccharides Feeding Enhances Bioavailability of Soy Isoflavones in Rats.

Mariko Uehara[1], Atsutane Ohta[2], Shaw Watanabe[1], Kazuharu Suzuki[1], Herman Adlercreutz[3].

[1] Department of Nutritional Science, Tokyo University of Agriculture, Tokyo, Japan

[2] Bioscience Laboratories, Meiji Seika Kaisha, Ltd., Saitama, Japan

[3] Department of Clinical Chemistry, University of Helsinki and Institute for Preventive Medicine, Nutrition and Cancer, Folkhälsan Research Center, Helsinki, Finland

Most flavonoids and the isoflavonoids in foods are glycoside conjugates. Lactobacilli, Bacteroides and Bifidobacteria in the intestinal flora hydrolyze glycosidic bonds to yield aglycones for absorption. Fructooligosaccharides (FOS) stimulate the growth of Bifidobacteria, so they may result in increased absorption of phytoestrogens. The effect of dietary FOS on the absorption of soybean isoflavones was studied by measuring portal, central and tail venous serum and urine.

SD male rats (6 week-old) were fed a control AIN-93G diet or a 5% FOS supplemented diet for 7 days. A single dose of soy isoflavone (Fuji Flavone P40), 15mg genistein and genistein and 60mg daidzein and daidzein/kg body wt, was given by a stomach tube and the blood was collected at 0,1,3,6,12,24 and 48 hrs through the catheters from portal and central vein, and puncture of tail vein. Urine was also collected during 0-24h and 24-48h after dosing. Isoflavones in the samples were analyzed by time-resolved fluoroimmunoassay.

The genistein concentration reached a peak (4,300nmol/l in the control and 3,500nmol/l in the FOS) in the portal vein at 1h and declined thereafter. The concentrations in the central and tail vein were nearly half of those in the portal vein. Daidzein remained high until 6h after dosing in the portal vein. Both genistein and daidzein delayed to appear in the tail venous serum of the FOS fed rats. The recovery in urine was 24% in the control and 27% in the FOS fed rats. Both of the isoflavone excretions in the 24-48h urine were significantly higher in the FOS fed rats than in the control.

Pharmacokinetics of bioavailability of isoflavones were clarified. These results suggested FOS treatment was effective to enhance the absorption in the large intestine, specially for genistein (about 20% high in the FOS).

Poster Abstract # 58

Long Chain Inulin Suppresses AOM-Induced Aberrant Crypt Foci in Colon of Retired Male Fisher 344 Rats

Verghese, M.[1], Chawan, C.B.[1], Rao, D.R[1]. and Van Loo, J.[2]

[1]Nutrition and Carcinogenesis Laboratory, Department of Life Sciences,
Alabama A & M University, Normal, AL 35762
[2]Orafti, Belgium

Colorectal cancer is the second leading cause of death in the U.S. Carcinogenesis is a degenerative disease that afflicts older populations at much higher frequencies than younger ones. Rat model studies, however, generally include younger rats and there are no studies using adult rats. In this study, Inulin a known suppressor of colon carcinogenesis in younger rats, has been tested for its ability to suppress azoxymethane (AOM)-induced preneoplastic aberrant crypt foci(ACF) in the colon of adult Fisher-344 male rats. After a 2 wk acclimatization period, 48 Fisher 344 retired male breeder rats of 52 wk. age were assigned to 4 diets: AIN 93M diet (C) and AIN 93M containing 2.5%, 5% and 10% long chain inulin (RAFTILINEÒ HP, Orafti, Belgium). All the rats received two s/c injections of AOM dissolved in saline @ 10 mg/kg body weight, one each at 55 and 56 wk. The dose rate of AOM was based on the results of a preliminary experiment on mortality, morbidity and ACF induction. The animals were sacrificed after 9 wk following 2nd injection of AOM. There were no significant differences in weight gain between control and experimental groups. There was a significant increase in cecal weight and a decrease in cecal pH from 7.17 in control group to 6.87, 6.61, 5.76 in the groups fed inulin at the level of 2.5%, 5% and 10%, respectively. Long chain inulin reduced ACF in the colon significantly ($p < 0.01$) in a dose-dependent manner. Compared to control diet, the percent reductions of ACF in 2.5, 5.0, 10% inulin diets were 25.3, 51.3 and 65.3, respectively. The results of this study indicate that dietary long chain inulin suppresses AOM-induced ACF formation, an early preneoplastic marker in the process of colon carcinogenesis in adult Fisher 344 male rats.

Poster Abstract # 59

Regulation of Uterine Gene Expression by Daidzein and Genistein in vitro and in vivo

Gunter Vollmer, Patrick Diel and Horst Michna
Molecular Cell Physiology and Endocrinology
Technical University
Dresden
Department of Morphology and Cancer Research
DSHS
Cologne, Germany

Possible adverse or beneficial effects of phytoestrogens and their potential impact on human health are conversely debated. Therefore, the aim of this study was to assess the estrogenic potency of phytoestrogens, predominantly daidzein (DAI) and genistein (GEN), in experimental uterine models in vitro and in vivo. In vitro we measured the relative binding affinity of DAI and GEN to the estrogen receptor (ER) of the rat endometrial adenocarcinoma cell line RUCA-I and their effects on the expression of the complement C3 gene. In vivo the impact of 500 mg/kg/d of DAI and of 100 mg/kg/d of GEN was assessed in comparison to ethinlestradiol (EE) in a three day uterotrophic assay. The substances were administrated p.o. The uterine wet weight and the mRNA expression of the estrogen sensitive genes of c-fos, ER, progesterone receptor (PR) and clusterin (CLU) were analyzed. The relative binding attinity of GEN to the ER of RUCA-I cells was 1% of estradiol. The binding affinity of DAI was 20 fold lower. However, 10^{-6} M concentration of both substances led to an equally potent induction of complement C3 expression in RUCA-I cells. In vivo a significant increase of uterine wet weight resulted from administration of 100mg/kg/d DAI. The analysis of uterine gene expression revealed a complex pattern of regulation. In contrast to DAI but administration of GEN, like EE, led to a significant induction of c-fos mRNA expression, correlating to the uterotrophic potencies of these substances. In contrast, the mRNA expression of CLU and PR was significantly down regulated by DAI, GEN and EE. In summary, both DAI and GEN are potent regulators of the expression of estrogen-dependent genes in rat uterine models in vivo and in vitro. Additionally, the relative potency of phytoestrogen action clearly differs if individual genes or cellular processes are examined. Finally, neither does the relative binding affinity necessarily predict the potency of phytoestrogens on gene expression, nor does in vitro potency correlate with the relative potency in vivo.

Poster Abstract # 60

Dose-dependent Reduction in DNA Damage in Peripheral Blood Lymphocytes of Dogs by Dietary Selenium Supplementation

Shen S[1], Glickman LT[2], Oteham C[1], Tice RR[3], Waters DJ[1]

[1]Dept of Veterinary Clinical Sciences & [2]Veterinary Pathobiology,
Purdue University, West Lafayette, IN
[3]Integrated Laboratory Systems, Research Triangle Park, NC.

It is likely that DNA damage contributes to at least two age-related processes: organismal senescence and cancer development. The purpose of this study was to determine if selenium supplementation would significantly reduce DNA damage in elderly dogs. Elderly (8 to 10 year-old) sexually intact male beagle dogs were randomly assigned to groups: no treatment (control group; n=5 dogs), 3(g/kg SelenoPrecise(High Selenium Yeast (low dose group; n=5 dogs), and 6(g/kg SelenoPrecise((high dose group; n=4 dogs). After five months of treatment, single cell gel electrophoresis (Comet assay) was used to measure basal DNA damage in peripheral blood lymphocytes. In all experiments, freshly harvested peripheral blood lymphocytes and 30 minute electrophoresis at pH > 13 were used. Extent of DNA damage was scored in 100 cells using a modification of Collins' method. Each cell was scored as follows: Type 0 = no damage, Type 1 & 2 = mild to moderate damage, Type 3 & 4 = extensive DNA damage. Mean percentage of extensively damaged cells (Type 3 & 4) were compared between treatment groups. Dogs in the low dose selenium group had significantly reduced basal DNA damage compared to age-matched controls. Mean ((SD) percentage of cells with extensive DNA damage was 25 (3% and 12 (2% for control dogs and selenium supplemented dogs, respectively ($p<0.01$). In contrast, the mean percentage of cells with extensively damaged DNA in the high dose selenium group was 28 (12%, which was not significantly different from the control group. In conclusion, using the Comet assay, we found that elderly male dogs receiving 3(g/kg SelenoPrecise(had significantly reduced basal DNA damage detectable in their peripheral blood lymphocytes compared to unsupplemented dogs. The influence of selenium supplementation on DNA damage, stromal senescence, and epithelial carcinogenesis within the dog prostate is currently being investigated.

Poster Abstract # 61

Green Tea Flavonoids Inhibit TCDD-Induced CYP1A1 and CYP1A2 Gene Expression in Human Liver Cancer Cells

SN Williams[1], H Shih[2], and LC Quattrochi[2].
[1]Department of Pharmaceutical Sciences, [2]Department of Medicine
University of Colorado Health Sciences Center, Denver, CO

Green tea contains several flavonoids, also known as catechins, which have been identified as potential dietary chemopreventive agents. Some dietary flavonoids have been shown to alter the expression and/or activities of some carcinogen-metabolizing enzymes, including members of the cytochrome (CYP) P450 family. We examined the effects of commercial green tea extracts (GTEs) and individual catechins on the expression of human CYP1A mRNA, which is mediated by the aryl hydrocarbon receptor (AhR). Pretreatment of primary human hepatocytes or human HepG2 hepatoma cells with GTEs, followed by addition of the AhR ligand 2,3,7,8-tetrachlorodibenzo-p-dioxin (TCDD) resulted in a concentration dependent decrease in the level of induced CYP1A1 and CYP1A2 mRNA. To determine if the observed inhibition of induced CYP1A mRNA was due to an inhibition of gene transcription, we used a stable cell line derived from HepG2 cells that contains the 5' flanking DNA and the promoter of the human CYP1A1 gene linked to the luciferase reporter gene. Pretreatment with GTEs resulted in a concentration-dependent inhibition of TCDD-induced promoter activity. To determine if this was due to a single component in GTEs, we investigated the individual catechins. We found that pretreatment with individual catechins had little or no effect, but if we combined the catechins into a mixture that mirrored the amounts of each found in the commercial extracts, the same inhibition of TCDD-induced CYP1A1 promoter activity was observed. Using electrophoretic gel mobility shift assays, we found GTEs inhibited the TCDD-induced activation of the AhR to a DNA-binding species. These results suggest that the combination of catechins found in green tea, as opposed to a single component, is effective in altering CYP1A expression and this occurs at the level of transcription, most likely due to alterations in the biochemical and/or functional properties of the AhR.

Poster Abstract # 62

Adriamycin multidrug resistance: modulation b α-tocopherol succinate

Heng-Kuan Wong, Jacqueline Riondel, Marie-Jeanne Richard, Alain Favier
Laboratoire de Biologie du Stress Oxydant
Biochimie
Faculte de Pharmacie
Domaine de la Merci
38706 La Tronche cedex
FRANCE

Chemoresistance of human malignant tumors causes the failure of anticancer agents for most cancers. It is due to various cellular and molecular mechanisms. Previous studies conducted in our laboratory, proposed a radical or oxidant involvement in the cancer process with alteration of the malignant cell redox-state and implication of the glutathione redox-cycle in acquired multidrug resistance (mdr 1).

RRR-α-tocopheryl succinate was studied for effects on sensitive (IGR-OV1) and multidrug resistant (IGR-OV1-DXR) human ovarian carcinoma cell line proliferation. As expected, doxorubicin (DXR) was more cytotoxic in IGR-OV1 cell line (IC 50 = 2 μM) than in IGR-OV1-DXR (IC 50 = 16 μM). α-tocopherol at 0.1-200 μg/ml had no effect on IGR-OV1 proliferation, whereas for the mdr 1 cell line α-tocopherol 12-200 μg/ml showed dose-dependent cytoxicity.

α-tocopherol had no effect on the cytotoxicity of doxorubicin in the drug-sensitive cell line without improvement of doxorubicin sensitivity, whereas α-tocopherol treatment enhanced the cytotoxicity of doxorubicin in the mdr cell line, reversing partially the chemoresistance.

In conclusion, α-tocopherol, an essential antioxidant, acts probably by modulation of the cell redox-state and escape multidrug resistance in a human ovarian carcinoma, indicating that doxorubicin resistance could be modified by redox-state changes, i.e. by intracellular glutathione content modulation.

Immunoblotting conducted on nuclear protein extracts from drug sensitive and mdr 1 cell lines, confirms the alteration of mdr cell line redox-status compared to sensitive cell line, with a decreased expression of Sp1 (a redox-sensitive transcription factor) in the mdr cell line, whereas NFκB, a transcription factor inducible by an oxidative stress, showed an increase of its expression.

Poster Abstract # 63

Mechanistic studies of the role of cyclooxygenase (COX) in cell growth inhibition induced by tea flavonoids in human colorectal cells

Anita Xu Wei Xin
Department of Community, Occupational and Family Medicine
National University of Singapore
SINGAPORE

It is well known that tea, one of the most popular beverages in the world, has lots of beneficial effects on human body. Recently, substantial evidence has been shown that the beneficial effects are mainly due to its flavonoids. Tea flavonoids can effectively scavenge reactive oxygen species (ROS), such as hydrogen peroxide, superoxide anion, which are closely associated with chronic degenerative diseases, such as cardiovascular diseases and cancer.

Among the various beneficial effects of tea, anti-carcinogenic activity is the most noteworthy. Since the relationship between tea drinking and cancer risks in humans is rather complicated, so far the evidences based on epidemiological investigations are not consistent, although a favorable effect is generally suggested. In contrast, evidences obtained from animal studies concerning potentially protective effects of tea are compelling and encompasses several important mechanisms that suggest possible beneficial effects of tea and tea flavonoids at most stages of cancer development. It is found that green tea polyphenols can significantly lower the incidence of colon carcinomas in rats ingesting water extract of green tea (WEGT).

Colorectal cancer is one of the leading cancers in Western countries. Numerous studies have demonstrated that human colorectal cancer (CRC) is closely related to high level of prostaglandin E2 (PGE2) and over expression of cyclooxygenase-2 (COX-2), the inducible isoenzyme of COX. PGE2 is the main product of COX-2 in colorectal tumor tissues. The venous blood draining from colon tumors contains large amounts of PGE2 and the larger the tumor, the higher the PGE2 output. In human studies, COX-2 was shown to increase in 80-90% of CRC tumors and in 40% of premalignant colorectal adenomas. Given the existing evidence, COX-2 may promotes cancer cell proliferation through different pathways: inhibiting apoptosis (suicide), inhibiting cell immunity (homicide), increasing mitogenesis of cancer cells as well as other mechanisms, for example, induction of ornithine decarboxylase (ODC) activity, which is considered to be closely associated with tumor promoting activity of a variety of tumor promoters.

It has been demonstrated that catechin and epicatechin, the predominant components of green tea flavonoids, have potent inhibitory effect against purified cyclooxygenase in vitro. It also has been showed that (-)-epigallocatechin gallate (EGCG), the most abundant and most potent epicatechin in green tea, blocked epidermal growth factor (EGF) binding to its receptor (EGFR) in A431 cells, a human epidermoid carcinoma cell line , and subsequently inhibited EGFR kinase activity. Blockade of the EGFR may result in decreased COX-2 expression. It was also found that quercetin can inhibit cyclooxygenase (Kim et al., 1998). Evidence from antioxidants supports the possibility that tea flavonoids may inhibit COX-2 expression and reduce PGs production in colorectal cancer cells for tea flavonoids have been considered potent antioxidants, though no direct evidence has been shown. It was demonstrated that antioxidants dose-dependently decreased endogenous H_2O_2, an event that correlated with a decrease in

PGE2 levels. These cellular changes (H2O2 production and PGE2 levels) were significantly correlated with the observed decrease in cellular proliferation (P<0.001.) This statistically significant correlation demonstrates a link between the ability of antioxidants to alter intracellular redox status, PGE2 production and cellular proliferation. On the other hand, the fact that ROS induce COX-2 expression further confirms the inhibitory effects of antioxidants on COX expression.

It is obvious that COX is one of the key factors that regulate tumor proliferation. Since so far, there is no direct evidence correlating the anti-proliferative effect of tea flavonoids with the inhibition of COX , especially COX-2 expression in colon cancer cells, it is expected to elucidate the link between these two in colon cancer cell lines. Further investigation of whether or not it is due to the antioxidant activities that tea flavonoids may inhibit COX-2 expression would be done.

Poster Abstract # 64

Effect of Dietary Supplementation with High-Selenium Soybean on Experimental Metastasis of Melanoma Cells in Mice

D. Li[1], G.L. Graef[2], J.A. Yee[1], and L. Yan[1]

[1]Creighton University School of Medicine, Omaha, NE 68178
[2]University of Nebraska-Lincoln, Lincoln, NE 68583

The present study investigated the effect of dietary supplementation with high-selenium (Se) soybean on experimental metastasis of melanoma cells in mice. Plants of soybean cultivar "Colfax" were treated with selenate by foliar application at R1 (beginning flowering) and R5 (beginning of pod fill) stages of the development. After harvest, the seeds of Se-treated soybean (hereafter referred to as high-Se soybean) and untreated soybean (hereafter referred to as low-Se soybean) were dehulled and defatted, and soybean protein isolate (SPI) was extracted. Three-week old male C57Bl/6 mice were assigned to five groups of 18 each. Five diets were compared. They were a basal AIN-93G diet, a basal diet supplemented with 10% low-Se SPI, 5% low-Se SPI plus 5% high-Se SPI, 10% high-Se SPI, and a 10% low-Se SPI diet supplemented with Se as selenomethionine. Selenium added to the diet was equivalent to that provided in the 10% high-Se SPI diet. Mice were given free access to the experimental diets for two weeks before and after the intravenous injection of 0.5×10^5 B16BL6 melanoma cells. At necropsy, the number of tumors that developed in the lungs was determined by counting the black foci using a dissecting microscope. Tumor size was analyzed using a Quantimet 500 image analysis system (Leica Cambridge, Cambridge, UK).

The number of tumors that formed in the lungs was illustrated in two ways. First, all mice were classified into two categories: 1 to 50 tumors and >50 tumors. Our results show that the number of mice that had >50 tumors was 13, 8, 7, 3, and 6 in the control group and the groups fed a diet containing 10% Low-Se SPI, 5% Low-Se SPI plus 5% high-Se SPI, 10% high-Se SPI, and 10% low-Se SPI plus Se. The difference between the control group and the group fed the 10% high-Se SPI diet or the 10% low-Se SPI plus Se diet was significantly different. Second, the difference in the number of lung tumors between groups was compared. Dietary supplementation with low-Se SPI and high-Se SPI significantly reduced the number of lung tumors. The greatest inhibition was observed in mice fed the 10% high-Se SPI diet.

Tumor size was analyzed by determining the tumor cross-sectional area and tumor volume. The median tumor cross-sectional area was 0.15, 0.08, 0.09, 0.06, and 0.04 mm^2, and the median tumor volume was 0.05, 0.02, 0.02, 0.01, and 0.01 mm^3 in mice fed the respective diets described above. Both tumor cross-sectional area and volume of mice fed the 10% high-Se SPI diet were significantly smaller than those of mice fed the basal diet and the diet containing 10% low-Se SPI or with 5% low-Se SPI plus 5% high-Se SPI.

It is concluded that dietary supplementation with high-Se soybean has a greater inhibitory effect on experimental metastasis than that with low-Se soybean.

(Supported by American Institute for Cancer Research, Nebraska Department of Health, and Health Future Foundation).

Poster Abstract # 65

Agonistic Steroid Hormone Activity of Flavonoids and Related Compounds in an In Vitro Tissue Culture System

Rachel S. Rosenberg Zand[1,2], David JA Jenkins[1] and Eleftherios P Diamandis[2,3]

[1] Dept of Nutritional Sciences, University of Toronto, Toronto, Canada

[2] Dept of Pathology & Laboratory Medicine, Mount Sinai Hospital Toronto, Canada;

[3] Dep't of Laboratory Medicine & Pathobiology, University of Toronto, Toronto, Canada.

Introduction: High fruit and vegetable consumption, (>5 servings/ day) is associated with reduced risk of cancers of all types. Researchers are investigating components of these plant foods, to determine which are responsible for this protection. One family, collectively known as flavonoids, are polyphenolic compounds found in fruits, vegetables, legumes, tea and red wine. In North America, consumption of flavonoids has been approximated at 45-100 (g/day). Isoflavones, a class of flavonoids found in soy, have been demonstrated to possess estrogenic and antiestrogenic activity, and are indicated as one explanation why populations who consume high amounts of soy (Asians) have significantly lower rates of breast and prostate cancer than populations who consume low amounts (North Americans). Much less work has been focused on other flavonoids.

Objectives: Because control of steroid hormone activity is believed to be important in the prevention of these cancers, we assessed the steroid hormonal activity of 75 flavonoids and structurally-related compounds. This entailed measuring the estrogenic, androgenic and progestational activity of these compounds. Methods: Flavonoids and related compounds were tested on BT-474 human breast cancer cells at concentrations of 10^{-8} to 10^{-5} M, with estradiol, norgestrel and dihydrotestosterone used as positive controls, and anhydrous ethanol as a negative control. pS2, an estrogen-regulated protein, and prostate-specific antigen (PSA), regulated by androgens and progestins, were quantified using immunosorbent assays developed in-house. Results: Of the 75 compounds tested, 9 showed estrogenic activity at 10^{-5} M. Of this subset, 7 showed progestational/androgenic activity at this concentration. The soy isoflavones, Biochanin A, Genistein and Daidzein, showed greatest estrogenic activity (550-1000 ng/mL pS2), followed by Naringenin and Luteolin (580 and 400 ng/mL, respectively). Apigenin showed greatest progestational/androgenic activity (>3000 ng/L PSA).

Conclusion: Several flavonoids demonstrate steroid hormone activity. This effect may implicate flavonoids in the modification of cancer risk by diet.

Poster Abstract # 66

Resveratrol and Piceatannol Inhibit Mitochondrial F0F1-ATPase Activity by Targeting the F1 Complex

Jianbiao Zheng and Victor D. Ramirez
Department of Molecular and Integrative Physiology
University of Illinois at Urbana-Champaign
Urbana, IL 61801

Resveratrol and piceatannol are stilbene phytochemicals that possess antitumor activity. We recently reported that red wine constituent resveratrol and soybean isoflavone genistein inhibited mitochondrial F0F1-ATPase/ATP synthase activities. Here, we demonstrate that piceatannol also potently inhibited the rat brain mitochondrial F0F1-ATPase activity in both digitonin-solubilized mitochondrial preparations and submitochondrial particles (IC50 of 8-9 microM), while having relatively small effect on the Na+, K+-ATPase activity of porcine cerebral cortex (no effect up to 7 microM). The inhibition of F0F1-ATPase by the stilbenes was of mixed type, and that of genistein was noncompetitive. Both resveratrol and piceatannol inhibited the ATPase activity of the purified rat liver F1 with IC50 of about 14 and 4 microM, respectively. On the other hand, genistein was much less effective in F1 (10% inhibition at 50 microM) than in F0F1-ATPase (IC50 of 55 microM). Piceatannol at microM concentrations also inhibited the [3H]estradiol binding to a rat uterine cytosol preparation rich in nuclear estrogen receptors with Ki similar to resveratrol (about 14 microM). Our results indicate that piceatannol and resveratrol inhibit the F-type ATPase by targeting the F1 sector, which is located to the inner membrane of mitochondria and in the plasma membrane of normal human umbilical vein endothelial cells and several cancer cell lines. This novel mechanism could potentially contribute to the multiple effects of these chemopreventive phytochemicals.

INDEX

Abberant crypt formation	12
Allicin	85-87
Alliin	83, 85, 86
Allyl sulfur compounds	69, 71, 73, 74, 83, 85, 86, 88, 89, 91, 93-96, 99, 124
Angiogenesis	127, 132, 137, 139
Antioxidants	29, 36, 48, 172, 198, 219, 224
Antiproliferative effects	48
Apoptosis	124, 131-134, 136, 139, 168
Arsenite	122
Aryl hydrocarbon receptor	183, 184, 190
Atherosclerosis	163, 165, 167
Azoxymethane	12-14, 16, 42, 147
Bioavailability	6, 30, 45, 120, 121, 175, 176
Biomarkers	15, 243, 251, 256
Biotransformation	45, 71, 72, 75, 76, 97
Botanicals	196-198, 211
Bowman-Birk trypsin inhibitor	2, 5, 6
Breast, cancer	20
Caffeine	40, 42, 44, 47, 48
Calcium	95
Cancer, breast	20
colon	11, 13-16, 235
inhibition	42, 47, 197
lung	24
prevention	1, 5-7, 70, 84, 99, 107, 119, 151, 234, 247
prostate	4
selenium compounds	109, 119, 121, 123, 126
stomach	23-25
Carcinogens	72, 73
Carotene, carotenoids	29-32, 35, 219-228, 238
Catechins	40, 41, 177
Cell cycle, regulation	44
Cell signal	36
Chymotrypsin	5
Clinical trials	221-225
Colon, crypt cell	15, 16
Crambe meal	14
Crambene	238
Cyclooxygenase	48, 75, 76, 147, 151-155, 159, 163, 164, 198
Daidzen	23
Daidzin	12
Diallyl sulfide	90
Diet	237-239
Dietary, intervention	233, 234, 237-240, 243, 244
supplements	203, 204, 210, 243, 250, 251
7,12-Dimethylbenz(a)anthracene	43, 56, 242
1,2-Dimethylhydrazine	14, 42
Dioxin	169, 183, 190, 191

Epidemiologic studies	220
colon cancer	11
garlic and	70
hormones	19, 20
lycopene and prostate cancer	21, 30
tea	40
Epidermal growth factor	44
Epigallocatechin	40, 43-46, 59
Epigallocatechin-3-gallate	40, 43-46, 48, 59, 61, 62
Equol	21
Estrogens, isoflavones similarity	7, 8
Estrogenic activity	174, 175
Fat, dietary	20
Fatty acids	75
Flavones	40
Flaxseed	240
Food supplements	249, 250
Garlic	69-76, 83, 84, 94, 99, 258, 259
Genistein	13, 20, 23
Genistin	12-14
Glutathione-S-transferase	73, 197
Glycitin	16
Herbal medicines/supplements	195, 198, 211, 259
Hormones, mechanism	98
metabolism	96, 97
responsiveness	89, 96
Human, intervention study	14-16
Iberin	238
Immunohistochemical test	15
Immunostimulant	211
Indole-3-carbinol	238
Inflammation	163
Information source	214
Inositol, hexaphosphate	7
Intervention, human	14, 15
Isoflavones	6, 7, 12, 20
Kunitz trypsin inhibitor	2, 5
Labels, for dietary supplements	206
Lipids, metabolism	167
Lipoxygenase	48, 76, 77, 165
Lung cancer	19, 24, 42, 234
Lycopene	29, 30, 33-36, 226
Lutein	234
Lyase	121
Mammary gland, tumorigenesis	43
4-(Methylnitrosamino)-1-	
(3-pyridyl)-1-butanone (NNK)	42, 43
Methylnitrosourea	138
Methylselenol	136
Nitric oxide	96, 166, 172, 173
Nitroso compounds	47, 70-72, 90
NSAID	199
Nuclear factor kappa B	91, 92
Nutrition and selenium	108
Oncogene expression	92

Phenylethylisothiocyanate   238
Phorbol ester   148, 151-154, 171
Phytoalexins   160
Phytochemicals   12, 21, 29, 84, 196, 200, 255-257, 260
Phytoestrogens   21, 174, 240
Phytic acid   7, 8
Polyamines   88, 90
Polycyclic aromatic hydrocarbons   183
Polyphenols   41, 55
Prevention   142
Proliferation   36, 60, 88, 89
Proliferative cell nuclear antigen   15
Promotion   88
Prostaglandins   147-149, 151, 164
Prostate cancer   4, 22, 23, 29
Prostate specific antigen   97, 98, 170, 256, 257
Protease, inhibitors   5, 6
Protein binding   41
Protein kinases   57, 61, 84, 89, 93, 94, 150, 153-155
Quercetin   40, 173, 177
Rapeseed meal   14
Resveratrol   147-178, 185-191, 197, 258-261
Retinoic acid   221
Salt, stomach cancer   23
Saponins   6, 8
Selenium and compounds   75, 109-113, 115, 119-127, 131-133, 135, 222
Signal transduction   55, 58, 60, 62, 63, 84, 87, 96, 98
Silymarin   213
Soy   1-16, 19, 21, 22, 208
Stomach cancer, and soy   19, 23, 25
Synergy, food components   238
Tea   39-43, 45, 48, 55, 59
Theaflavins   40, 42-44, 47, 60, 61
Tomato, carotenoid content   30, 34, 36
Toxicity, selenium compounds   120
Transcription, cell   56, 187, 188
Transformation, cell   60
Trypsin, inhibitor   2, 5
Tumor promotion   55-58, 88
Ultraviolet radiation, skin cancer   55, 57, 61, 62

Printed in the United States
1488900001B/85